A Colour Atlas of
Infectious Diseases

Second Edition

R. T. D. Emond
MB, ChB (St And), FRCP (Lond), DTM & H (Eng)
Consultant Physician, Infectious Diseases Department,
The Royal Free Hospital, London,
Honorary Associate Physician,
Hospital for Tropical Diseases, London,
Honorary Senior Lecturer, University of London

H. A. K. Rowland
MA, DM, PhD, FRCP, DTM & H
Department of Clinical Tropical Medicine,
London School of Hygiene and Tropical Medicine, Lond

Wolfe Medical Publications Ltd
Year Book Medical Publishers, Inc

Second edition published by Wolfe Medical Publications Ltd, 1987

Printed by W.S. Cowell Ltd, Buttermarket, Ipswich, England
ISBN 0 7234 0973 0 cased edition
ISBN 0 7234 0957 9 limp edition

General Editor, Wolfe Medical Atlases: G. Barry Carruthers, MD(London)

For a full list of other atlases published by Wolfe Medical Publications Ltd, please write to the publishers at: Wolfe House, 3 Conway Street, London W1P 6HE, England, or Year Book Medical Publishers, Inc., 35 East Wacker Drive, Chicago, Illinois 60601, USA.

Distributed in Continental North America, Hawaii and Puerto Rico by
Year Book Medical Publishers, Inc.

Library of Congress Cataloging in Publication Data

Emond, Ronald T.D.
A color atlas of infectious diseases.

Includes index.
1. Communicable diseases—Atlases. I. Title.
[DNLM: 1. Communicable Diseases—atlases. WC 17 E54c]
RC113.2.E46 1987 616.9 86-19203
ISBN 0-8151-3122-4

ACKNOWLEDGEMENTS

It would have been impossible to illustrate so many aspects of infection without the generosity and support of numerous friends and colleagues, who have provided photographs from their collections. We are most grateful to them for the following illustrations:

Dr June Almeida, **336**; Dr Isobel Beswick, **39**; Professor C.P. Beattie, Professor J.K.A. Beverley and the Department of Photography, The United Sheffield Hospitals, **442–4, 446, 448–9**; Dr A. Bloom, **41** and **57**; Dr Jean Bradley, **9**, **10**, **45–7**, **67**, **92–3**, **124**, **137**, **452**; the late Dr R.T. Brain, **293**; the late Dr E.H. Brown, **130**, **138**, **260**, **329**; Dr G. Laing Brown, **223–4**; Dr A.D.M. Bryceson, **150**, **153**; Dr D.C. MacDonald Burns, **201**; Dr K.C. Carstairs and the editor of the *Proceedings of the Royal Society of Medicine*, **229–30**; Dr L.S. Carstairs, **225–8**; Dr A.B. Christie, **231**, **407**; Mr C. Daniels, **411**; Professor S. Darougar, **184–5**; Mr D. Downton, **139**; Professor J.A. Dudgeon and the Hospital for Sick Children, London, who retain the copyright, **360–1**, **371**, **373**, **376**; Dr A.J. Duggan, **173**; Professor K.R. Dumbell, **268–9**; Dr G.J. Ebrahim, **437**; Dr Anne M. Field and Mr A. Porter, **205**, **311**, **320**, **378**, **404**; Dr W.J.D. Fleming, **299**; Dr T.H. Flewett, **112**; Dr J.A. Forbes, **160**; Dr W. Frain-Bell and the Department of Dermatology, University of Dundee, **50**, **419–20**; Dr G.A. Gresham, **163**, **415**, **453**; Mr N.D.F. Grindley, **91**; Dr S. Haider, **284**; Dr K.K. Hussain, **109**; Dr W.M. Jamieson, **20**, **87**, **131**, **133**, **165**, **343**, **405–6**, **408–10**, **418**; Mr J.J. Kanski, **181**; Dr T. Kawasaki, **470–5**, **477–8**; Dr S.G. Lamb, **15**, **34**, **210**, **251**, **286**, **300**, **355**, **447**, **465**; Professor H.P. Lambert, **377**, **450–1**; Dr J.H. Lawson, **171**; Dr J.J. Linehan, **344**, **352**, **368**; Dr S. Lucas, **147–8**, **431**, **440–1**; Dr J. Luder, **73**, **356**; Mrs S.D. Marston, **298**; Dr J.M. Medlock, **17–19**, **42**, **52**, **126**, **158**, **381**; Mr I. McCaul, **58**; Dr G.D.W. McKendrick, **60**, **78**, **159**, **199**; Dr W.F.T. McMath, Dr K.K. Hussain and the Editor and publisher of the *British Medical Journal*, **485–6**; Dr E. Montuschi, **84**; Dr J.McC. Murdoch and Dr J.A. Gray, **29** and **53**; Dr R.O. Murray, **107–8**, **110**; Professor I.C.S. Normand, **370**; Dr R.J. Olds, **48**, **85**, **121**, **123**, **125**, **141**, **157**, **168**; the late Dr E.P. O'Sullivan, **55**, **56**, **86**, **88**, **215**, **359**, **374**, **393**; Dr G. Pampiglione, **358**; Dr J.D.J. Parker, **290–1**; Dr H.G. Prentice, **297**; Dr J.I. Pugh, **272–3**, **277**, **487**; Dr C.S. Ratnatunga, **188**, **200**; Dr G.H. Ree, **203–4**; Dr D. Taylor-Robinson, **206–7**; Dr G. Sangster and Dr J.A. Gray, **95–6**; Dr I. Sarkany, **43**; Professor P. Schever, **425**; Professor C. Scully, **398**; Mr J.C. Smale, **399**; Dr O.D. Standen, **172**; Dr H. Stern, **294–5**, **482**; Dr J. Stevenson, **382–4**; Dr R.N.P. Sutton, **270–1**, **182**, **322**, **324**, **326**,

337–8, **379–80**, **401**; Dr Frances Tatnell, **491**; Dr M.M. Esiri and Dr A.H. Tomlinson and the Editor of the *Journal of The Neurological Sciences*, **236**; Dr A.H. Tomlinson, **275–6**; Dr J.M. Vetters and the Department of Pathology, University of Glasgow, **40**, **51**, **101–2**, **134–5**, **169**, **208–9**, **235**, **237**, **274**, **296**, **312–14**, **323**, **339–42**, **445**, **484**, **488**; Dr R.V. Walley, **170**; Dr J.F. Warin, **117–18**; Dr D.A. Warrell, **161**, **400**, **402–3**; Dr D.I. Weiss and the Editor, *American Journal of Diseases of Childhood*, **375**; Dr P. Welsby, **396–7**; Department of Pathology, Whittington Hospital, **69**; Dr P.H.A. Willcox, **416–17**; Dr I. Zamiri, **127**, **129**.

We wish to express special thanks to our colleagues, Dr A.M. Ramsay and Dr Hillas Smith, in the Infectious Diseases Department of The Royal Free Hospital, and to Dr J.I. Pugh of The City Hospital, St Albans, for their help and advice in preparing this atlas. We are also indebted to Dr C.S. Ratnatunga of The Royal Free Hospital and to Mr Martin Jones of the Photographic Department of the North London Group of Hospitals. Many of the colour reproductions have been obtained from members of the Association for the Study of Infectious Disease, to whom we are most grateful. We would also like to thank Dr Susan Young for her assistance in reading and criticising the proofs. Every endeavour has been made to identify the source of the illustrations, but if any mistakes have been made we offer our sincere apologies.

CONTENTS

PREFACE

The twentieth century has witnessed tremendous advances in the understanding of infectious disease, but many problems remain. With the natural ebb and flow of infection some old plagues have vanished, while others have been routed by rising standards of living and great advances in preventive medicine. Yet experience teaches that there is no final victory over infection, for elimination of one problem highlights another, and the delicate balance between man and micro-organism remains. Moreover, the speed of air travel is such that banished infections can readily invade from distant lands. Constant vigilance is essential, but few undergraduates have the opportunity to study infectious diseases at the bedside and most enter their profession ill-equipped to recognise even common infections, which form such an important part of everyday practice.

This atlas endeavours to provide the student and newly qualified doctor with a guide to the diagnosis of the common exanthemata, and the experienced physician with clinical photographs of less common though important diseases. It is not feasible to encompass the whole of the subject in one atlas, for many conditions are rare and others do not lend themselves to photographic illustration. Emphasis has been placed on the clinical aspects of disease, but this would be incomplete without a brief account of the causative organism and the relevant pathology. The texts accompanying the illustrations are of necessity short, but, when read in sequence, are intended to give a simple, coherent account of each disease. When size is important in an illustration the relevant information is provided in the text.

COMPONENTS OF RASHES

Rashes are a prominent feature of many infectious, as well as toxic and allergic, states. A skin eruption occurring as an integral part of an infectious disease is termed an exanthem, and corresponding changes in mucous membranes constitute an enanthem. Accurate diagnosis of an exanthem is not always possible on preliminary examination and, if necessary, judgment should be deferred until the rash develops. Most mistakes arise from assessing the rash as an independent entity instead of one feature in a disease process. It should be appreciated that many communicable diseases are not accompanied by an exanthem.

In making a diagnosis based on the nature of a rash many factors must be considered: the duration of the prodromal period between the beginning of the illness and the onset of the rash, the site at which the rash starts, the distribution and density of the skin lesions, and finally the primary elements from which the rash is composed.

1 Components of rashes — macule. A macule is a circumscribed discoloration of the skin, not raised above the surface of the surrounding skin. Macules often evolve into papules, and many rashes consist of a combination of both. Rashes of this intermediate type are designated maculopapular.

2 Components of rashes — papule. A papule is a small nodular elevation of the skin. Such lesions are common in chickenpox.

3 Components of rashes — vesicle. A vesicle is a small blister containing clear fluid. These may be scattered irregularly over the skin, as in chickenpox, or grouped in clusters, as in herpes zoster and herpes simplex.

4 Components of rashes — pustule. A pustule is a small elevation of the skin containing pus. It may form directly as a result of local sepsis or evolve from a vesicle.

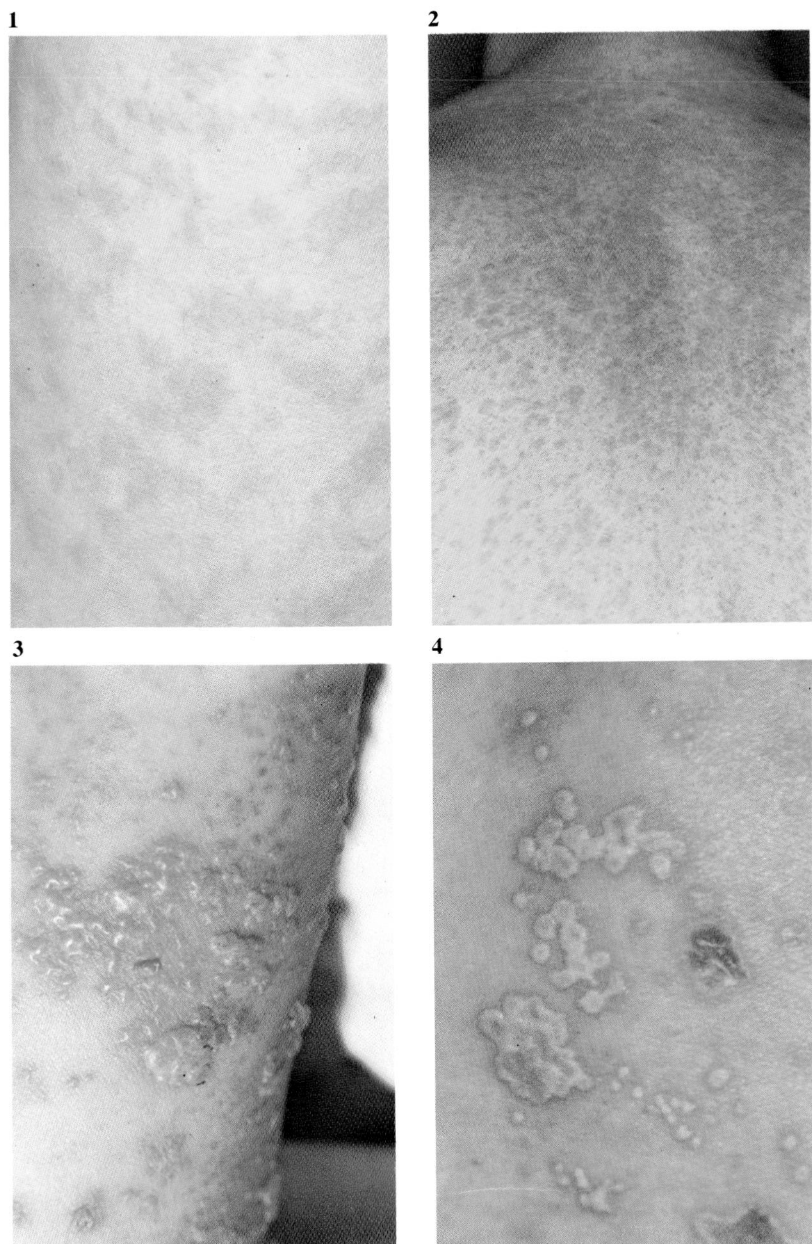
1
2
3
4

5 Components of rashes — crust. A crust or scab is a congealed exudate on the skin. Crusts are a prominent feature in impetigo and are a terminal stage in the evolution of vesicular eruptions.

6 Components of rashes — wheal. A wheal is a localised effusion of fluid into the skin causing a raised, white or pinkish-white zone with a halo of erythema. Wheals vary in size and never rupture. They are characteristic of allergic rashes and are especially florid in serum sickness.

7 Components of rashes — erythema. An erythema is a diffuse or localised redness of the skin. The character of an erythema varies considerably with different diseases. An erythematous patch with a pale centre and intensely red margin is described as circinate. In gyrate rashes the borders are scalloped. Erythematous rashes blanch on pressure.

8 Components of rashes — petechiae and ecchymoses. Purpuric rashes consist of petechiae and ecchymoses. A petechia describes a small haemorrhage beneath the epidermis while an ecchymosis is a larger area of haemorrhage. In infectious diseases haemorrhages into the skin may precede the specific eruption or appear during the evolution of the exanthem. When an erythema is intense there may be no focal bleeding, but red cells may leak through dilated capillary vessels and cause pigmentation or staining of the skin.

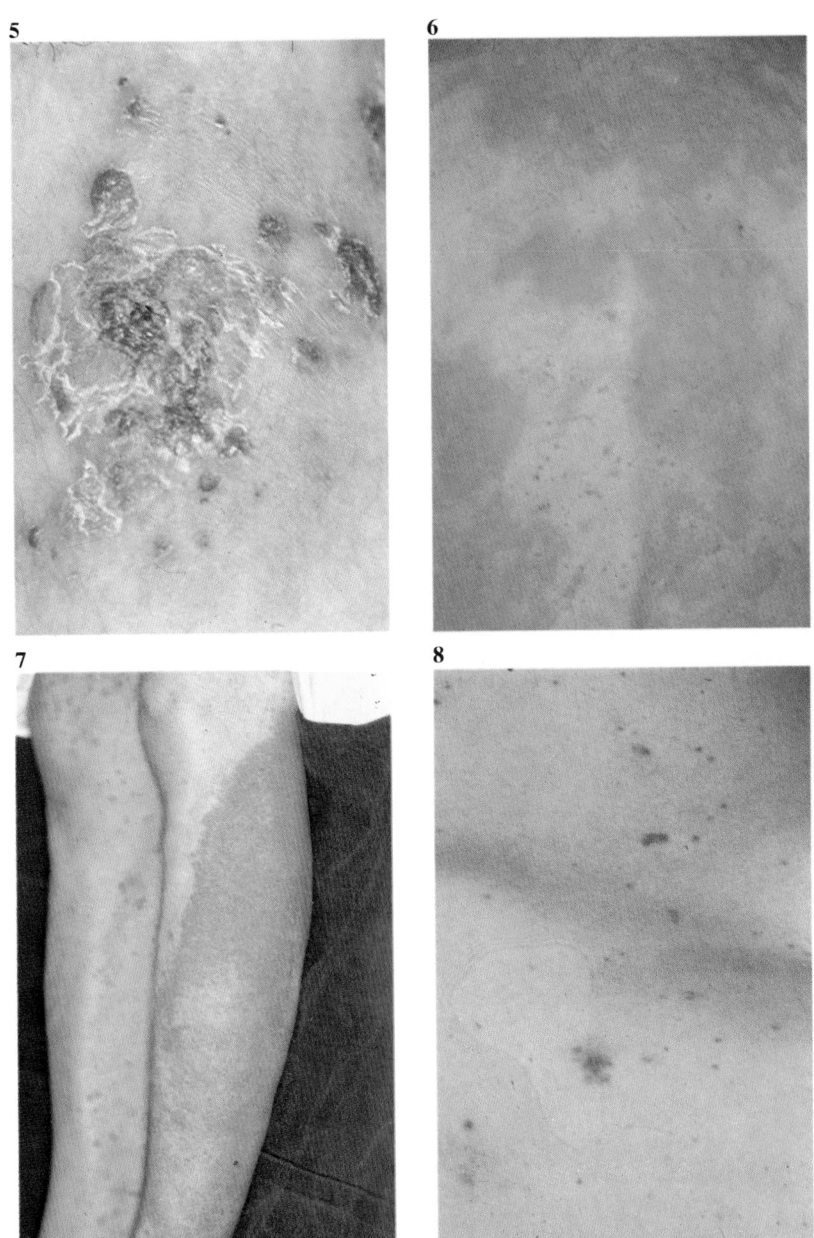
5
6
7
8

BACTERIAL AND FUNGAL INFECTIONS

Streptococcal infection

Streptococcus pyogenes causes many human and animal diseases. The source of human infection may be a carrier or a patient suffering from streptococcal disease, especially of the upper respiratory tract. Children are more likely to transmit infection than adults. Convalescent carriers are more infectious than chronic carriers. Nasal carriers are less common than throat carriers but shed large numbers of organisms and are more dangerous.

Infection is usually spread by droplets of secretions sprayed from the air passages by sneezing, spluttering, or coughing, but the organism may also be transmitted indirectly by dust or fomites. Outbreaks of tonsillitis or scarlet fever may originate from contaminated milk.

The outcome of streptococcal infection depends on the virulence of the organism and the resistance of the host. When antibacterial immunity is high the streptococcus may fail to become established or may be confined to the surface of the mucosa or skin of the host. When antibacterial resistance is low or the streptococcus is highly virulent, surface invasion may cause tonsillitis or impetigo and deeper penetration to lymphadenitis or septicaemia. If the invading organism produces large amounts of erythrogenic toxin, and antitoxic immunity is also low, then scarlet fever results.

Most human infections are caused by *Streptococcus pyogenes*, the organism associated with such varied diseases as tonsillitis, scarlet fever, erysipelas, and impetigo. Sensitisation to this organism gives rise to acute rheumatic fever or to acute glomerulonephritis. *Streptococcus viridans* is a major cause of bacterial endocarditis, and anaerobic streptococci play an important part in surgical and puerperal sepsis.

Organism

9 Smear of pus showing streptococci (Gram stain). Streptococci are Gram-positive, spherical or oval cells, measuring 0·5 to 0·75μm in diameter, and are arranged in pairs or chains of varying lengths. They are non-motile and do not form spores. Capsules may be seen in young cultures but are not prominent; most are aerobes or facultative anaerobes, but some are anaerobic or microaerophilic.

10 Blood agar culture showing ß-haemolysis. Some aerobic streptococci produce a soluble haemolysin which creates a clear zone of haemolysis on fresh blood agar. This is termed ß-haemolysis. ß-haemolytic streptococci may be classified in the Lancefield system according to the carbohydrate C antigen in the body of the organism. There are 15 Lancefield groups and those ß-haemolytic streptococci belonging to Lancefield Group A are also known as *Strep. pyogenes*. Colonies are less than 1mm in diameter and are surrounded by a clear, colourless zone within which the red cells are completely lysed. Haemolysis is more striking when *Strep. pyogenes* is cultured anaerobically and may occasionally be absent on aerobic culture. Several exotoxins may be produced including haemolysins, fibrinolysin, hyaluronidase, and erythrogenic toxin.

Surface infections

Streptococcal infection of the upper respiratory tract

11 Appearance of the lips and mouth in streptococcal tonsillitis. Streptococcal infection of the throat is often accompanied by changes in the appearance of the lips, which become glazed and cherry-red in hue. Moist cracks may be found at the angles of the mouth.

12 Cervical lymphadenitis. Infection may spread from the tonsils to the cervical lymph nodes causing suppurative lymphadenitis. In young children the swelling of the neck may be disproportionate to the degree of inflammation in the throat and this may be confused with mumps; however, careful examination will show that the swelling lies inferior to the salivary glands.

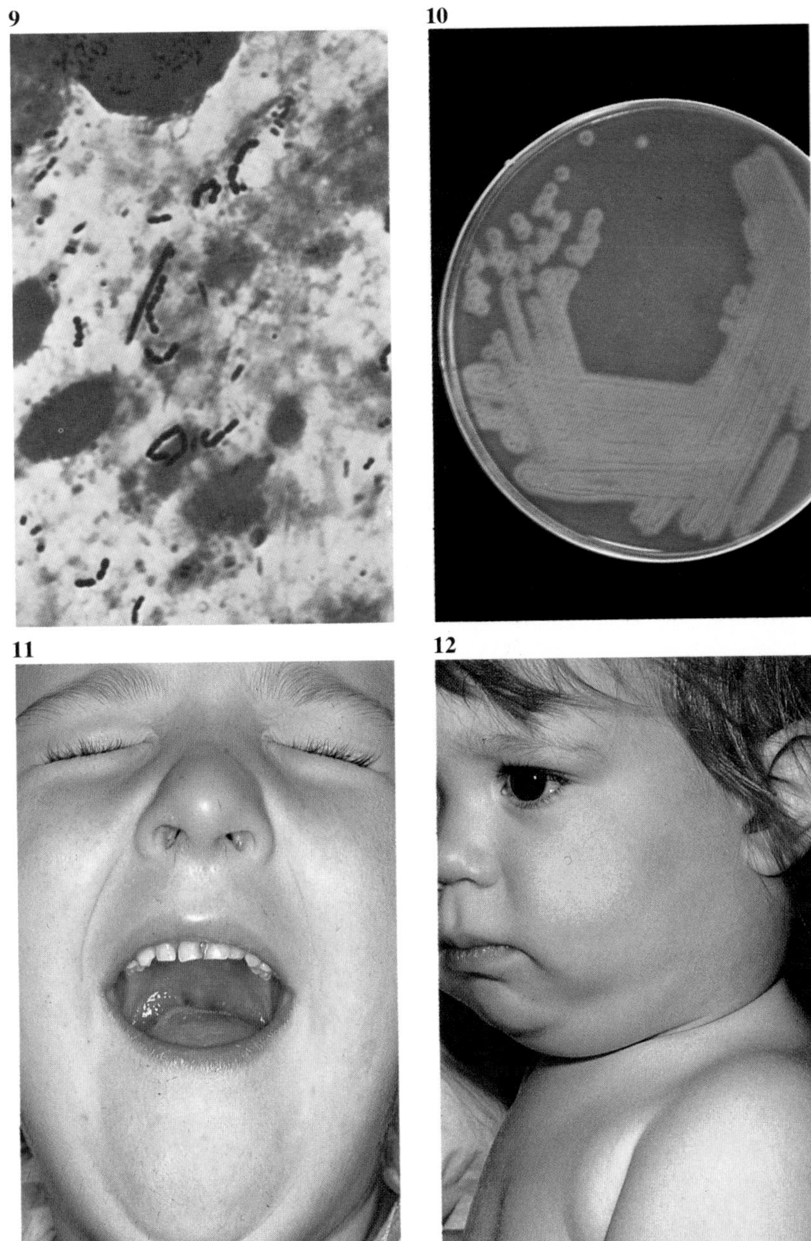
9
10
11
12

13 Inflamed tonsils without exudate. Without laboratory tests it is difficult to be certain about the aetiology of mild tonsillitis. The appearance of the throat may be identical in both viral and streptococcal infections. Redness and congestion extend along the arch of the soft palate to the oedematous uvula.

14 Inflamed tonsils with exudate. When an attack is more severe the congestion of the fauces increases, and patches of white or yellowish exudate appear on the surface of the tonsils. Swallowing is painful.

13

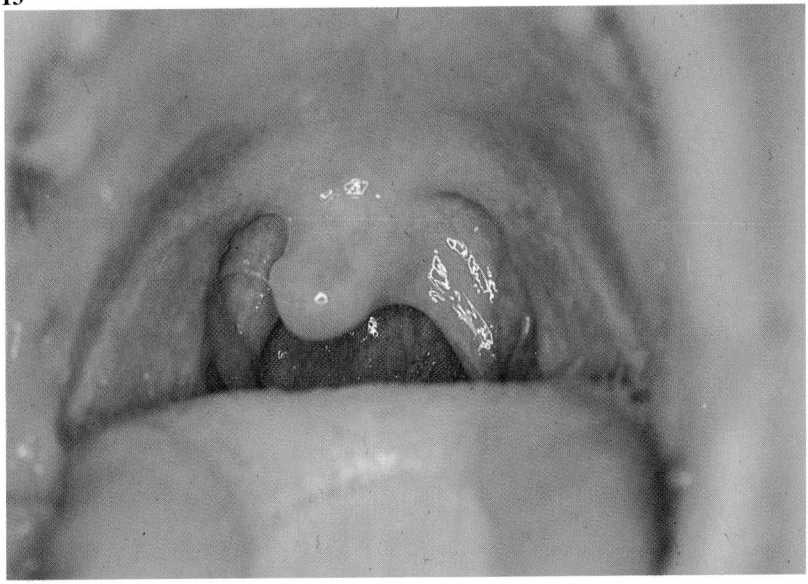

14

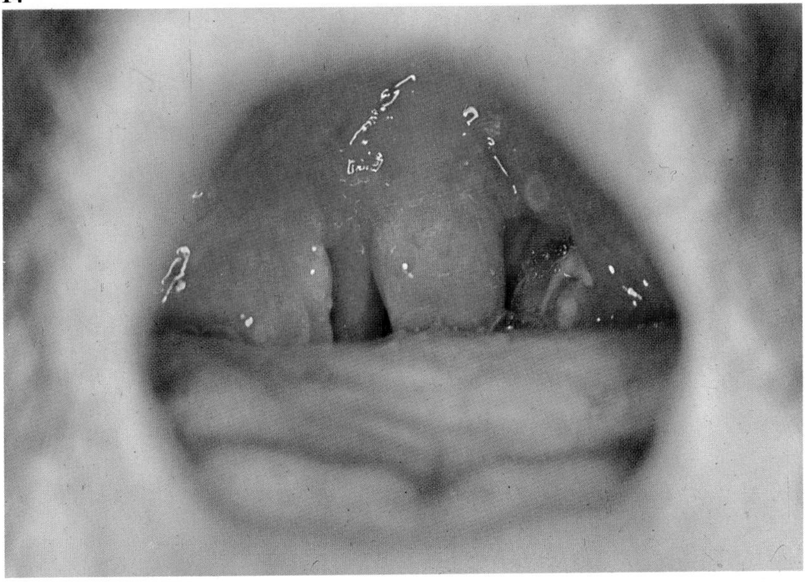

15 Follicular tonsillitis. The degree of congestion varies considerably, and follicular exudate may be present on the tonsils with minimal reaction in the surrounding tissues.

16 Peritonsillar abscess (quinsy). When a streptococcus spreads from the tonsil into the adjacent soft tissues congestion and swelling increase rapidly and suppuration usually follows. The patient experiences great difficulty in opening his mouth, swallowing becomes exquisitely painful, and the voice develops a nasal intonation. The anterior wall of the fauces bulges and displaces the uvula to the opposite side. Pus forms and tracks to the surface, where it points as a yellow spot through which it eventually discharges.

15

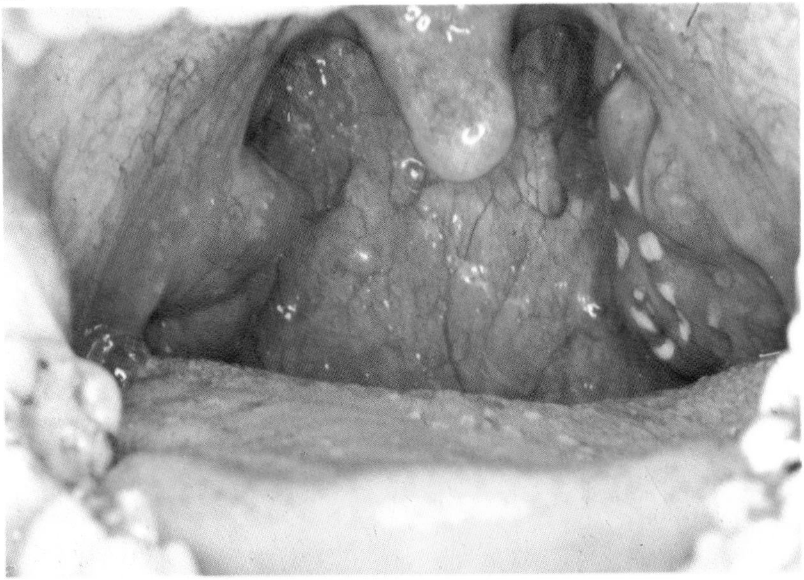

16

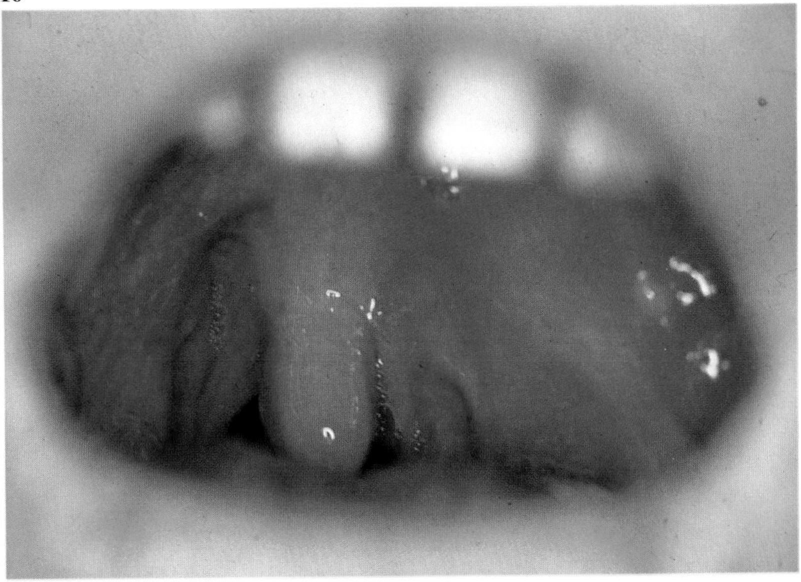

17 Ludwig's angina — front view. Ludwig's angina is the term generally applied to severe forms of cellulitis in the region of the submaxillary gland. It is usually caused by infection of the connective tissue planes from a suppurating lymph node, secondary to tonsillitis or dental infection. A streptococcus is often responsible, but there may be mixed infection with anaerobes.

18 Ludwig's angina — side view.

19 Ludwig's angina — floor of mouth. Inflammatory oedema distorts the floor of the mouth and makes swallowing difficult. Oedema of the glottis may arise suddenly and cause dangerous respiratory obstruction.

17

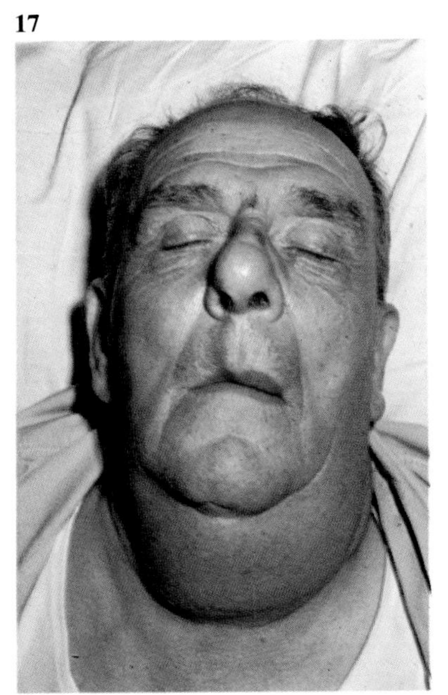

18

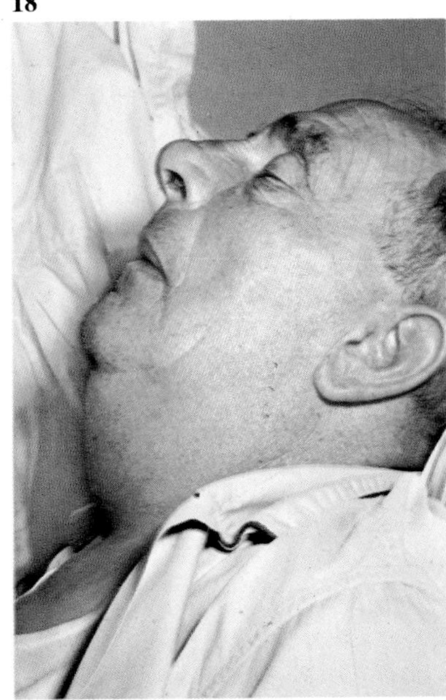

19

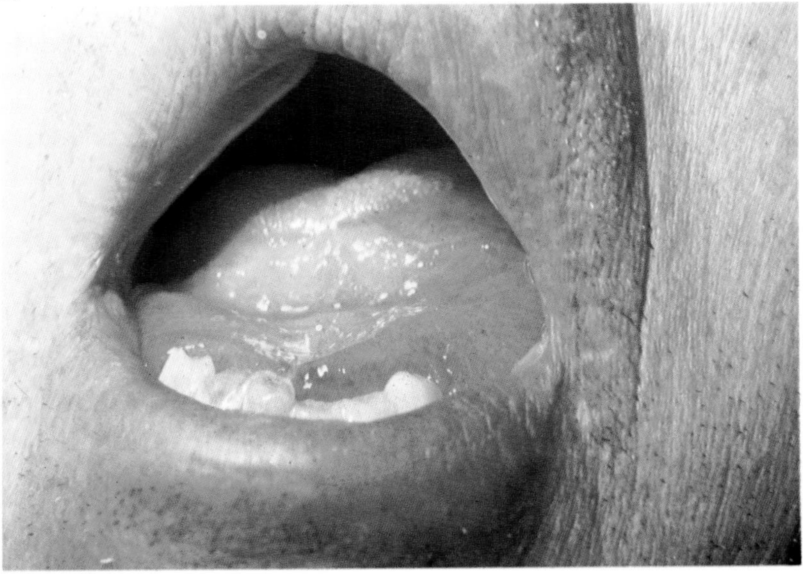

Scarlet fever

20 Circum-oral pallor and rash on trunk. Scarlet fever is caused by an erythrogenic strain of streptococcus invading a susceptible host. The portal of entry is usually the throat, but scarlet fever may follow infection of a wound, burn, or other skin lesion, such as a chickenpox vesicle. This type is commonly designated 'surgical scarlet fever'. Infection of the genital tract may give rise to 'puerperal scarlet fever'.

The onset of scarlet fever is sudden with a sharp febrile reaction, soreness of the throat, and vomiting. In mild attacks vomiting may be absent and some children may not complain of a sore throat. The exanthem follows within 24 to 36 hours and evolves from above downwards. There is a bright flush on the cheeks and chin, which contrasts vividly with the pallor round the mouth. Elsewhere there is an erythematous background of varying intensity with tiny superimposed red spots or puncta. This punctate erythema is most prominent over the neck and upper chest. Over the distal parts of the limbs the rash may condense into discrete macules. Pallor around the mouth is seen in many other conditions, especially lobar pneumonia.

20

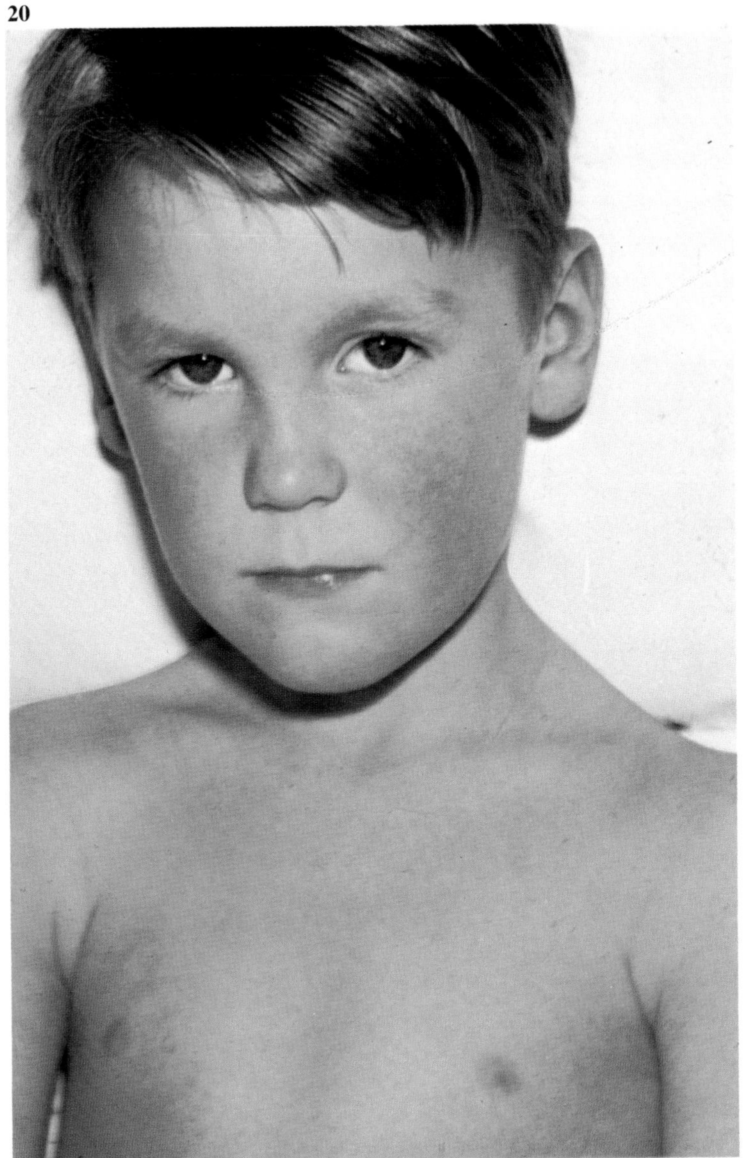

21 Punctate erythema on trunk. The punctate erythematous rash is most prominent over the neck and upper chest, where it resembles flushed goose-flesh.

22 Rash on thigh. The rash on the limbs is blotchy and may condense into discrete macules over the distal portions. It may be difficult to differentiate the rash from rubella, but the characteristic appearance of the mouth and throat will indicate the correct diagnosis (see **364**).

21

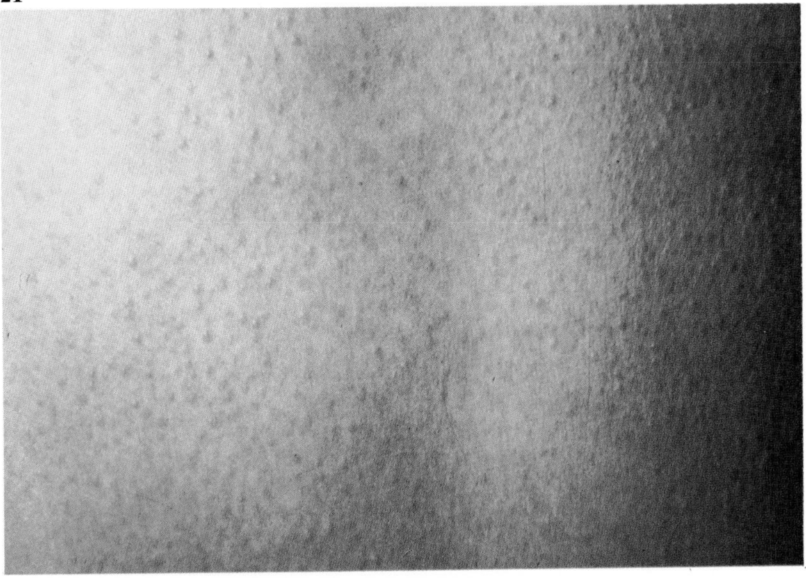

22

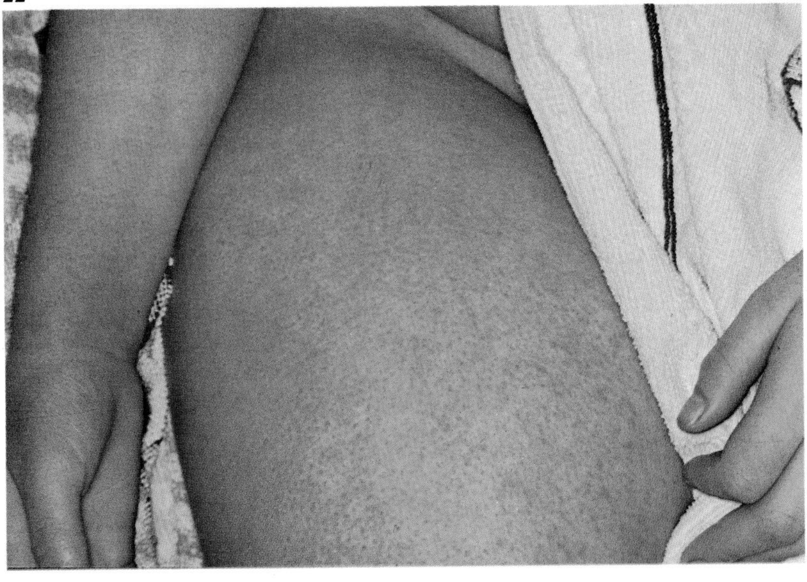

23 'Surgical scarlet fever' from an infected cut. Absorption of erythrogenic toxin from an infected wound or skin lesion gives rise to scarlet fever in a susceptible person. The typical enanthem is present even when the streptococcus is confined to the skin lesion. (See also scarlet fever in chickenpox — **223** and **224**.)

24 Pastia's sign. Petechiae may be found in the antecubital fossa when the rash is heavy. The pigmentation persists after the erythema has faded and is called Pastia's sign, which is mainly of historical interest.

25 Desquamation on hand. About four to five days after onset of the rash the skin begins to peel. Small patches of desquamation appear on the neck and thorax and spread downwards to the hands and feet by the end of the second week. The amount of peeling varies greatly but tends to be pronounced when the erythema has been intense. After the rash has faded desquamation is a helpful diagnostic clue but is not pathognomonic of scarlet fever. Desquamation begins with a minute central pinhole surrounded by a small collar of epidermis which separates to form flakes.

26 Desquamation on hand. Towards the end of the second week the skin splits round the nail folds, and coarse strips may peel from the thick skin of the hands and feet.

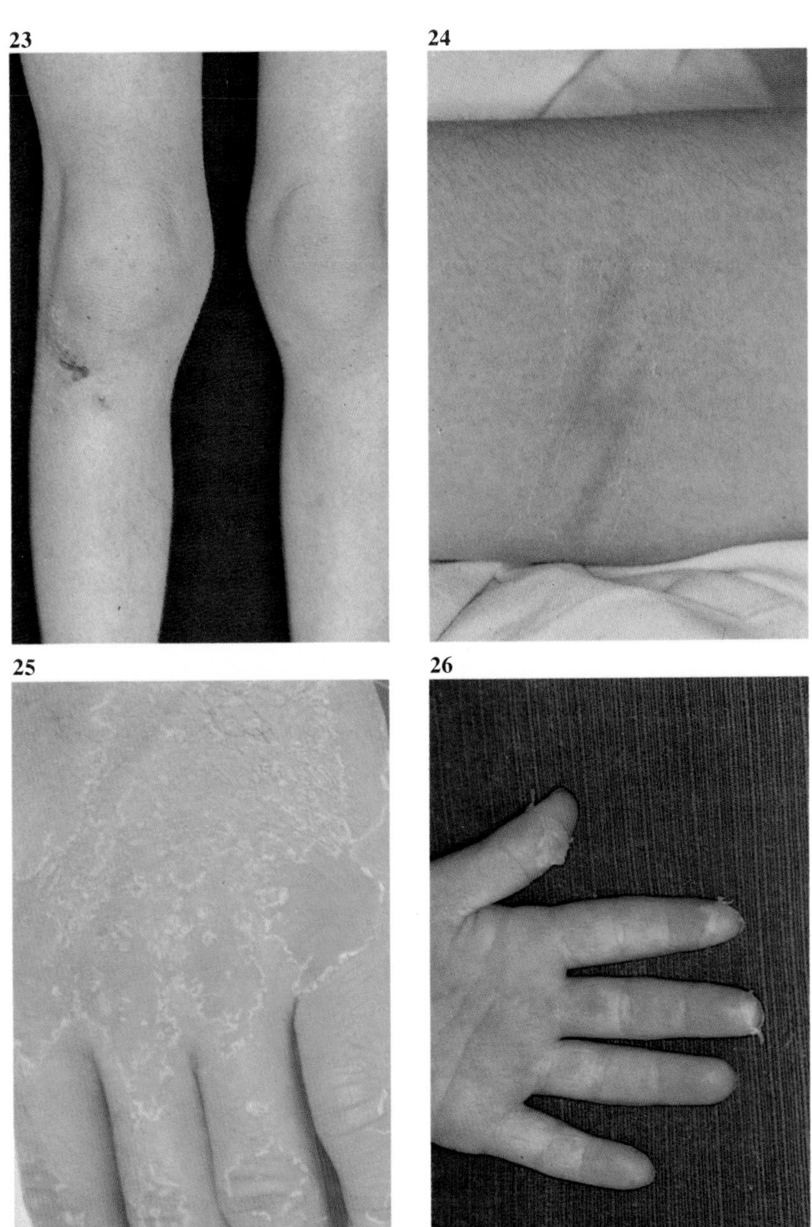
23
24
25
26

27 White strawberry tongue. During the first day or two the tongue is covered with a thick white fur through which the enlarged red papillae protrude. The palate is stippled with dark red macules and occasionally a few petechiae. The fauces are vividly red and swollen, and there may be patches of white exudate on the tonsils.

28 Red strawberry tongue. Within a few days the fur peels from the tip and edges of the tongue to produce the red strawberry stage. The illustration shows the red, glazed surface with prominent papillae and the remnants of white fur.

27

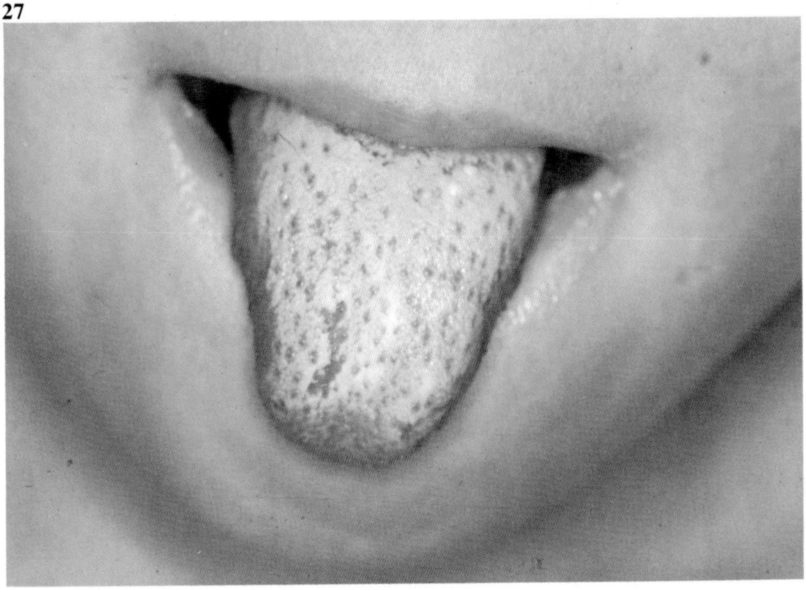

28

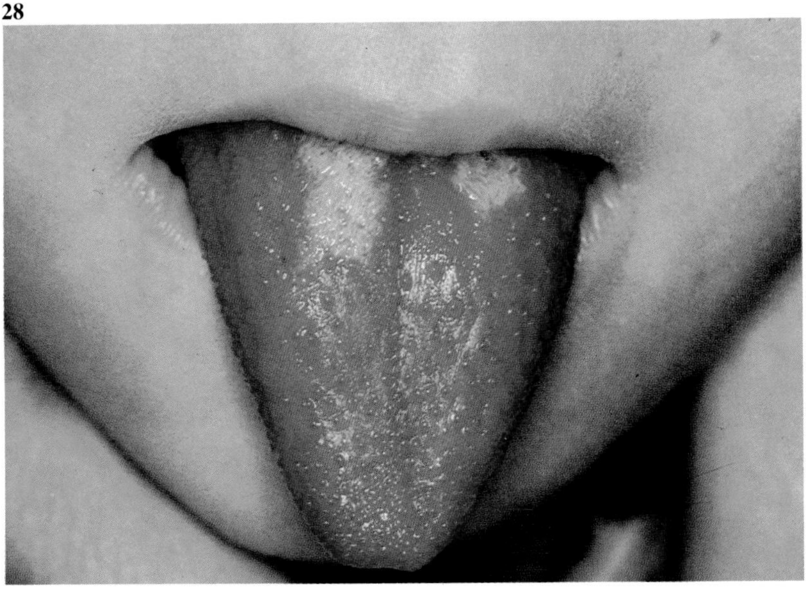

Erysipelas

29 Butterfly-wing rash on face. Erysipelas is often preceded by an upper respiratory infection and is more common in older age groups with degenerative skin changes which allow easy penetration by the streptococcus. It usually affects the face or legs, and infection may possibly be transferred on the patient's fingers to these 'scratch areas' of the body. The streptococcus generally invades through an invisible breach in the skin and spreads centrifugally from the point of entry through the lymphatics. Infection may be confined to the skin or extend into the subcutaneous tissues. Occasionally the streptococcus may gain access through a surgical wound, leg ulcer, or the umbilical stump in a newborn infant.

After a short incubation period of less than a week, the illness starts abruptly with general symptoms. Within a few hours an unpleasant sensation of tightness and burning develops at the site of invasion, followed quickly by a patch of erythema which rapidly extends outwards. The spreading edge is sharply defined as a palpable ridge. Bullae may form in the central erythematous zone and rupture, leaving raw weeping areas.

Erysipelas of the face often starts on one cheek and spreads across the nose to the other side producing a characteristic butterfly-wing appearance. Occasionally it may be confined to one side.

29

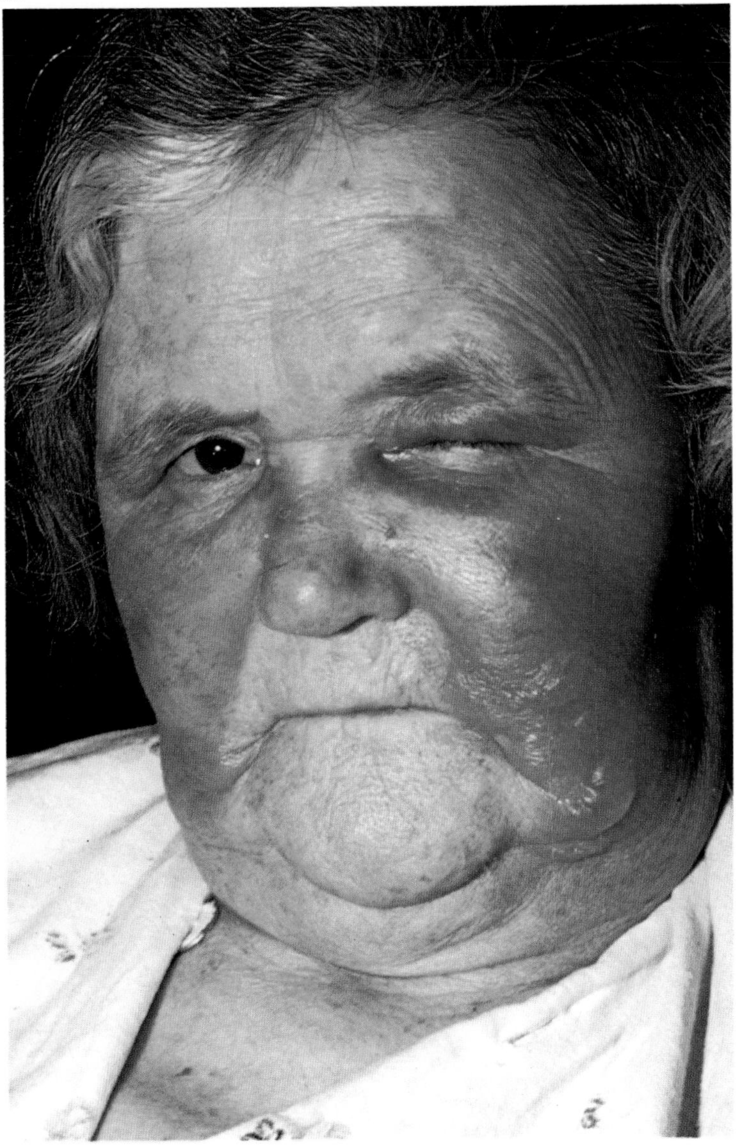

30 Erysipelas of the face — acute stage. During the acute stage the eyelids may become so swollen that they cannot be opened, and the eyelashes may be matted by purulent discharge. This is commonly confused with herpes ophthalmicus, but the hemicranial distribution of herpes should prevent error (see **239**).

31 Erysipelas of face — convalescent stage. Once infection has been overcome the inflammation subsides, leaving pigmentation and desquamation in the affected area. For some months afterwards exposure to cold wind or strong sunshine may cause local flushing.

32 Erysipelas of leg — acute stage. Infection may spread into the subcutaneous tissues to produce an erysipelo-cellulitis. Bullae are common and may rupture with discharge of seropurulent fluid. Necrosis sometimes occurs.

33 Erysipelas of leg — convalescent stage. Pigmentation and desquamation are prominent features. Damage to lymph vessels may obstruct lymphatic flow and cause persistent oedema, which predisposes the patient to further attacks.

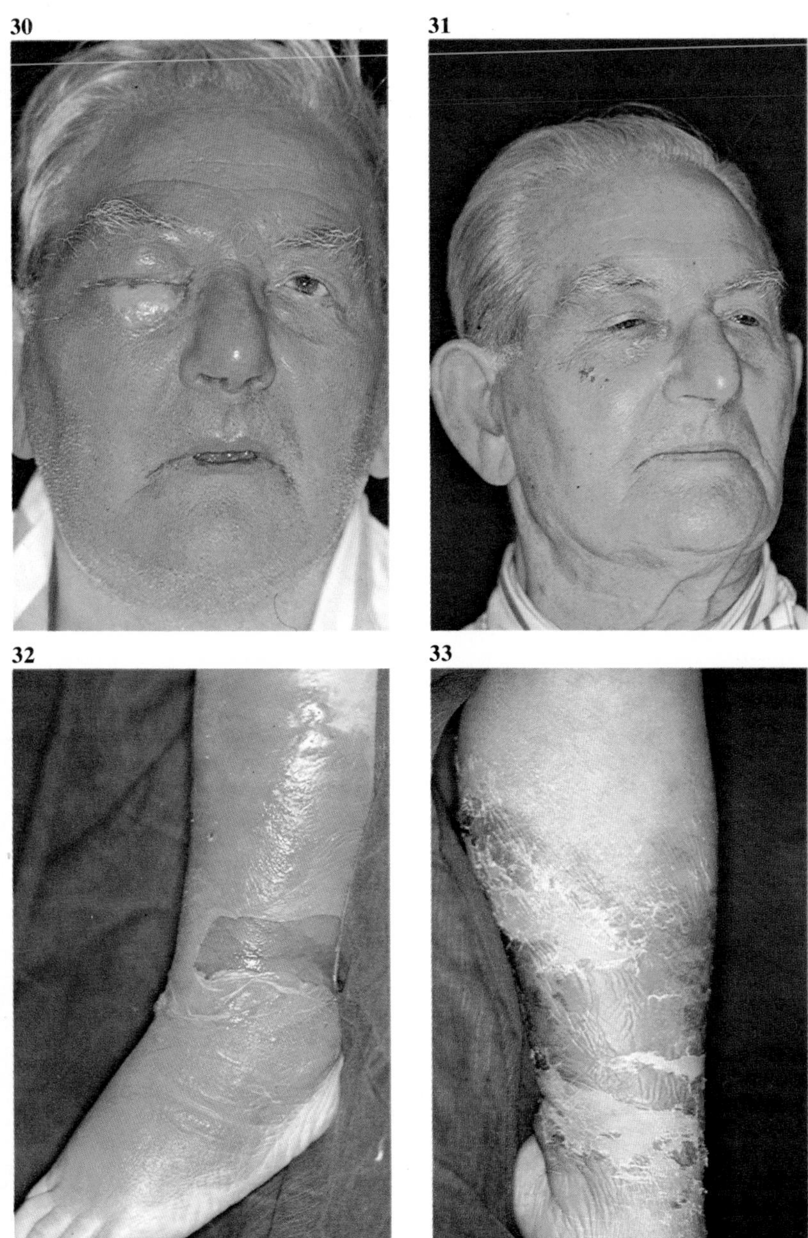
30
31
32
33

Impetigo

34 Impetigo contagiosa of face. Impetigo is a highly contagious superficial infection of the skin caused either by streptococci or by staphylococci. The disease may affect an apparently normal skin or complicate some underlying skin condition, such as pediculosis, scabies, eczema, or acute fungus infection. It commonly starts on the face round the mouth or nose, spreading with alarming rapidity to other parts of the body. In streptococcal impetigo the exudate dries to form a thick crust with a golden-yellow colour. (Contrast with staphylococcal impetigo — **52** to **54**.)

35 Impetigo contagiosa of leg. The thick crusts protect the underlying streptococci from local applications. Skin infection with nephritogenic strains of streptococci may cause outbreaks of acute nephritis.

Invasion of deeper tissues

Cellulitis

36 Cellulitis. When a streptococcus enters through a breach in the skin or mucosa it may provoke a local reaction of cellulitis or spread into the bloodstream causing septicaemia. The zone of inflammation is less sharply demarcated in cellulitis than in erysipelas, and suppuration occurs more often.

34

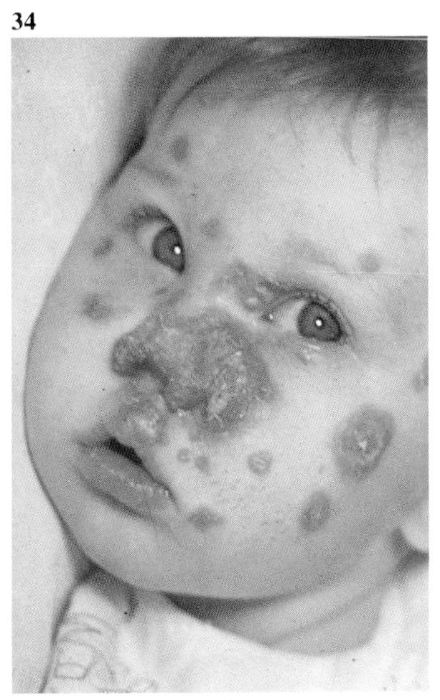

35

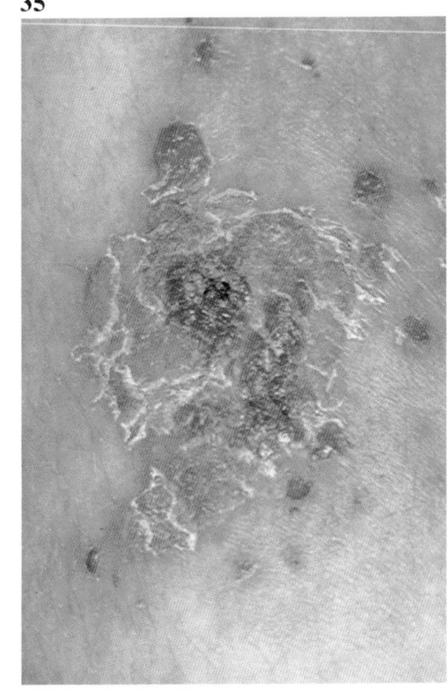

36

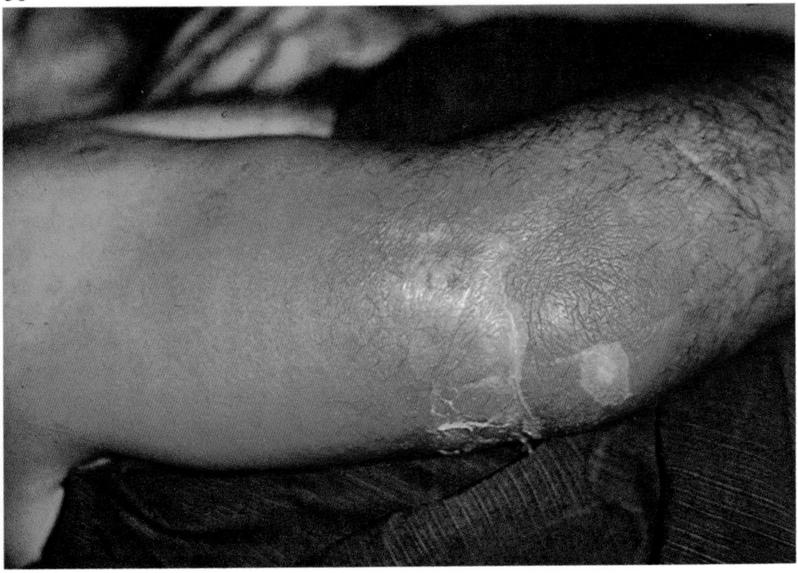

Septicaemia

37 Septicaemia. Invasion of the bloodstream by *Strep. pyogenes* may produce metastatic lesions with haemorrhages and focal cellulitis. The local reaction is overshadowed by the general disturbance.

38 Brain abscess. Streptococci of low virulence, entering the bloodstream in small numbers, produce minimal general disturbance but may lodge in an organ, such as the brain, causing local damage and abscesses. These streptococci are usually microaerophilic or anaerobic. There may be a long interval before clinical signs appear.

37

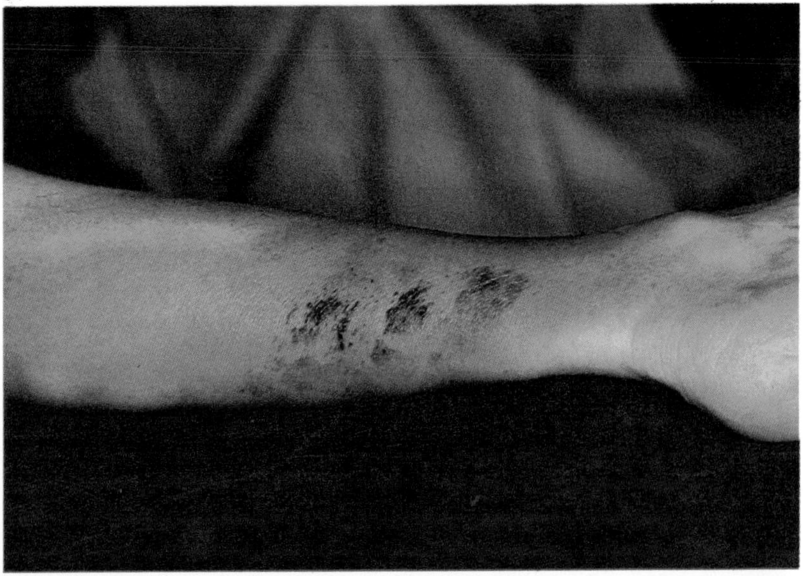

38

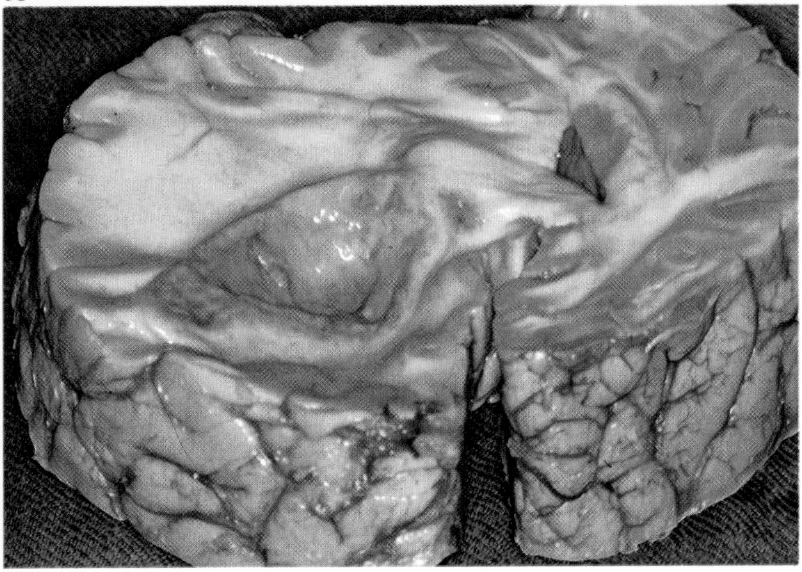

39 Subacute bacterial endocarditis. Most streptococcal infections in man are caused by ß-haemolytic strains, but other streptococci may be responsible for serious disease. Viridans streptococci, normal inhabitants of the mouth, may gain access through the teeth or gums into the bloodstream and cause endocarditis, particularly if a heart valve is already defective. The illness manifests as an unexplained fever which can only be diagnosed with certainty during life when the organism is recovered from blood cultures.

The vegetations formed on the heart valves are larger, softer, and more crumbling in character than those found in rheumatic heart disease. They tend to spread on the endocardial surface, but there is less destruction of the valves than in acute bacterial endocarditis. Emboli are common, but the infarctions do not suppurate. The arrows indicate vegetation.

40 Subacute bacterial endocarditis — histology of heart valve. The vegetation has three layers. The outer layer or cap has an eosinophilic granular appearance and consists of platelets in a matrix of fibrin. Streptococci occupy the middle zone, and the base is formed by the inflamed cusp. Most small emboli, so common in subacute bacterial endocarditis, are shed from the outer layer. (A = myocardium, B = cusp, C = cap.)

41 Subacute bacterial endocarditis — splinter haemorrhages. The small emboli thrown off the outer layer of the vegetation seldom contain organisms and therefore cause bland infarcts. A high proportion terminate in the kidneys and brain, but some lodge under finger nails, where they produce linear haemorrhages.

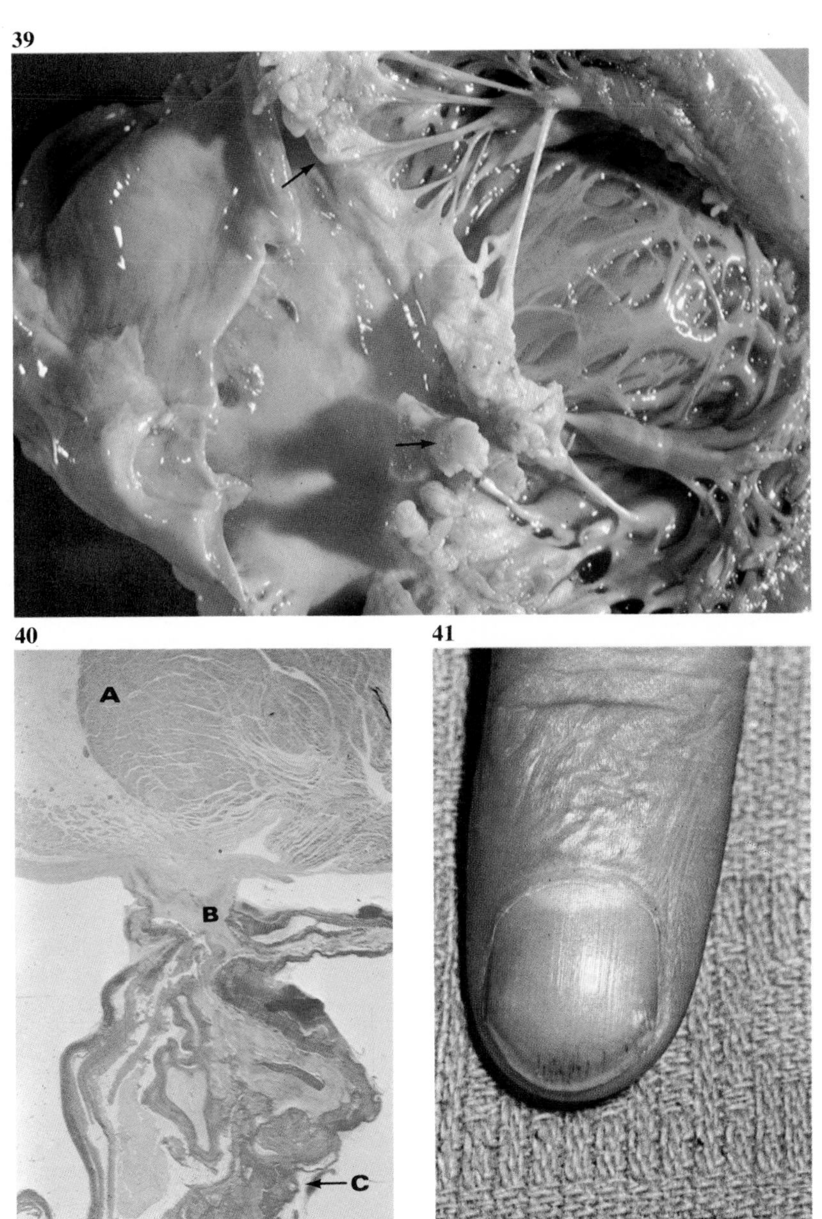
39
40
A
B
C
41

Sensitisation reactions to streptococci

42 Erythema nodosum — distribution of rash. The rash of erythema nodosum consists of tender nodules, ranging in diameter from 1 to 5cm. The eruption is prominent on the anterior surface of the legs but may also be present on the arms or face. The disease occurs mainly in young adults and may follow sensitisation to a number of agents including ß-haemolytic streptococci. Constitutional disturbance is variable, but fever is often present and lymph nodes may be enlarged.

43 Erythema nodosum — rash on legs. During the acute stage the nodules are red and painful, but as the rash subsides the nodules pass through the range of colours seen in a fading bruise. The nodules never ulcerate, and there is no residual scarring.

44 Erythema marginatum. Erythema marginatum, also known as rheumatic erythema, is a circinate erythema resulting from streptococcal sensitisation. This fluctuating rash is found mainly in children and is most prominent on the trunk. It is sometimes associated with subacute rheumatic fever.

42

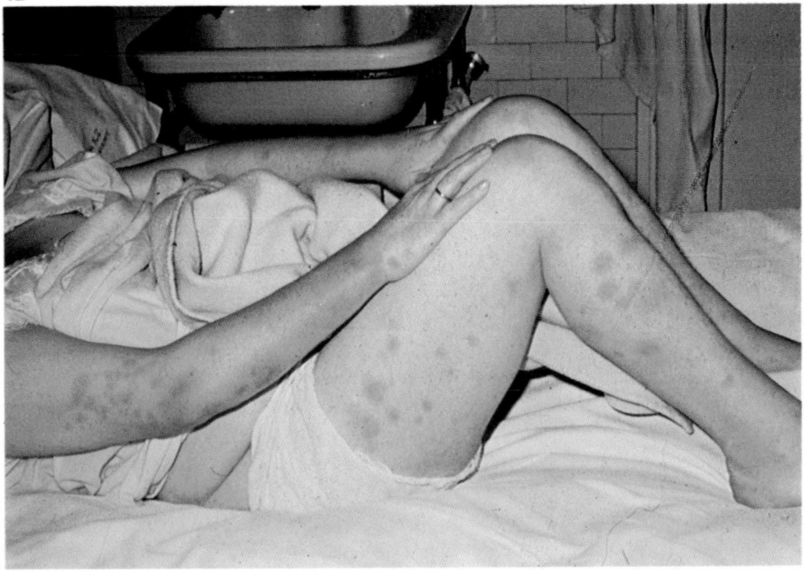

43

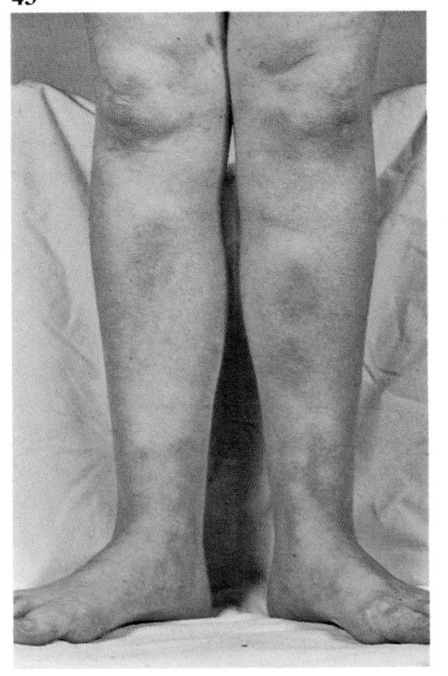

44

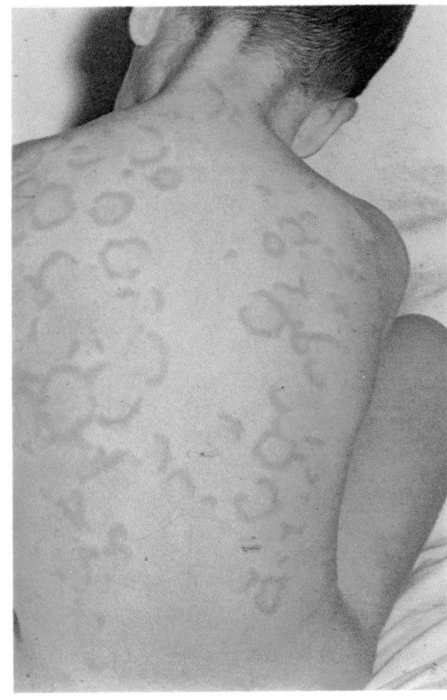

Staphylococcal infection

Staphylococci are widely distributed. Many are saprophytic and can be isolated from water and soil; others are parasitic and may be found as commensals or pathogens in human beings or animals. When freshly isolated most pathogenic staphylococci produce a golden pigment and therefore belong to the species *Staphylococcus aureus*. Pigment production is not an infallible guide to pathogenicity because some pathogenic staphylococci grow as white or creamy colonies. Pathogenic strains may be identified by their ability to clot blood plasma.

Staph. aureus may be recovered from the body surface of 30 to 40% of healthy people. The sites most heavily colonised are the nasal vestibule, the perineum, groin, axilla and umbilicus. Individuals with dry, scaly skin conditions tend to shed large numbers of organisms. Invasion of the skin may produce impetigo or boils, while spread to deeper tissues may result in cellulitis or pneumonia. Invasion of the bloodstream is a serious complication causing septicaemia and metastatic abscesses. Some strains of staphylococci produce an enterotoxin responsible for outbreaks of food poisoning. Certain staphylococci resistant to antibiotics spread readily in hospitals and maternity units causing serious outbreaks.

Organism

45 Smear of pus containing staphylococci (Gram stain). Staphylococci are Gram-positive, spherical cocci measuring roughly 1 μm in diameter. They are grouped in clusters resembling bunches of grapes, but single forms and pairs may also be found.

46 *Staphylococcus aureus* — culture on blood agar. Staphylococci grow readily on blood agar forming relatively large colonies, with a diameter of 2 to 4mm after 24 hours. Mature colonies are opaque, convex, circular discs with a shiny surface and golden colour. Zones of haemolysis appear on sheep or rabbit blood agar, but are minimal or absent on horse blood agar.

45

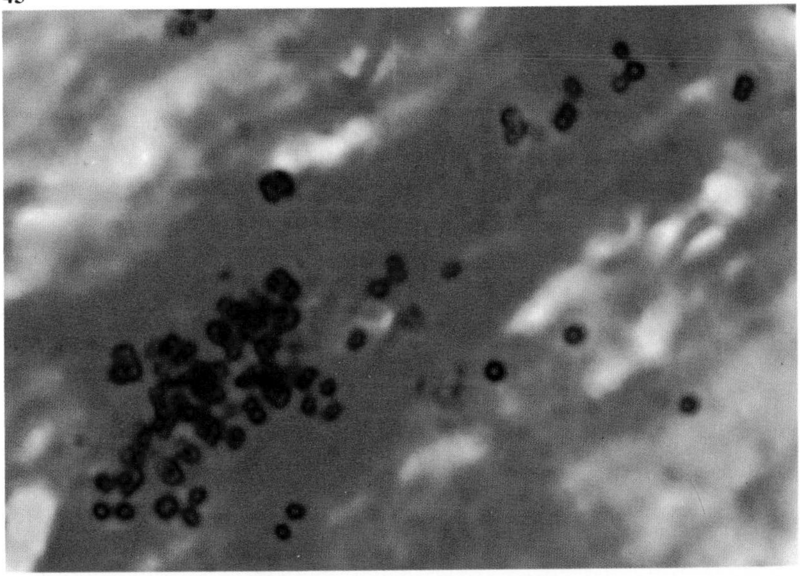

46

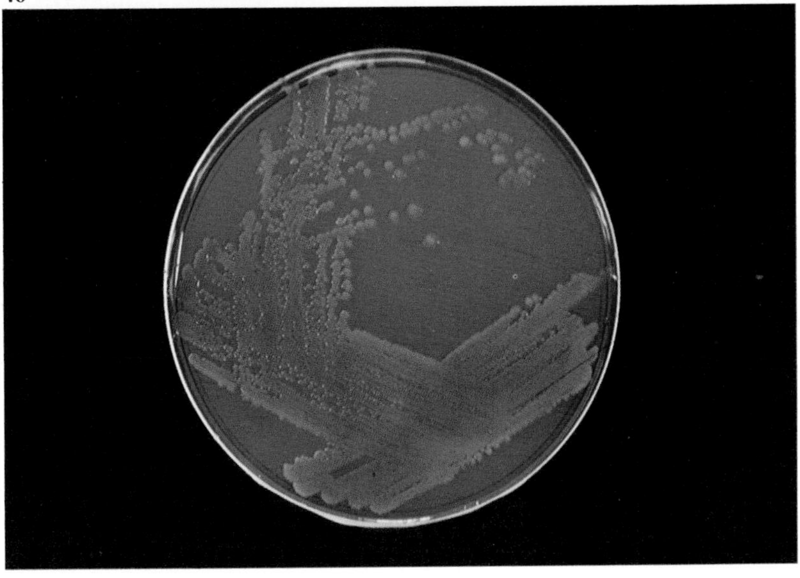

47 Coagulase test. Pathogenic strains may be identified by their ability to clot blood plasma. The production of coagulase is probably the most reliable in vitro guide to pathogenicity. Many other toxins are elaborated by staphylococci, but little is known of their part in producing disease. Some strains of *Staph. aureus* produce an enterotoxin responsible for outbreaks of food poisoning.

In the two tubes of plasma shown in the illustration the control has remained fluid, but that inoculated with *Staph. aureus* has clotted.

48 Phage typing — typical pattern using standard phages. Bacteriophages are viruses capable of growing in bacterial cells and producing lysis. Most strains of *Staph. aureus* may be destroyed by several distinct phages, but some strains are untypable. Using a combination of typing phages it has been possible to identify several hundred strains, and phage typing has proved a useful epidemiological tool.

Drops containing each of the typing phages have been placed in a prescribed pattern on the surface of the medium after it has been evenly inoculated with the staphylococcus. Lysis has occurred where the organism has been attacked by particular phages.

Staphylococci may be allotted to a number of groups by the pattern of lysis. Those in group II cause minor sepsis outside hospital. Those in groups I and III, especially when lysed by phages 80 and/or 81, are associated with hospital sepsis and are commonly resistant to many antibiotics.

Staphylococcal infection of skin

49 Stye (hordeolum). Staphylococcal invasion of a hair follicle gives rise to a small abscess or boil. When this affects the sebaceous gland of an eyelash follicle the resulting abscess is called a stye or hordeolum. The term furunculosis is applied to recurring crops of boils. Diabetes mellitus is an important, though uncommon, predisposing factor in furunculosis.

50 Carbuncle. When several adjacent hair follicles are affected the abscesses merge to form a carbuncle. The central necrotic core sloughs, leaving a large ulcer and disfiguring scar. The possibility of underlying diabetes mellitus should always be excluded.

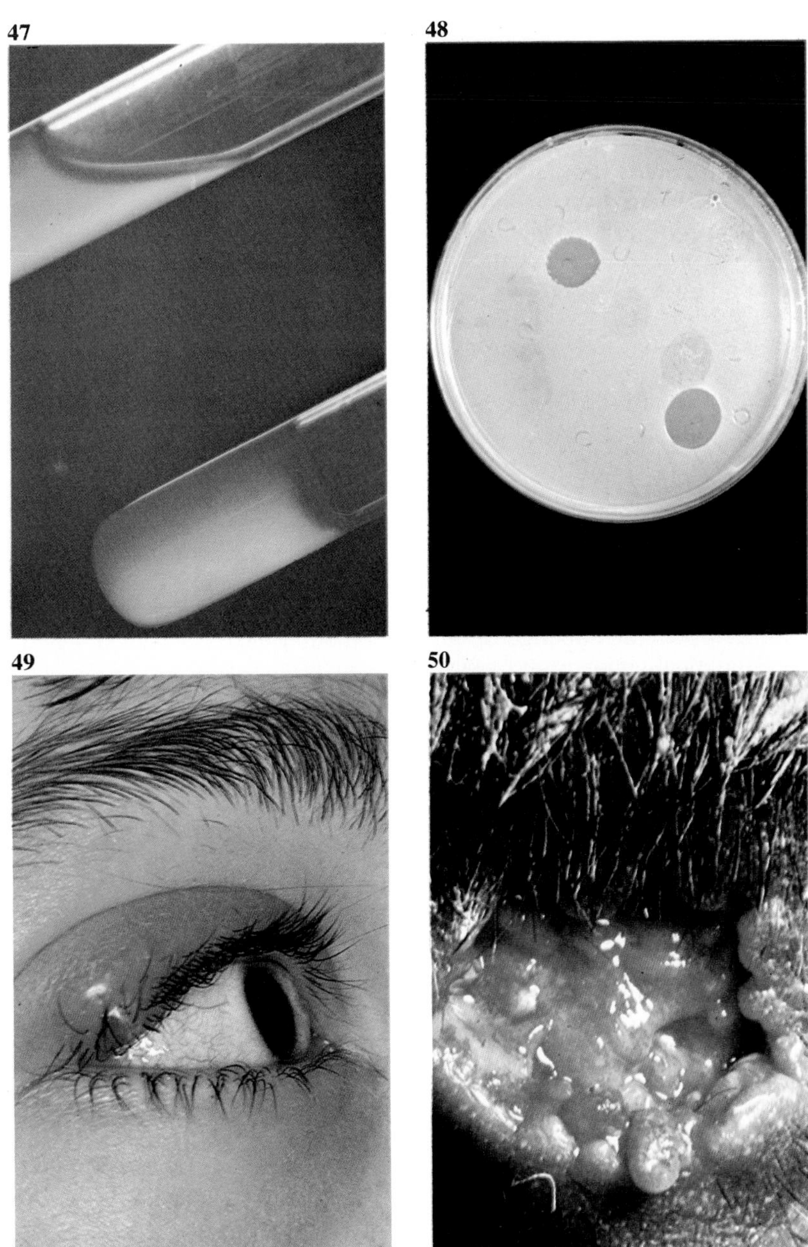
47 48 49 50

51 Histology of skin abscess (H and E). Local invasion of the skin is rapidly followed by an inflammatory reaction with infiltration of pus cells and the formation of a sharply demarcated abscess. The outer wall consists of a layer of fibroblasts that provides an effective barrier to the spread of staphylococci unless ruptured by squeezing or by surgery.

Coagulase-positive staphylococci are readily engulfed by phagocytes but are able to survive and multiply within these cells, ultimately destroying them and escaping. Antibody production does not seem to play an important part in preventing infection.

Note the striking contrast between staphylococcal infection that extends through the skin to involve the subcutaneous tissues and viral infections, such as varicella, where the changes are confined to the epidermis (see **208** and **209**). The arrow indicates the junction of the dermis with subcutaneous tissue.

52 Bullous impetigo of face. Superficial infection of the skin with *Staph. aureus* causes one variety of impetigo (see **34**). The rash usually begins around the nose or mouth and spreads rapidly to other parts of the body. Staphylococcal impetigo may take the form of bullae, containing pus, which rupture and produce crusts.

Staphylococcal impetigo is highly infectious in infants and young children; death may result from systemic invasion.

53 Pustular impetigo. In older patients pustular lesions predominate and systemic spread is rare. Phage group II staphylococci are commonly involved and many are resistant to benzylpenicillin.

54 Crusted impetigo. Bullae are usually succeeded by crusts within a few hours, but there may be a delay of a day or two before they form. Staphylococcal crusts lack the golden-yellow hue of streptococcal lesions (see **34**).

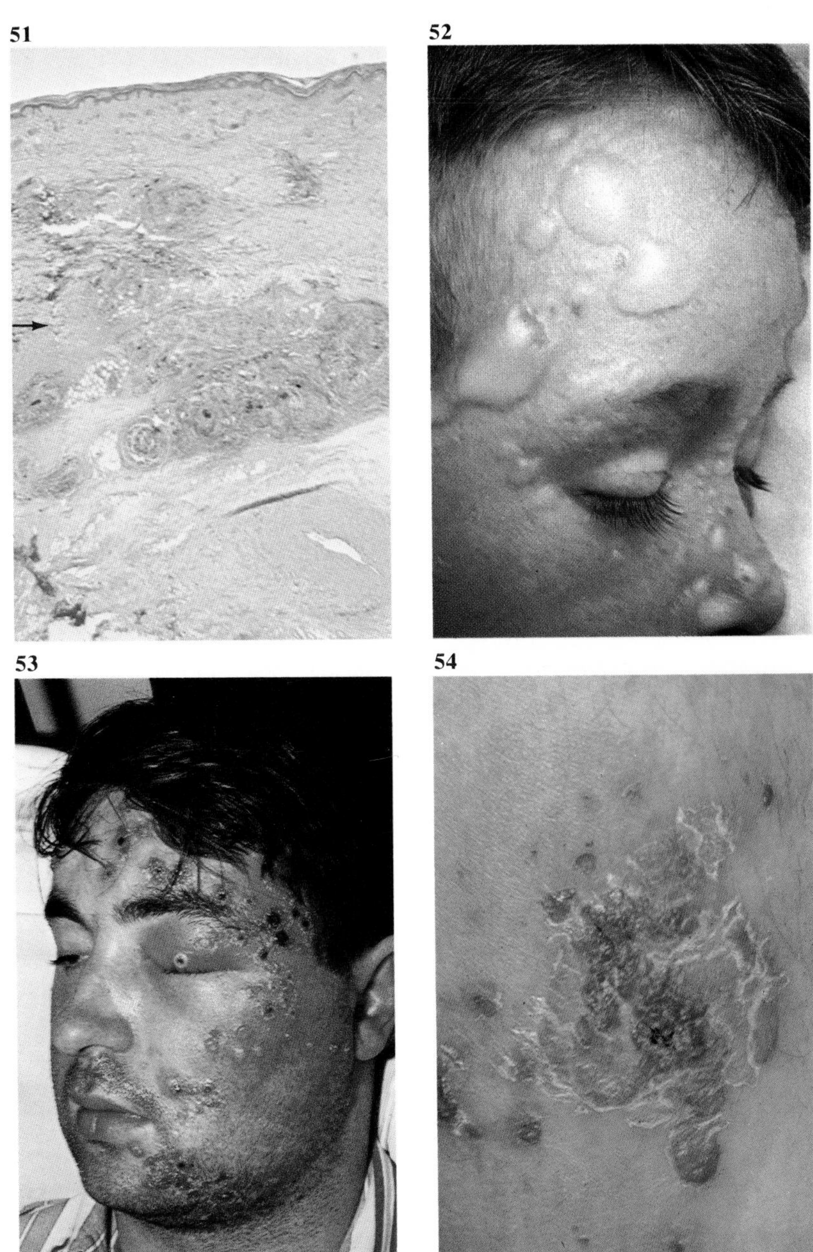
51
52
53
54

55 Acute epidermal necrolysis (Lyell's syndrome; scalded-skin syndrome). Acute epidermal necrolysis closely resembles Stevens–Johnson syndrome. Both conditions are characterised by conjunctivitis, stomatitis, urethritis, and a rash, but the skin lesions differ. In Lyell's syndrome the skin is extremely painful and large patches of necrotic epidermis slide off the underlying layers at the slightest pressure leaving extensive raw areas (Nikolsky's sign). The appearance closely resembles a severe scald. There seem to be two varieties of epidermal necrolysis; one associated with group II staphylococci, especially phage type 71, and the other with hypersensitivity to drugs. The staphylococci, growing on the surface of the skin or mucosae, produce an epidermolytic exotoxin, exfoliatin, which damages the skin, resulting in cleavage within the epidermis (see **462**).

56 Ritter's disease. Ritter's disease appears to be the neonatal form of toxic epidermal necrolysis. The illness begins abruptly with redness and crusting around the mouth followed within a day or two by a generalised erythematous rash. The skin is painful, and flaccid bullae develop. The slightest pressure rubs the surface off the skin leaving raw areas. During the acute stage there is systemic disturbance with fever. Mucous membranes are seldom affected. After several days the erythema begins to subside and is followed by desquamation. The skin is restored to normal within 7 to 10 days. Occasionally systemic invasion leads to death.

Toxic-shock syndrome

57 Rash. Most cases of toxic shock syndrome have been associated with the use of tampons during menstruation. *Staph. aureus* in the vagina elaborates enterotoxin F, which is absorbed and causes widespread tissue damage. The illness is characterised by fever, an erythematous rash, diarrhoea, myalgia (accompanied by high blood levels of creatinine phosphokinase), tachycardia, and hypotension. The illness may be fatal. There are no characteristic features of the rash.

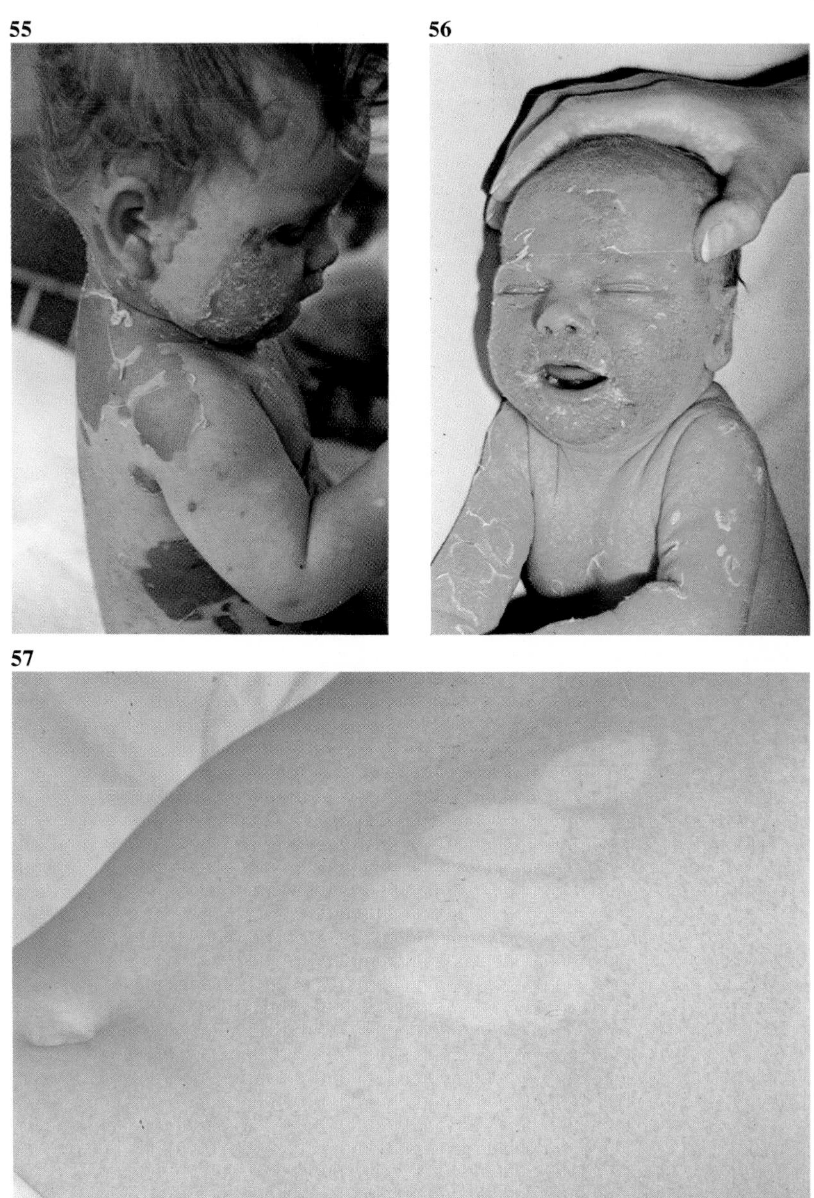
55
56
57

Staphylococcal septicaemia

58 Haemorrhages under nails. Staphylococcal septicaemia may follow sepsis in the skin or genital tract. Often, however, there is no obvious portal of entry. In the early stages general symptoms dominate but, if the patient survives, metastatic abscesses usually appear. Toxic damage to capillary endothelium or multiple emboli from acute endocarditis cause bleeding into the skin and under the nails. The lesions are more florid than in subacute bacterial endocarditis (see **41**).

59 Haemorrhage into toes. Skin haemorrhages are found in many types of septicaemia but are particularly common in staphylococcal and meningococcal infection.

60 Gangrene of feet. Massive emboli or arterial thrombosis may complicate overwhelming infection, especially in elderly or debilitated patients.

58

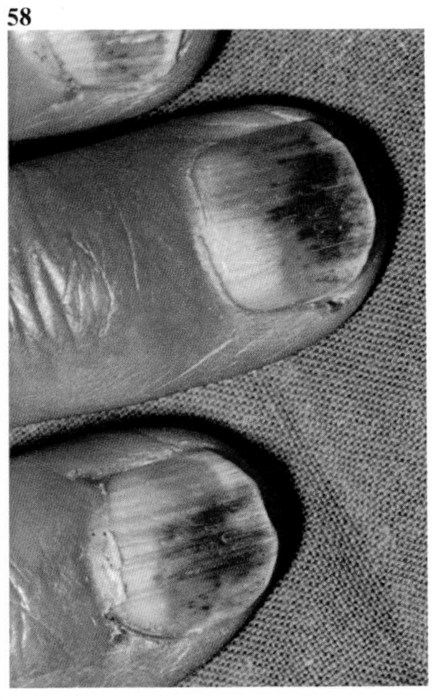

59

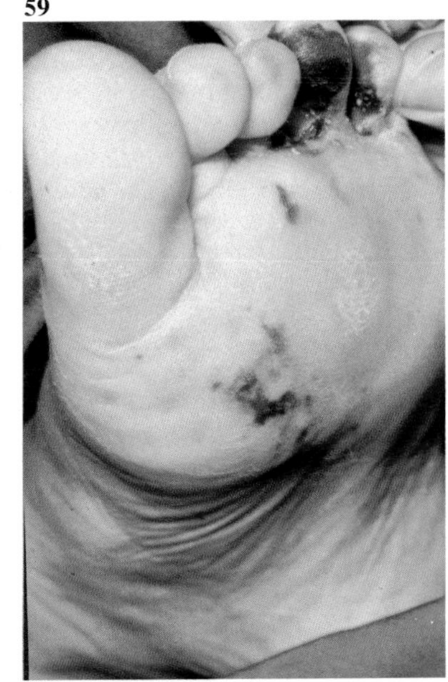

60

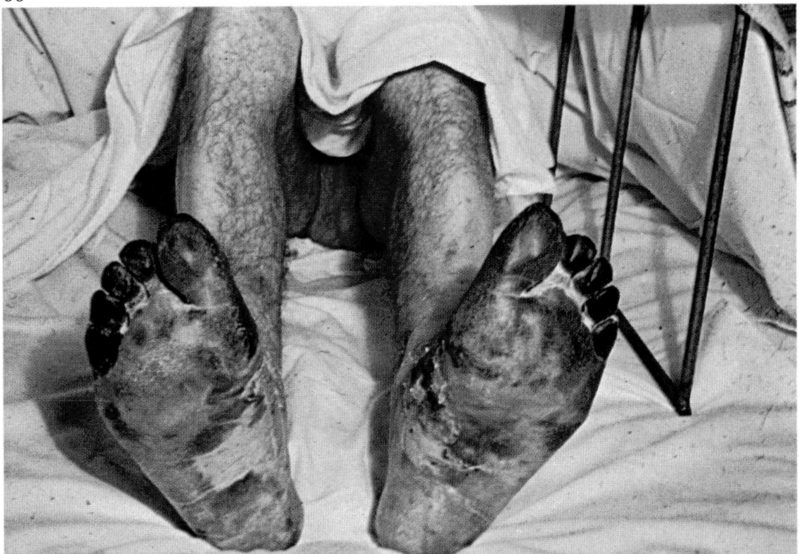

Staphylococcal scarlet fever

61 Septic hand. Some strains of staphylococci apparently produce an erythrogenic toxin which gives rise to the clinical picture of scarlet fever.

A pure culture of *Staph. aureus* was obtained from the septic lesions on this patient's hand. Throat and hand swabs yielded negative results for haemolytic streptococci, and the antistreptolysin O titre failed to rise.

62 Rash — close-up. The rash closely resembles that seen in streptococcal scarlet fever, but the puncta are not so pronounced. Desquamation follows.

63 Appearance of tongue. In the early stages of both staphylococcal and streptococcal scarlet fever there is circum-oral pallor and a white strawberry tongue (see **27**). Subsequently the fur peels leaving a typical red strawberry appearance.

Puerperal sepsis

64 Puerperal sepsis — staphylococcal mastitis. If an epidemic strain of staphylococcus is introduced into a maternity unit the brunt of the attack is borne by the babies. The cycle is continued from baby to baby with the older ones forming the reservoir of infection. The baby's nose is rapidly colonised and over 90% may be infected by the time of discharge. The sepsis rate among the neonates is generally 10 to 20%. Most of the infections are trivial, consisting of pustules and septic bullae, particularly around the nail folds, but occasionally the consequences are more serious, with invasion of the deeper tissues.

In nursing mothers staphylococci derived from the baby may invade the breast causing mastitis with suppuration. These breast abscesses commonly develop six to eight weeks after delivery and may be the first indication of a staphylococcal outbreak in a maternity unit. Note the superficial pustules on the skin around the inflamed breast.

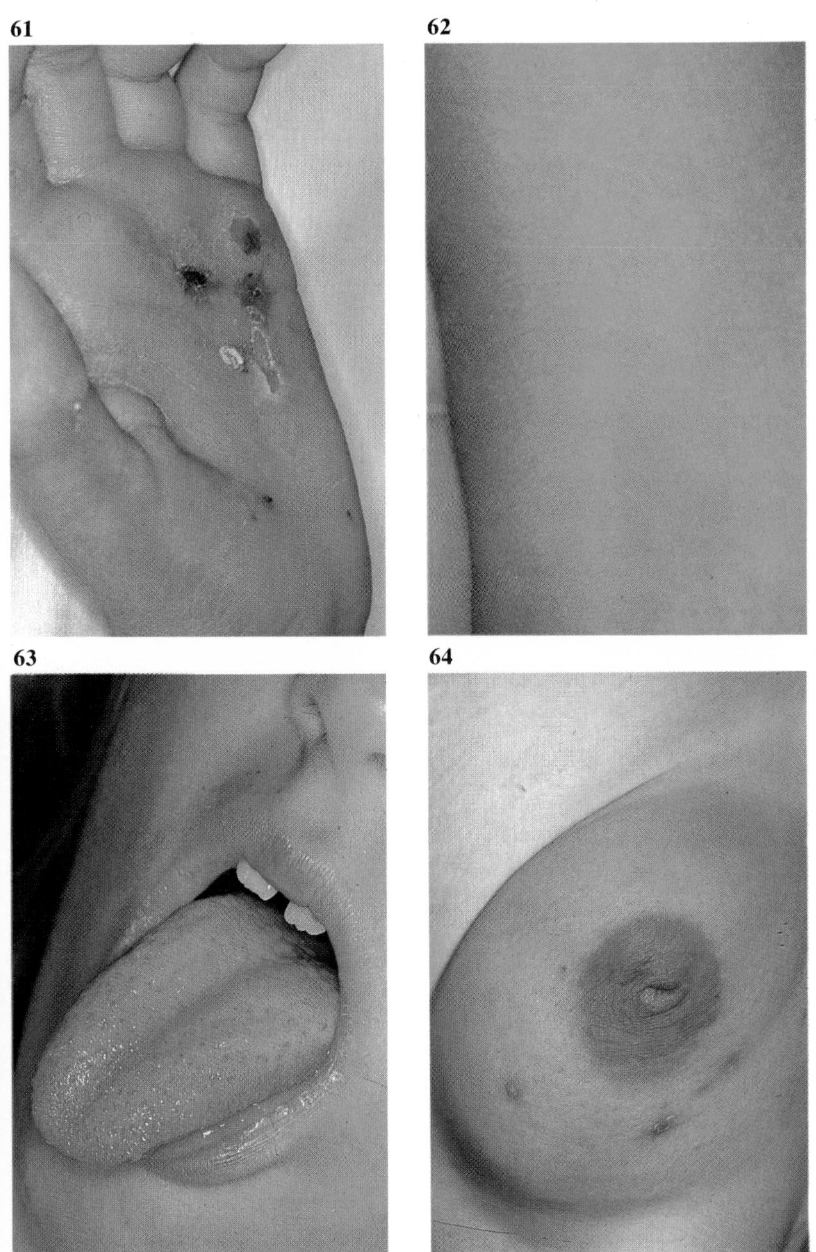

61
62
63
64

65 Osteomyelitis — x-ray of tibia. Invasion of the bloodstream may occur from a focal lesion on the skin or nasopharynx, but often there is no obvious portal of entry. In children with septicaemia, staphylococci may lodge in the metaphysis of a long bone producing osteomyelitis. Initially the illness is dominated by toxaemia with high fever and delirium, but later the affected bone becomes acutely tender and the slightest movement causes severe distress. During the early septicaemic phase the white blood cell count is often normal or even depressed, but as infection localises in bone a polymorphonuclear leucocytosis develops. Two or three weeks usually elapse before changes can be detected on x-ray examination.

Patchy decalcification and periosteal reaction with deposition of new bone are the characteristic findings. In untreated cases infection spreading to the periosteum and increased tension within the medullary cavity may interfere with blood supply causing necrosis of bone. Eventually a balance is reached between the formation of new bone and the destruction of old. In chronic staphylococcal osteomyelitis the anti-staphylolysin titre in the serum may be raised.

65

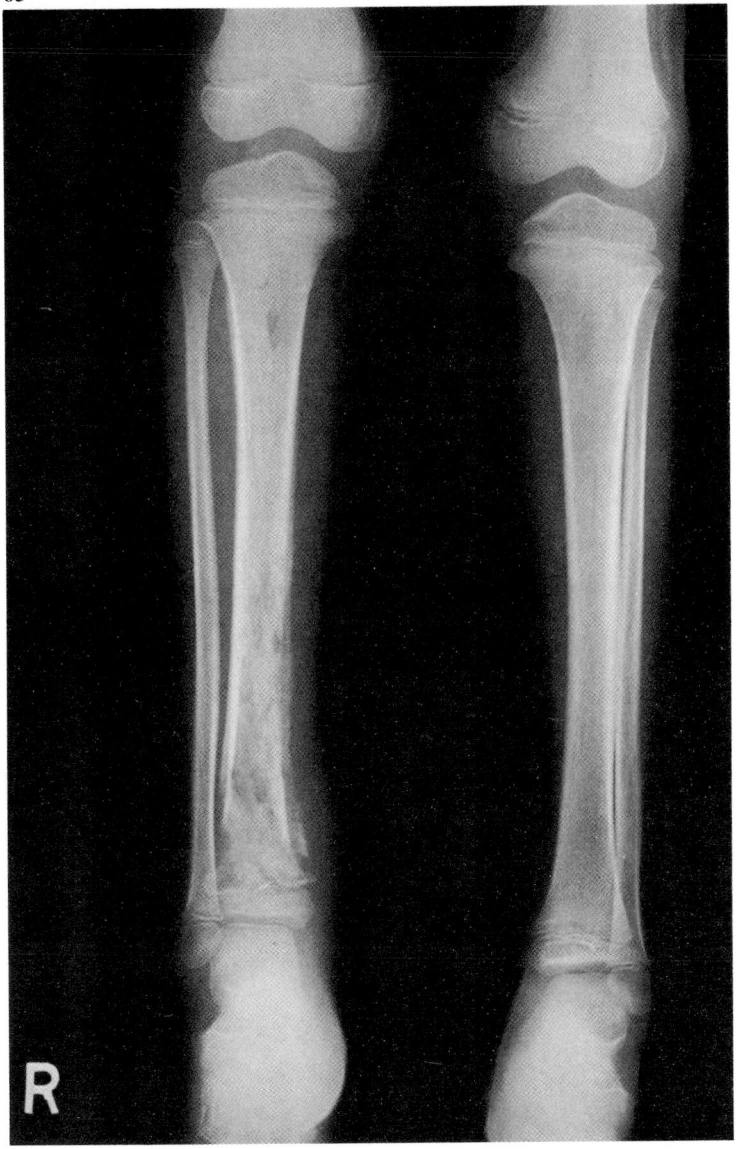

66 Staphylococcal pneumonia — chest x-ray. Staphylococcal pneumonia may complicate influenza and other viral infections, especially in patients with chronic bronchitis or uraemia. It may also follow surgical treatment or result from an outbreak of sepsis in a maternity unit. Invasion of the lungs from the upper respiratory passages may produce tracheobronchitis, bronchopneumonia, or multiple abscesses. Staphylococcal infection damages the walls of the smaller bronchi, which may rupture, allowing air to escape into the interstitial tissues. Air then accumulates under tension as a result of a ball-valve action and the typical pneumatoceles of severe staphylococcal pneumonia are formed. Rupture of a lung abscess into the pleural cavity produces an empyema or pyopneumothorax.

The radiograph of the child's chest shows collapse of the lung on the right and marked displacement of the mediastinum to the left as a result of a pyopneumothorax on the right side. Staphylococcal pus was aspirated from the pleural cavity (see **225**).

66

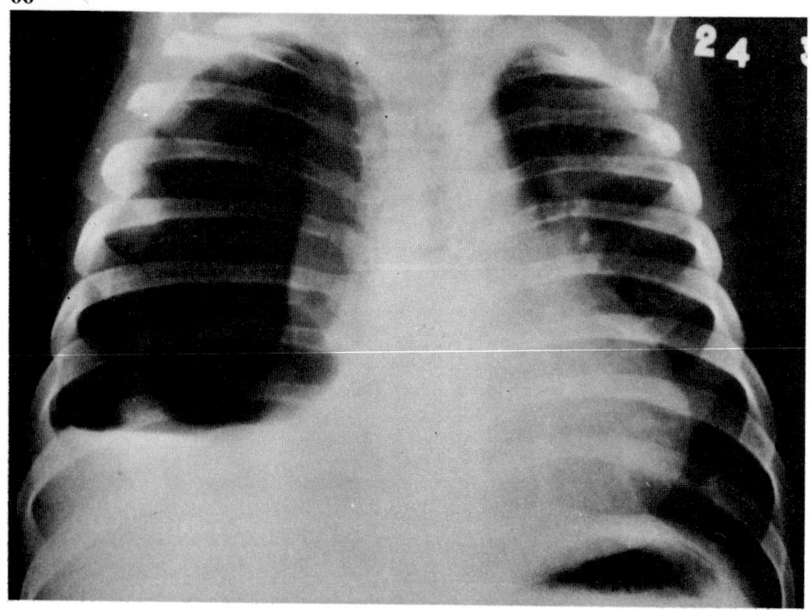

Meningococcal infection

Acute meningitis is an inflammation of the membranes surrounding the brain and spinal cord. A very wide range of micro-organisms, varying in complexity from viruses to protozoa, have been found in patients with meningitis, but clinically the disease may be classified simply into aseptic and pyogenic forms. Acute pyogenic meningitis is caused by pus-forming bacteria, particularly the meningococcus, pneumococcus, and *Haemophilus influenzae*.

Meningococcal meningitis may occur in epidemics, especially in over-crowded conditions. Children and young adults are principally affected, though no age group is exempt. The natural habitat of the meningococcus is the nasopharynx, where it may be found in a small proportion of healthy people. The carrier rate varies greatly and may reach 70 to 80% during epidemics, but high carrier rates are not invariably accompanied by outbreaks of meningitis. In most individuals the meningococcus remains confined to the nasopharynx, where there is little or no reaction, but occasionally it invades the bloodstream or spreads to the meninges with disastrous consequences.

Organism and pathology

67 Smear of purulent cerebrospinal fluid showing meningococci (Gram stain). The organism *Neisseria meningitidis* is a fastidious Gram-negative diplococcus with flattened adjacent sides. It does not have a demonstrable capsule. In cerebrospinal fluid from patients with meningococcal meningitis the organism is frequently present within cells. It is an aerobe, but primary cultures are obtained most readily in an atmosphere containing 10% carbon dioxide. Growth is enhanced by the addition of blood or serum.

68 Purulent cerebrospinal fluid. Meningococci are disseminated in droplets from the respiratory tract, the usual source being an unsuspected carrier. The organism may be classified serologically. Groups A, B and C are associated with epidemics. Sulphonamide-resistant strains usually fall into groups B and C.

A provisional diagnosis of pyogenic meningitis is confirmed by finding turbid cerebrospinal fluid on lumbar puncture. The nature of the infection may be suspected by the sudden onset of meningitis in a young person or the presence of a haemorrhagic rash, but a careful search should be made in a smear of cerebrospinal fluid or scrapings from skin lesions for Gram-negative intracellular diplococci. The meningococcus may be cultured from cerebrospinal fluid or blood.

69 Appearance of brain and meninges. It is commonly believed that the meningococcus spreads to the meninges via the bloodstream but direct spread from the nasopharynx has not been completely excluded.

Once the meninges have been invaded there is an acute inflammatory reaction with congestion and oedema, petechial haemorrhages and marked distension of the veins. Within 48 hours a thin layer of pus covers the brain, especially round the base, and the ventricles become distended with turbid fluid. The foramina may become blocked with viscous fluid and adhesions may further impair the free flow of cerebrospinal fluid.

Although the disease is essentially a leptomeningitis, changes are also found in the substance of the brain, where there is swelling, vascular engorgement and toxic damage to nerve cells.

67

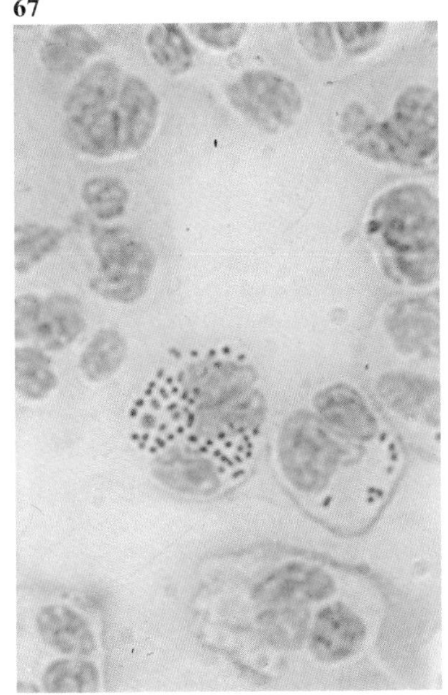

68

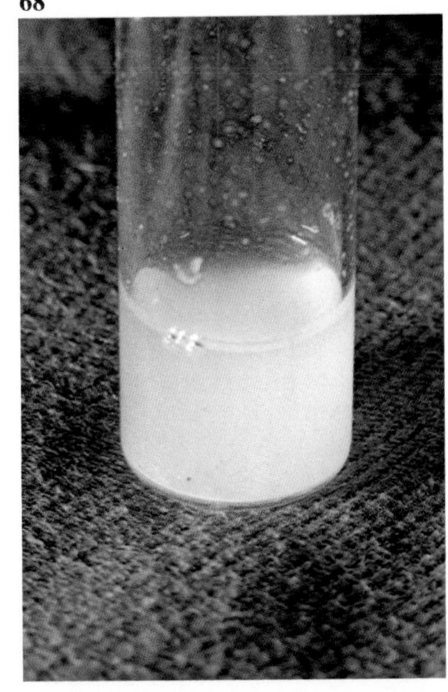

69

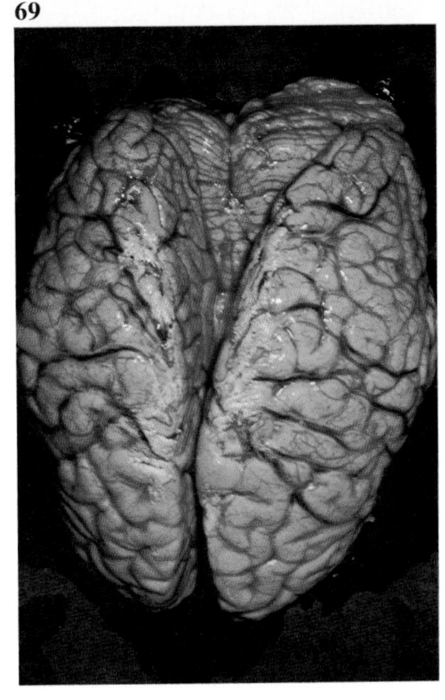

Clinical features

70 Meningitis — neck stiffness and head retraction. The onset of meningococcal meningitis in older children and adults is usually sudden with violent headache, feverishness and vomiting as the presenting symptoms. In the early stages of the illness it may be possible to flex the neck but stiffness quickly develops and the manoeuvre occasions great discomfort.

Neck stiffness is a feature of all forms of meningeal irritation and is found in such diverse conditions as meningitis, brain abscesses and tumours, subarachnoid haemorrhage and meningismus associated with infection of the respiratory passages or renal tract.

In infants under the age of two years the presenting features of meningitis are very variable and neck stiffness is seldom well marked.

This patient was highly irritable and preferred to lie undisturbed on his side with his back to the light. Minor degrees of head retraction are common, but the advanced state of opisthotonus is seldom seen when treatment is adequate. Increasing drowsiness, sometimes accompanied by convulsions, leads to coma.

71 Early rash. The incidence of rashes in patients with meningococcal meningitis varies considerably. During epidemics it may be as high as 50%, but in sporadic cases it rarely exceeds 20%. Fleeting macular or papular rashes are not uncommonly seen in young children in the early stage of the disease; these may occur alone or precede the haemorrhagic eruption by a few hours. In this child haemorrhages are just beginning to appear in the erythematous lesions. The rash quickly becomes haemorrhagic and consists of petechiae and small ecchymoses. The combination of purulent cerebrospinal fluid and a haemorrhagic rash is virtually diagnostic of meningococcal meningitis.

70

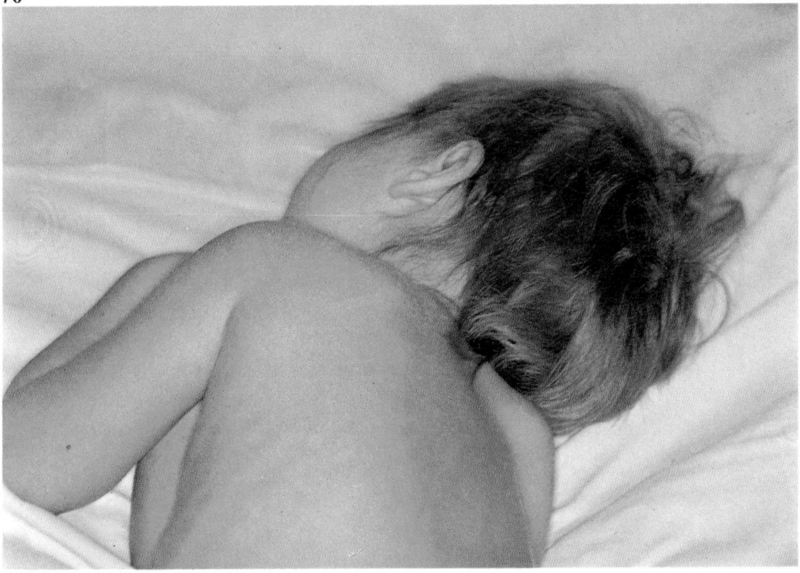

71

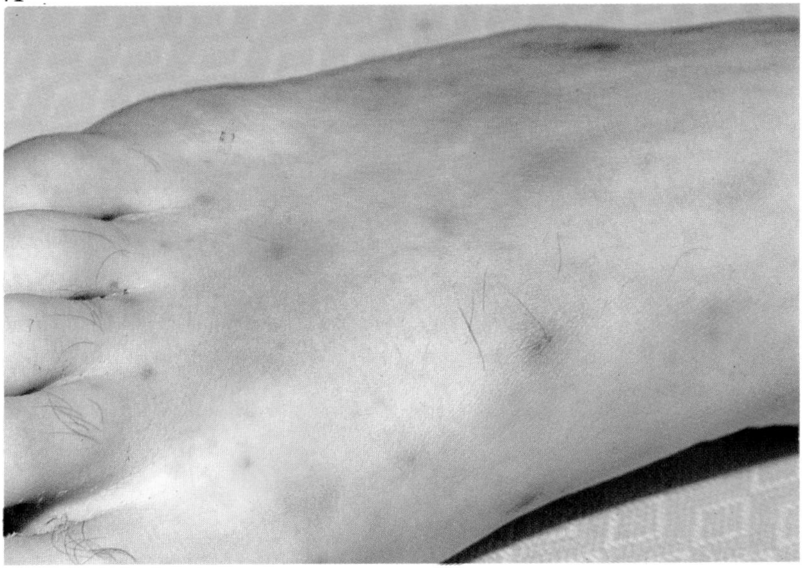

72 Meningitis — unconscious patient with rash. The child shown here was admitted to hospital unconscious and found to have a sparse rash of petechiae and small ecchymoses. *Neisseria meningitidis* was grown on blood culture and also from the purulent cerebrospinal fluid. Response to treatment was good and recovery uneventful.

73 Meningitis — haemorrhagic rash in young child. In very young children the onset of meningitis may be so insidious that the possibility may be overlooked for several days. Unexplained fever or vomiting, with or without diarrhoea, should always arouse suspicion of meningitis. Neck stiffness may be absent, but there is often some fullness of the anterior fontanelle. Convulsions occur in about a third of children with purulent meningitis, but are also common in other infections. The incidence of meningococcal meningitis is less in this age group, but the disease should be suspected whenever there is a haemorrhagic rash.

72

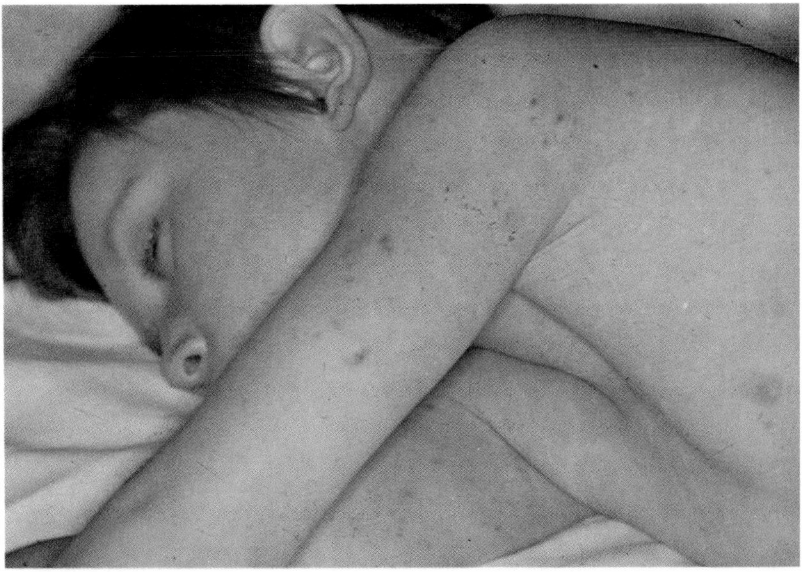

73

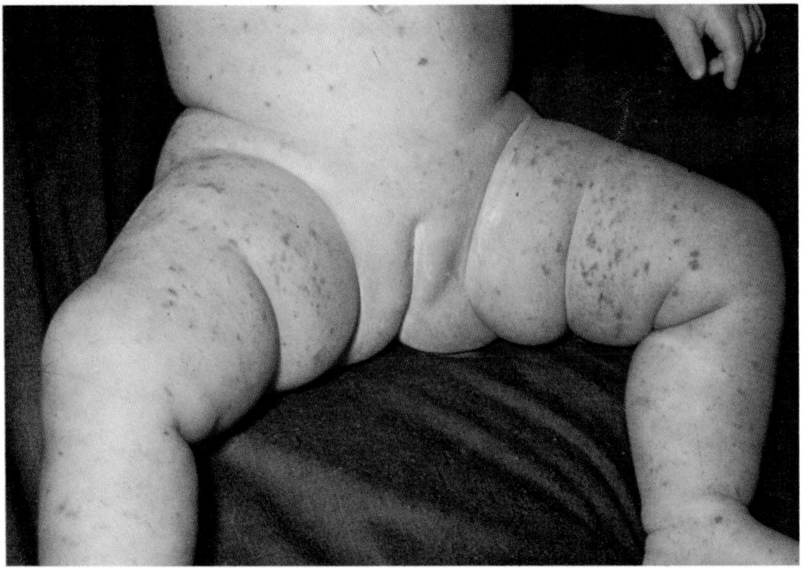

74 Meningitis — close-up of rash. Scrapings from the haemorrhagic skin lesions, when stained by Gram's method, may show meningococci and provide rapid confirmation of the clinical diagnosis.

On histological examination the capillaries and small arterioles in the skin lesions are dilated and engorged. The endothelial lining of the vessels is swollen, and the cells often packed with meningococci. Perivascular infiltration and haemorrhage complete the picture.

75 Fulminating infection. In about 10% of patients there is fulminating infection with overwhelming septicaemia and little or no evidence of meningitis. The illness is characterised by high fever, extensive purpuric lesions, especially over the face and extremities, shock and evidence of disseminated intravascular coagulation. Note the widespread haemorrhages into the skin of the face.

76 Disseminated intravascular coagulation (DIC). In fulminant cases DIC results in ischaemic damage to tissues, and extensive bleeding contributes to death; in less severe cases the clotting mechanisms are restored to normal as infection responds to treatment. Diagnosis is established by measuring a number of parameters. Fragmented, burred, microspherocytic and helmet-shaped erythrocytes are often seen on freshly made blood films, and the platelet count is reduced. Prothrombin and thrombin times are prolonged. Fibrin-degradation products are increased.

74

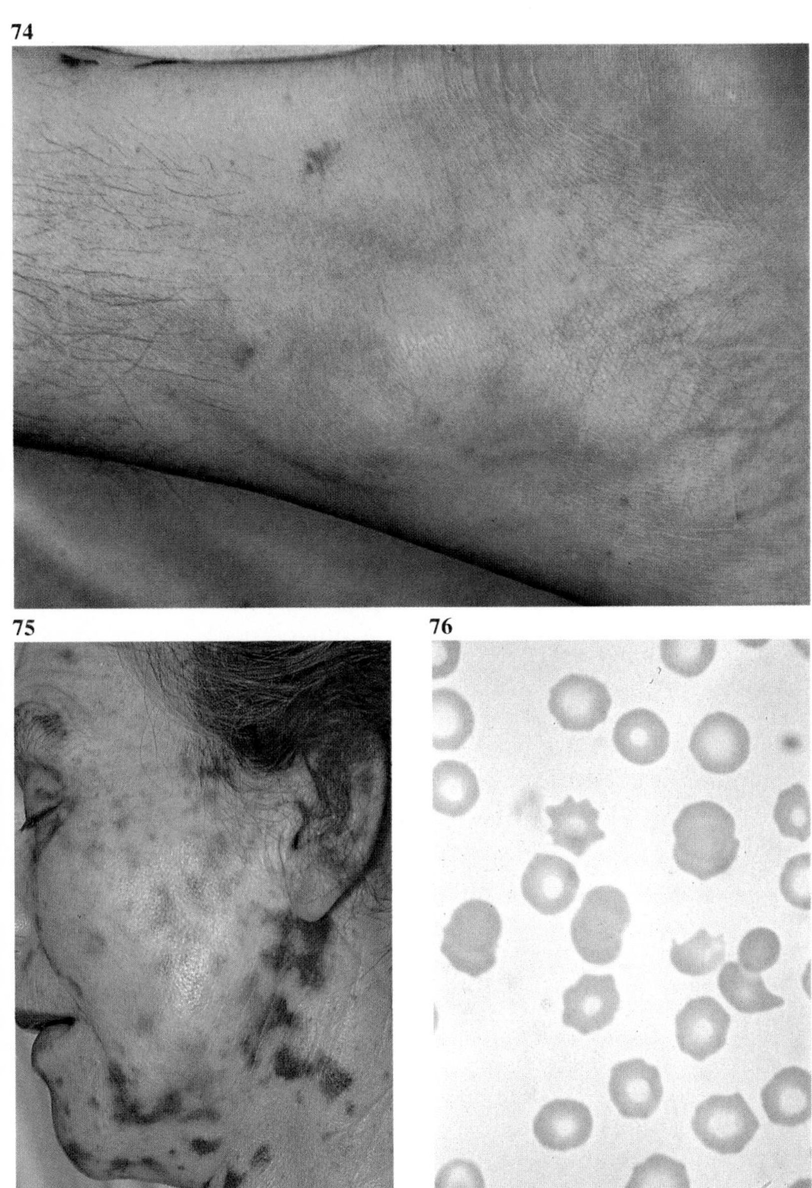

75

76

77 Chronic meningococcal septicaemia. The illness usually follows a prolonged benign course but may terminate in an attack of meningitis. The pattern of the illness is characterised by recurrent bouts of fever accompanied by fleeting joint pains and crops of spots. The rash is seldom profuse and consists of discrete macules, papules, petechiae, and even small vesicles or pustules. Occasionally there may be a rash on the legs resembling erythema nodosum. A similar picture may be produced by chronic gonococcal septicaemia (see **178**), but in this condition the skin haemorrhages are less prominent. The diagnosis is established by isolation of the meningococcus from blood, although repeated culture may be necessary.

Complications

78 Waterhouse–Friderichsen syndrome — haemorrhage into suprarenals. Patients with fulminating meningococcal septicaemia may develop signs of peripheral circulatory failure, advancing rapidly to profound shock and death. When the patient survives for sufficient length of time there is widespread bleeding into the skin, but when death is precipitate the rash may be scanty.

On postmortem examination there is often gross haemorrhage into the suprarenal glands accompanied by thrombosis of the large medullary veins. In some patients dying from septicaemic shock, frank haemorrhages may be absent, but degenerative changes may be found in the suprarenal cortex; in others there may be no evidence of damage. Waterhouse–Friderichsen syndrome may occur in other severe infections. The suprarenal lesion may sometimes be only one of many caused by widespread intravascular coagulation.

In the illustration the suprarenal glands have been replaced by two large clots of blood. (A = blood clots in suprarenal glands, B = kidney.)

79 Meningitis — arthritis. Arthritis may develop at a late stage of the illness. Large joints, such as the knee, are usually affected, and the effusion is viscous. Although pus cells predominate, the organism can seldom be found. Fleeting joint pains are common in chronic meningococcal septicaemia.

The patient in the illustration developed arthritis in both knees on the fifth day of illness, while undergoing treatment for meningococcal meningitis. The effusion contained pus cells but was sterile.

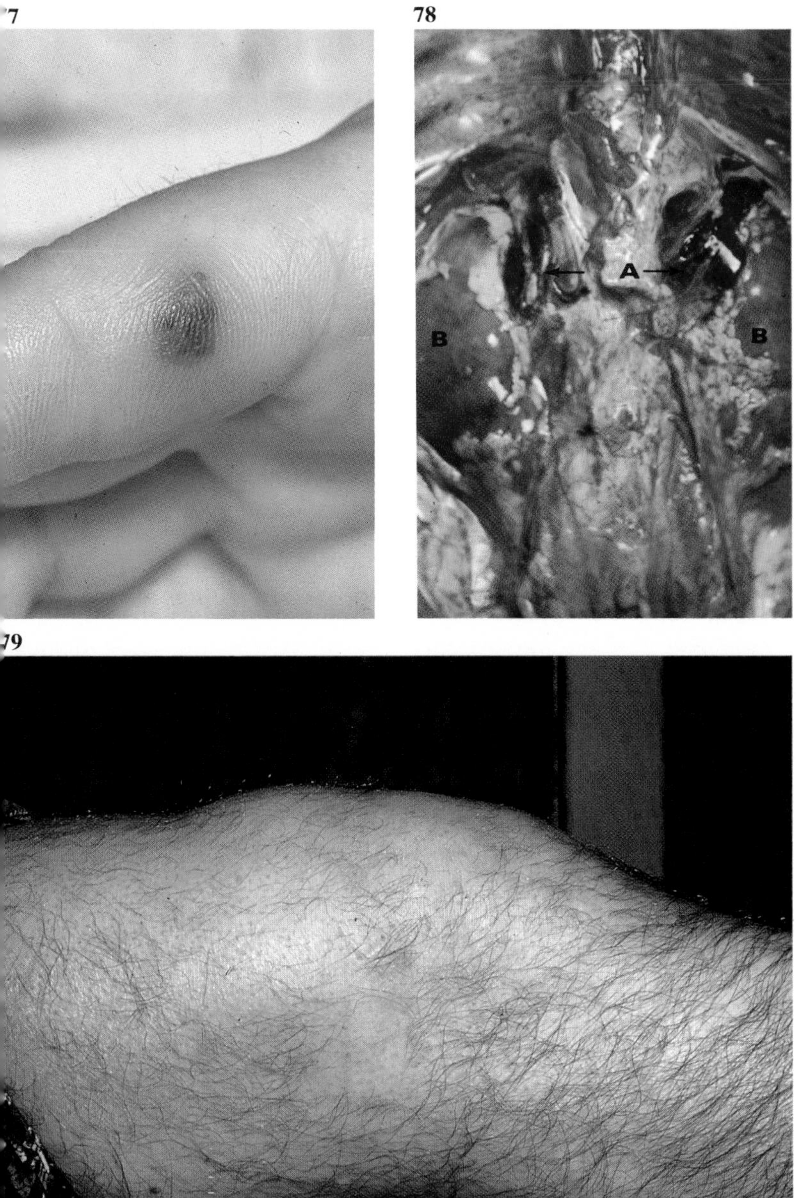
77
78
A
B
B
79

80 Meningitis — necrosis of skin (purpura necrotica). Profuse extravasation of blood into the skin may be followed by extensive necrosis, especially on the buttocks, where deep ulcers may result. The underlying lesion is thrombosis of the intensely inflamed blood vessels of the skin.

81 Meningitis — ulceration of skin. Healing of the resulting ulcer is often delayed, and skin grafting may be necessary. Keloid may form in the scar.

82 Squint following meningitis. Damage to cranial nerves can occur during the acute stage of the illness. The sixth cranial nerve, in its long course across the base of the brain, is particularly vulnerable, and paralysis of the external rectus muscle may be detected at an early stage. The weakness usually improves rapidly, and complete recovery takes place within a few weeks.

Extension of infection into the inner ear may cause partial or complete deafness.

83 Meningitis — iridochoroiditis. Serious damage to the eye is fortunately very rare with modern chemotherapy. Conjunctivitis, once common, resolves rapidly with treatment. Iridochoroiditis is more serious and may progress to panophthalmitis with risk of permanent blindness.

80

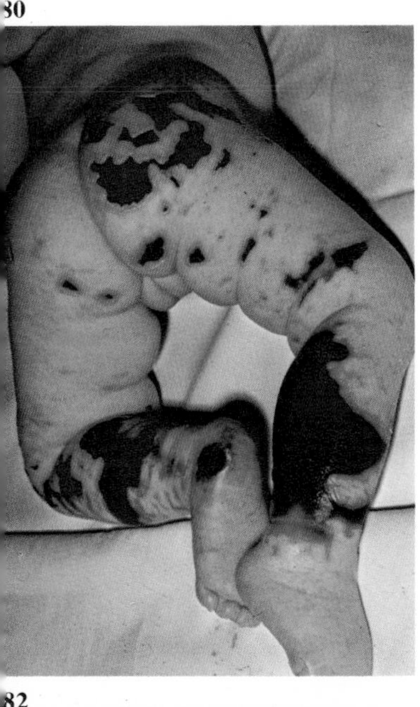

81

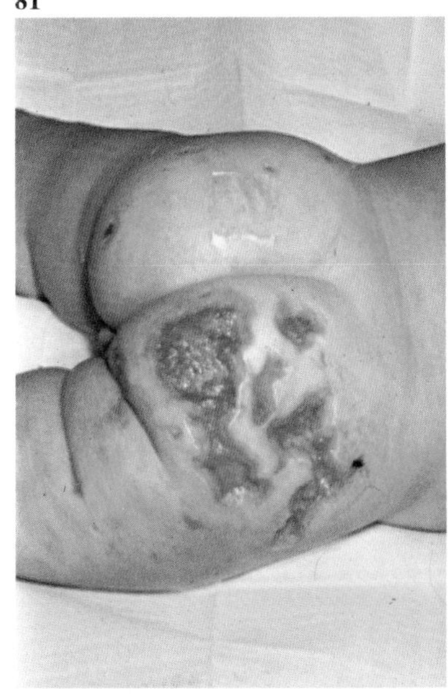

82

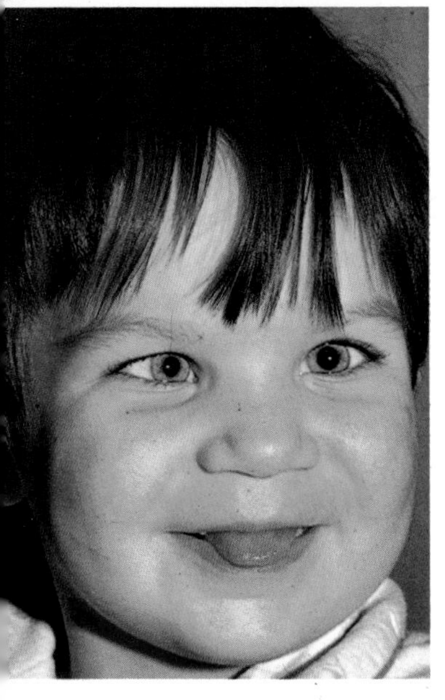

83

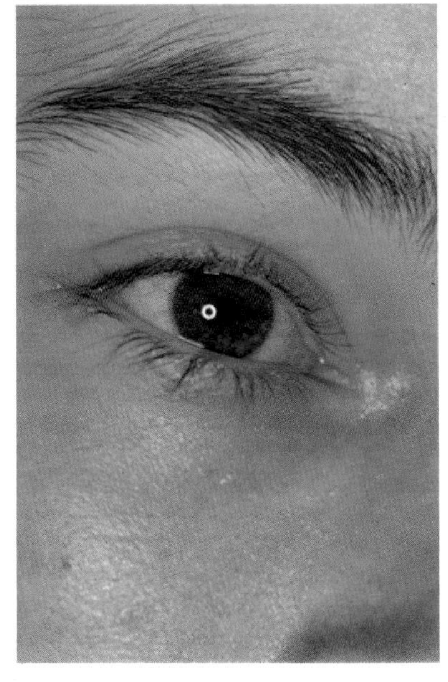

84 Pericarditis — chest radiograph. Endocarditis, myocarditis, and pericarditis may occur during the course of acute meningococcal infection. Pericarditis is a rare complication and may be an unexpected finding at necropsy of patients dying from sudden overwhelming infection. In some patients pericarditis may develop during the course of treatment and bears a close resemblance to arthritis occurring at the same stage of the illness.

The chest radiograph shows the typical globular shadow of a pericardial effusion that developed during the early convalescent stage of meningitis while the patient was still under treatment. Treatment was continued and the pericarditis subsided.

84

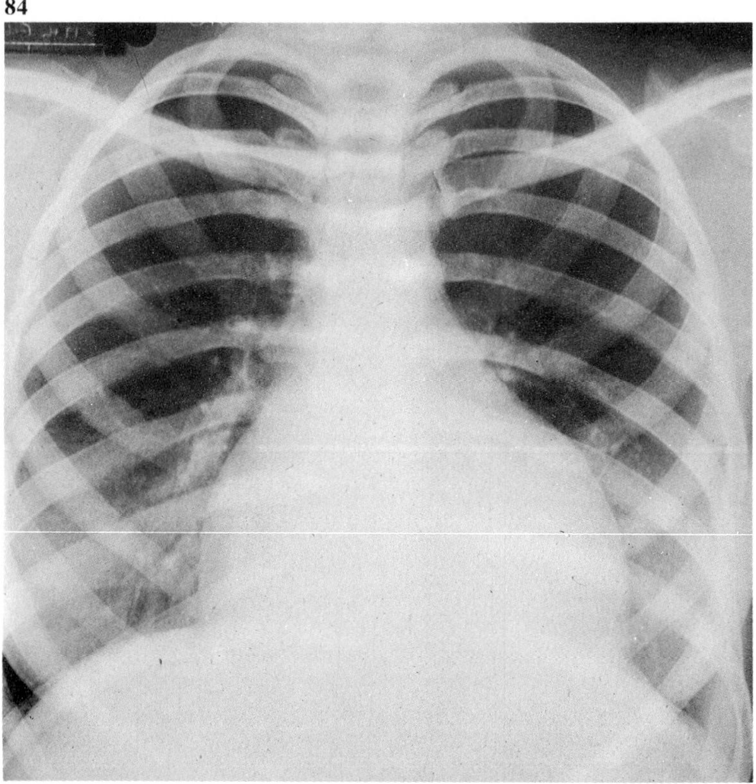

Whooping cough (pertussis)

Whooping cough has long ranked among the most serious of the common infectious diseases of childhood. Permanent disability and even death may follow complications such as bronchopneumonia, lung collapse, and encephalopathy. Apnoeic attacks in infants may cause brain damage and may end fatally.

Bordetella pertussis and *Bordetella parapertussis* are usually regarded as the causative organisms, though certain viruses, notably adenoviruses, parainfluenza, and respiratory syncytial virus have been associated with clinical states indistinguishable from whooping cough. Whooping cough is endemic and occurs throughout the year. Epidemics occur unpredictably every few years and may be related to the emergence of new or virulent strains of the organism. Any age group may be affected, but the disease predominantly involves young children.

The illness varies greatly in severity, though tends to run a protracted course. The initial catarrhal phase is accompanied by a simple cough, which alters in character as the illness progresses gradually into the paroxysmal stage. When fully developed the paroxysms consist of a series of coughs terminating in a characteristic whoop, often accompanied by vomiting. Abatement of the paroxysmal stage is gradual, and a residual cough with whoop may continue for many months.

Organism

85 ***Bordetella pertussis*** **colonies on Lacey's modification of Bordet–Gengou medium. Three days' incubation at 37°C (× 4·4).** The usual shape of *Bordetella pertussis* is a short, thick, oval rod, but filamentous forms may be found in old cultures. The organism is Gram-negative and a strict aerobe. Enriched media are required for primary isolation. After 24 hours small transparent colonies may be detected. These grow larger on further incubation and become opaque and greyish. There are three serotypes.

Bordetella pertussis is recovered most readily from per-nasal swabs taken during the first two weeks of illness. Cough plates give less successful results.

Clinical features

86 Subconjunctival haemorrhage. The subconjunctival collections of blood retain their bright red colour because oxygen diffuses easily across the thin membrane and saturates the haemoglobin. The blood is absorbed after a week or two, and no permanent harm results.

87 Subconjunctival haemorrhages. During a violent paroxysm of coughing the intrathoracic pressure rises sharply and affects the venous return to the heart. The sudden surges in capillary pressure may rupture the poorly supported subconjunctival vessels and produce alarming haemorrhage. Secondary rise in intra-abdominal pressure may precipitate a hernia or rectal prolapse, but these complications are rare. Children with severe whooping cough often have a slightly cyanotic tinge owing to defective oxygenation of blood circulating through collapsed lung segments.

85

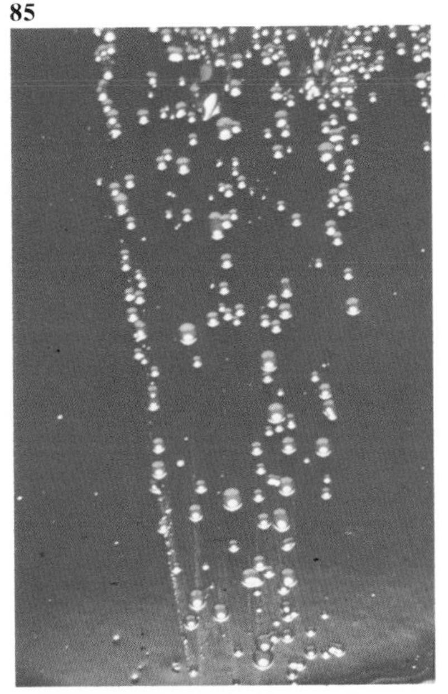

86

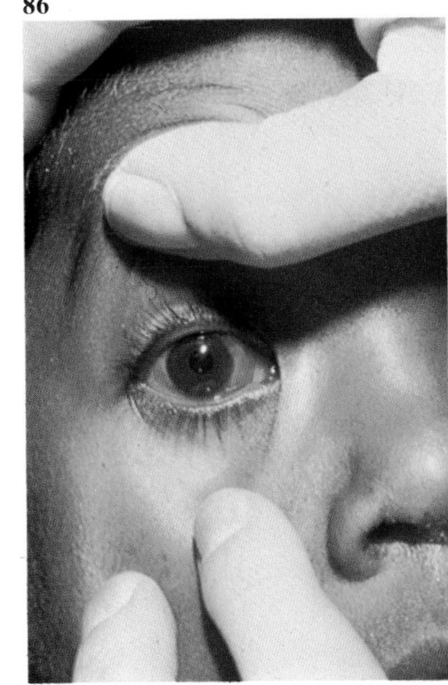

87

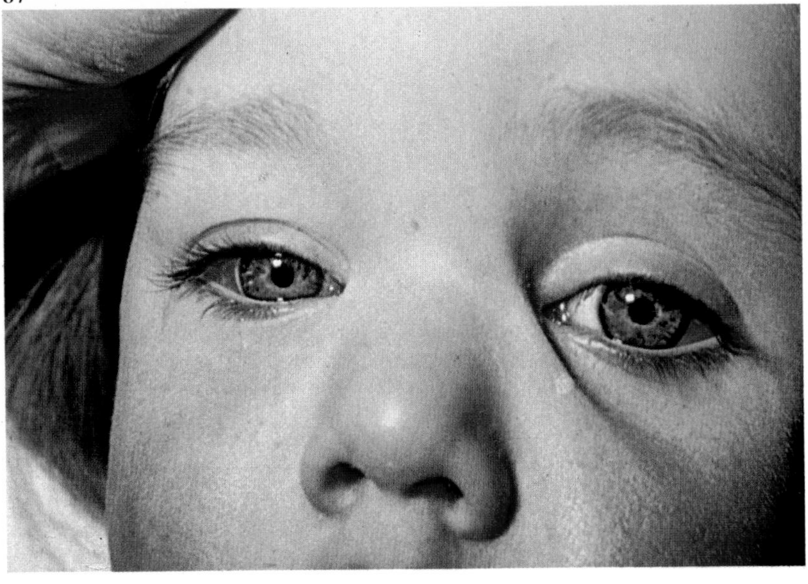

88 Frenal ulcer. During paroxysms of coughing in young children the tongue may be protruded against the sharp lower teeth causing a small traumatic ulcer on the frenum.

89 Chest x-ray showing patchy collapse and consolidation (postero-anterior view).

90 Chest x-ray showing patchy collapse and consolidation (lateral view). On its own *B. pertussis* may sometimes cause bronchopneumonia but more often it paves the way for secondary bacterial invasion from the upper respiratory tract. Plugs of sticky mucus may block the smaller bronchi and bronchioles producing lung collapse. Many patches of atelectasis are fleeting, but others become infected by pyogenic bacteria, and secondary pneumonia follows. The outlook has been greatly improved with modern chemotherapy, and collapse is seldom permanent. In prospective studies there is little evidence that lung damage in whooping cough commonly leads to bronchiectasis.

88

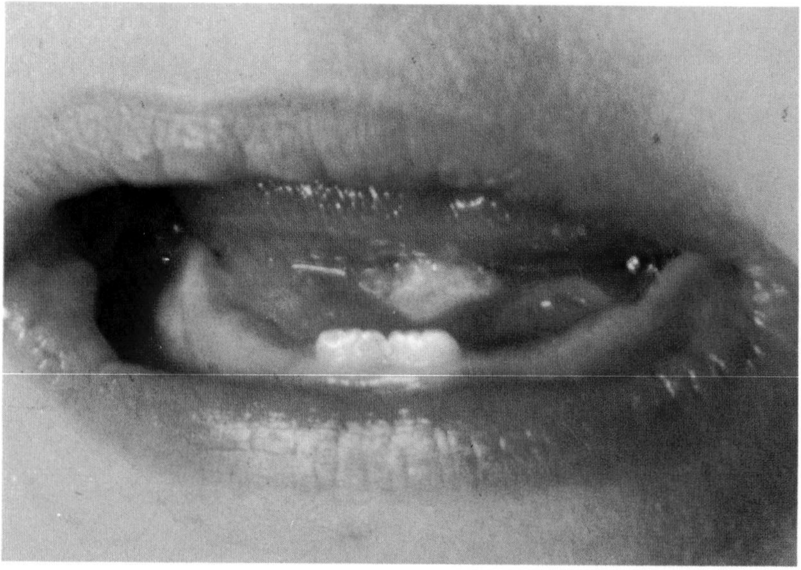

89

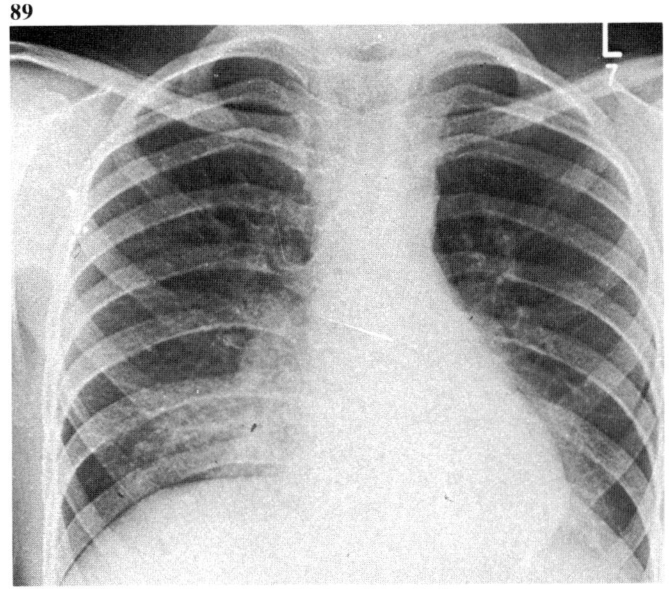

90

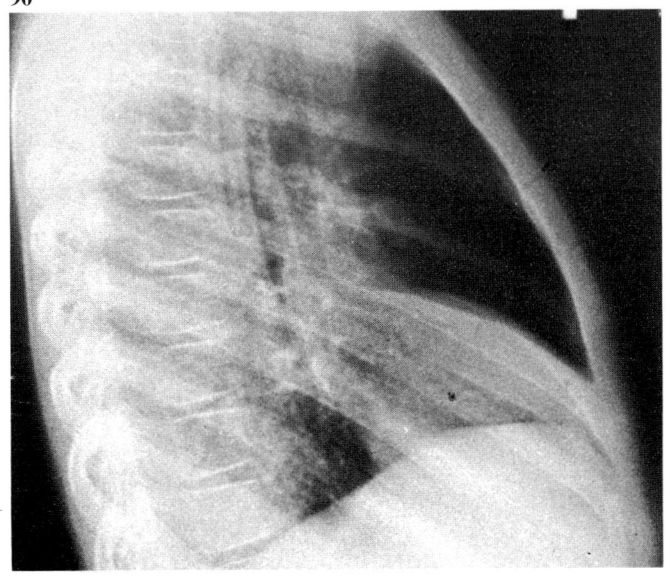

Salmonella infection

The genus *Salmonella* includes about 2,000 serotypes, which are distributed widely throughout the world. They are primarily intestinal parasites but are often found in sewage, water, and foodstuff. Members of the group have been detected in a great variety of hosts, including mammals, birds, amphibia, and reptiles. A few salmonellae are host specific but the majority are not. In man salmonellae are responsible for typhoid and paratyphoid fevers and for one variety of food poisoning.

Typhoid fever is a generalised infection caused by *S. typhi*. Paratyphoid fever may present as a generalised infection or as an acute gastroenteritis. The organisms causing paratyphoid fever are *S. paratyphi* A, B, or C. Both typhoid and paratyphoid infections are derived ultimately from the faeces or urine of a human case or carrier, and the organisms are transmitted by contaminated water or food.

Many salmonella serotypes have been found in outbreaks of food poisoning in man. These organisms usually come from animal sources, but may occasionally spread from human cases or carriers. In most attacks the salmonella is confined to the bowel, where it causes acute gastroenteritis. In some patients there may be local penetration of the bowel wall with suppuration; in others there is invasion of the bloodstream resulting occasionally in metastatic infection of meninges or bone.

Organism

91 Electron micrograph of a salmonella. Salmonellae are Gram-negative, non-sporing bacilli measuring 2 to 4 μm in length. They are actively motile and have numerous long peritrichate flagella. Most strains are fimbriate, and capsules are rarely formed.

91

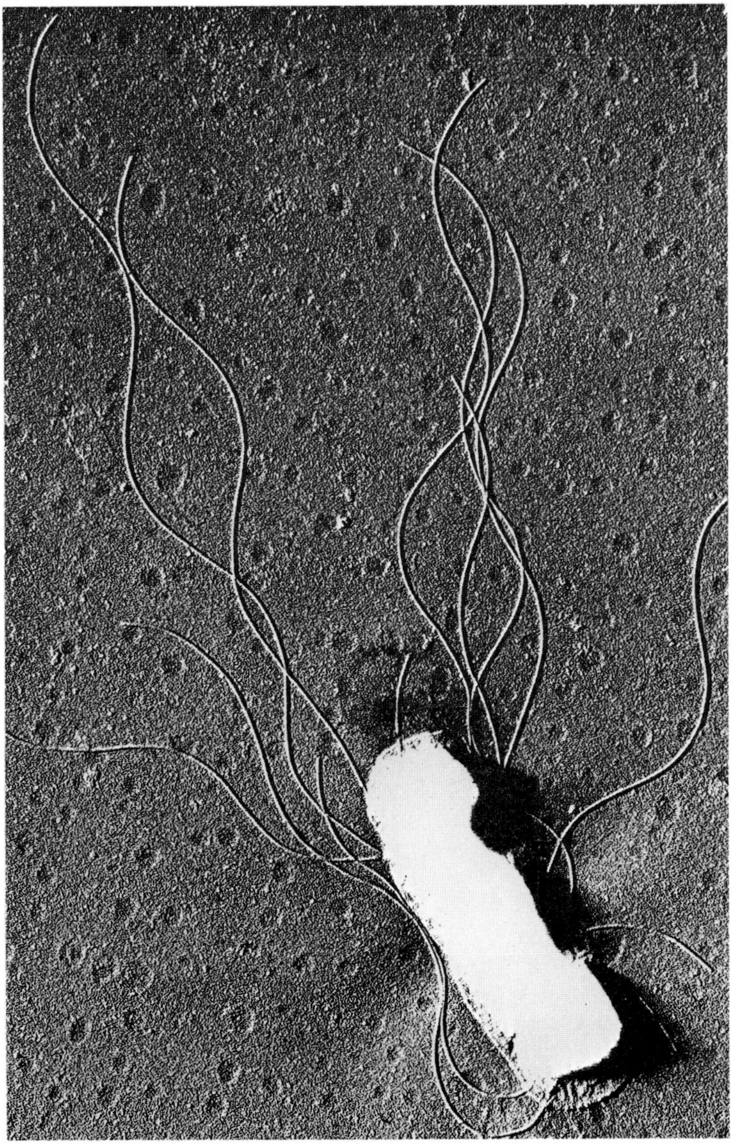

92 O agglutination. In agglutination of O type the clumps are small and granular. Inspection is facilitated by use of a hand lens and strong light. The bacteria in H agglutination are held together by entangled thickened flagella, whereas in O agglutination there is polar attachment.

93 H agglutination. Salmonellae contain flagellar antigens (H) and somatic antigens (O). The Kauffmann–White classification of the genus is based on the antigenic structure of the serotypes. Some members of the group, notably the typhoid bacillus, possess an additional somatic antigen, Vi, which is also present in some strains of *Escherichia* and *Citrobacter*. During the course of typhoid and paratyphoid fevers agglutinating antibodies develop in the patient's serum against H and O antigens. Detection of these antibodies forms the basis of the Widal test.

In agglutination of H type coarse flocculation can easily be seen by the naked eye in a good light. Note the contrast with the sediment in the control tube.

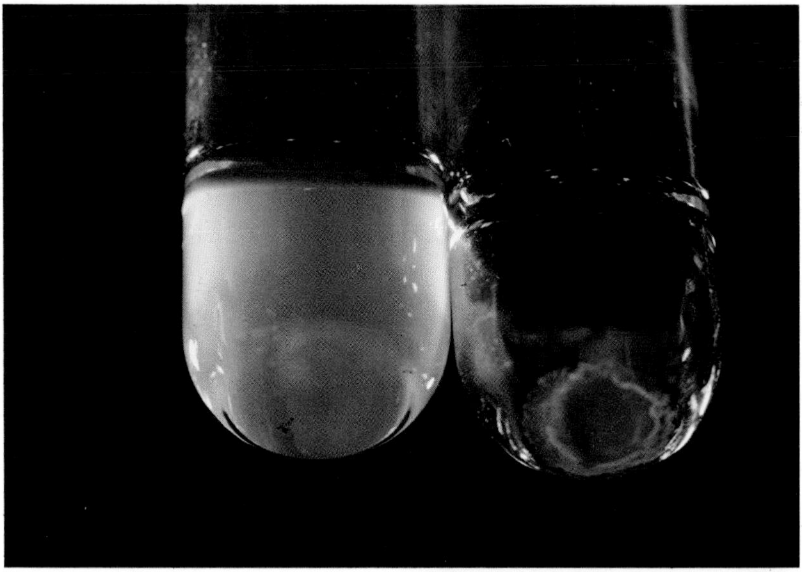

93

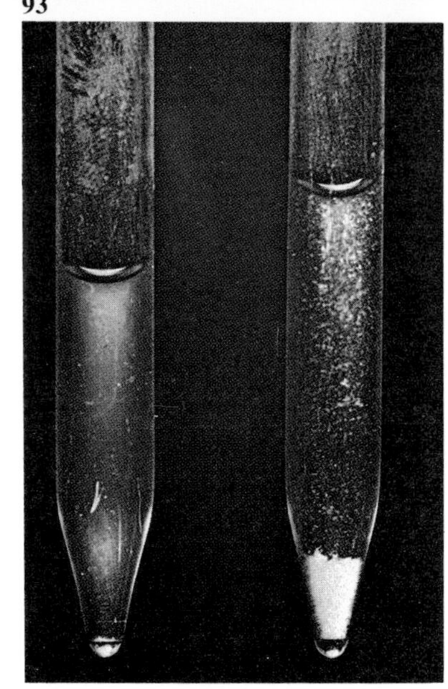

Clinical features of enteric fever

94 'Step-ladder' temperature chart of typhoid fever. The onset is generally insidious with lethargy, malaise, frontal headache, muscular aching, and joint pains. A dry cough is common. The temperature rises in step-ladder fashion, reaching its acme at the end of a week. The pyrexia continues unabated throughout the second and third weeks. When the outcome is favourable the temperature falls slowly by lysis, returning to normal in the fourth week. During the first week the pulse rate is not increased in proportion to the rise in temperature and rarely exceeds 100/min.

95 Distribution of rose-spot rash. The typical rash of typhoid fever may appear towards the end of the first week but it has been recorded as late as the 20th day. It is present in about half the adults with typhoid but is less common in children. Rose spots are difficult to detect on dark skins.

The rash is distributed over the abdomen and chest and may extend on to the back and proximal parts of the limbs but is rarely seen on the face, hands, or feet. To assist identification, the rose spots have been ringed on this patient.

94

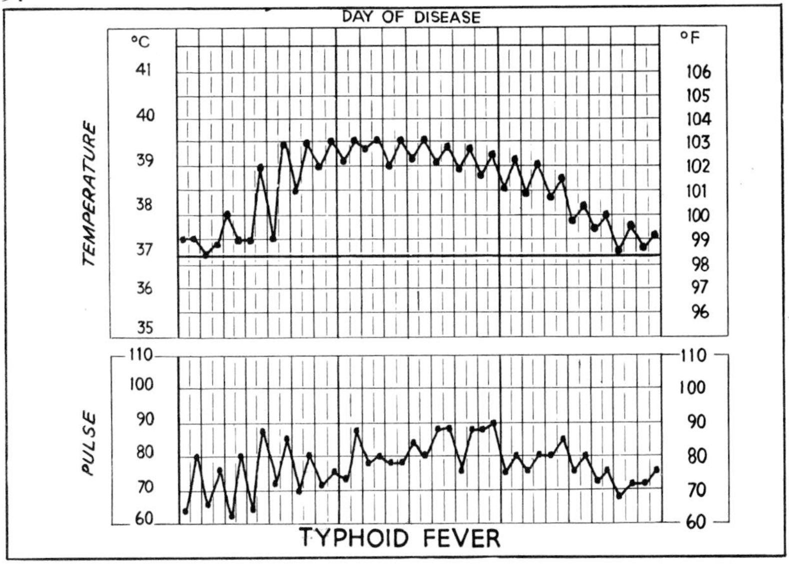

DAY OF DISEASE

TEMPERATURE

°C 41 40 39 38 37 36 35

°F 106 105 104 103 102 101 100 99 98 97 96

PULSE

110 100 90 80 70 60

TYPHOID FEVER

95

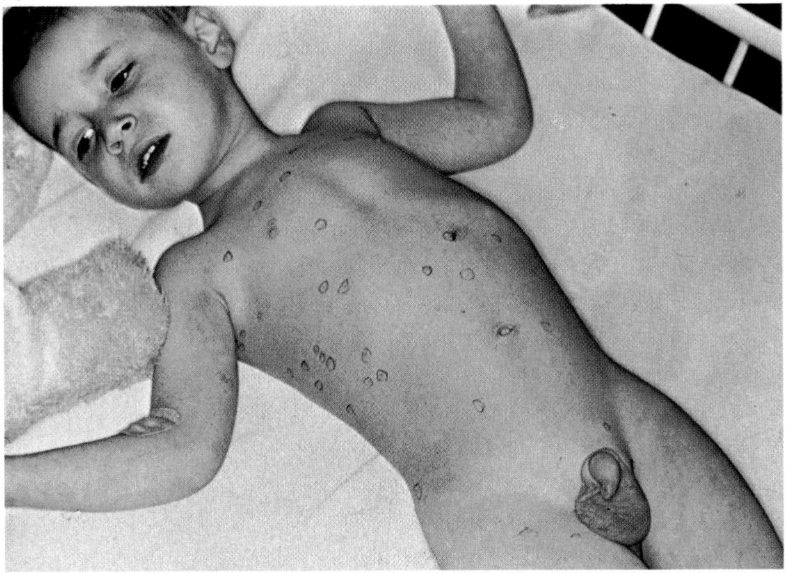

96 Rose spots in paratyphoid fever. The rose spots in paratyphoid fever tend to be larger than those found in typhoid, and the rash often has a maculopapular appearance. When the rash is heavy it may be mistaken for measles or infectious mononucleosis. Careful consideration of the history and other signs should prevent this error.

97 Rose spots on the abdomen in typhoid fever. The rash in typhoid fever consists of discrete pinkish macules or maculopapules 2 to 4 mm in diameter. The lesions appear in crops over a period of one to two weeks, and individual lesions persist for three to four days. The spots tend to reappear during relapses and have even been noted in convalescence.

Rose spots are nearly impossible to detect on dark skins and, when scanty, are easily overlooked on white skins. Two rose spots on the side of this patient's abdomen have been ringed, so that fresh lesions can be recognised when they emerge.

96

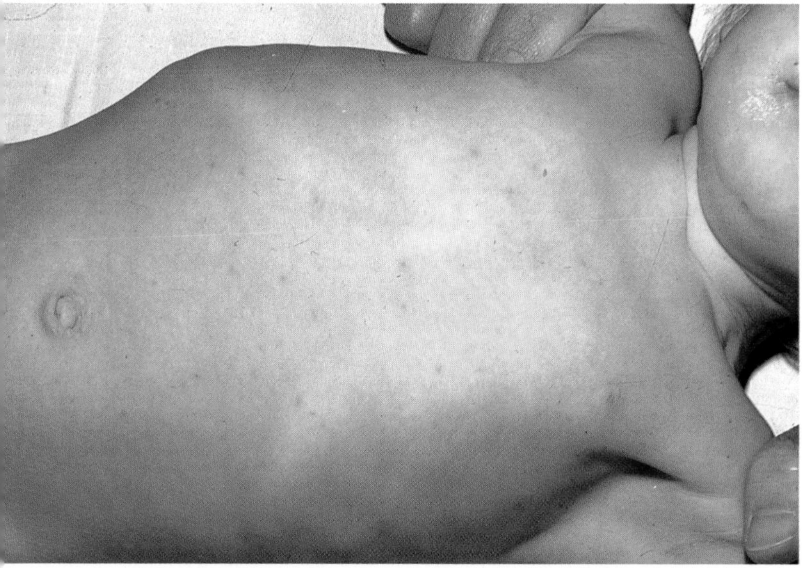

97

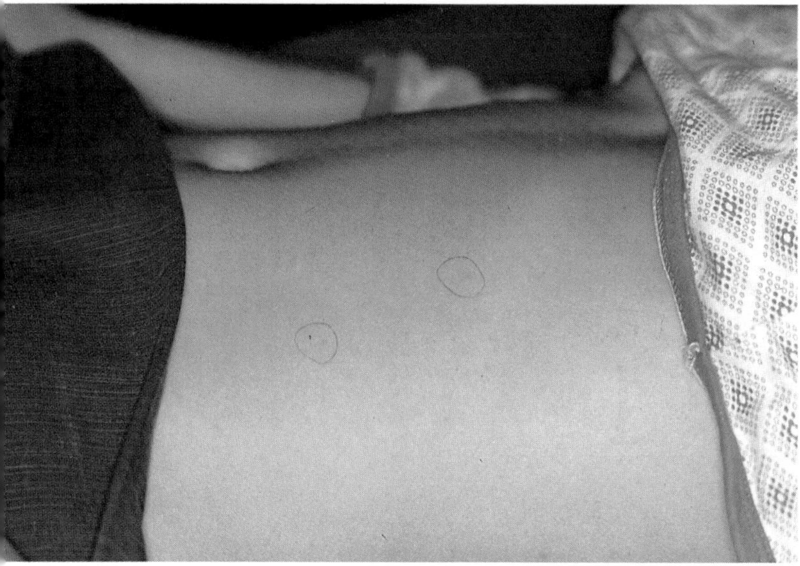

98 Close-up of rose spots. Rose spots consist of pinkish macules or maculopapules, measuring 2 to 4mm in diameter. They blanch on pressure. A drop of oil on a rose spot increases the intensity of the colour and renders it more prominent.

99 Typhoid abdomen. During the first week of the illness most patients complain of some abdominal discomfort. As the attack progresses the abdomen becomes distended, and is tender and tumid on palpation. The initial constipation gives way to diarrhoea in nearly a third of cases.

98

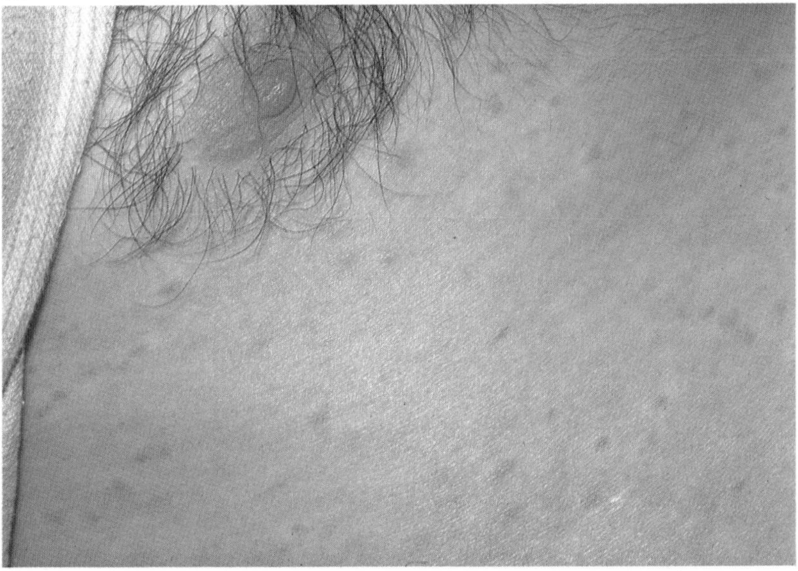

99

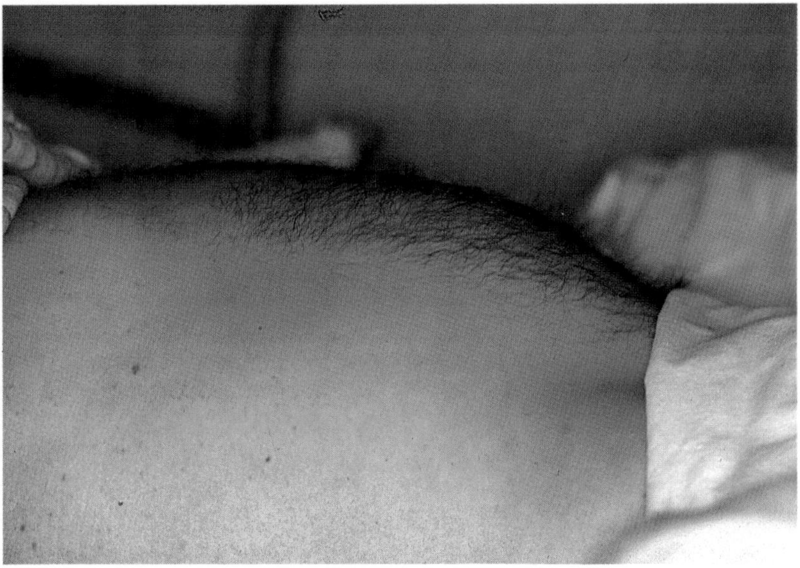

Complications of enteric fever and other salmonella infections

100 Plain x-ray of abdomen in paralytic ileus. In the second or third week of typhoid fever the patient may develop paralytic ileus with increasing distension of the abdomen and persistent vomiting. A plain x-ray examination of the abdomen may show dilated loops of bowel with fluid levels. This complication usually responds to standard medical treatment with gastric suction and intravenous infusion to maintain water and electrolyte balance.

101 Ulcerated Peyer's patches. During the first week of typhoid fever the Peyer's patches in the small bowel become swollen and hyperaemic. The lymphoid tissue is infiltrated by large numbers of macrophages derived from the reticuloendothelial system. The intervening mucosa usually appears to be normal but may sometimes be acutely inflamed.

In severe attacks the lymphoid tissue undergoes necrosis, and a slough forms that separates during the third week to leave a characteristic ulcer. These ulcers are most numerous in the terminal ileum and lie in the long axis of the bowel. Most are confined to the mucosa or submucosa, but some penetrate the muscular and serous layers giving rise to haemorrhage and perforation. In favourable cases the ulcers heal by granulation, with minimal scarring.

102 Histology of bowel in typhoid fever (H and E). Many large, rounded mononuclear cells are present. These modified histiocytes have abundant opaque cytoplasm and are sometimes referred to as 'typhoid cells'. In addition, there are moderate numbers of lymphocytes, but polymorphonuclear leucocytes are rare. (A = 'typhoid cell', B = lymphocyte.)

103 Plain x-ray of gallbladder. Chronic cholecystitis may follow an acute attack of typhoid fever, or may develop insidiously. It is often associated with cholelithiasis and may perpetuate the carrier state. Cholecystectomy alone may clear the infection in 68 to 90% of chronic faecal carriers. Acute cholecystitis is found in under 2% of cases of typhoid fever and is more frequently seen in women, particularly in older and obese subjects.

100

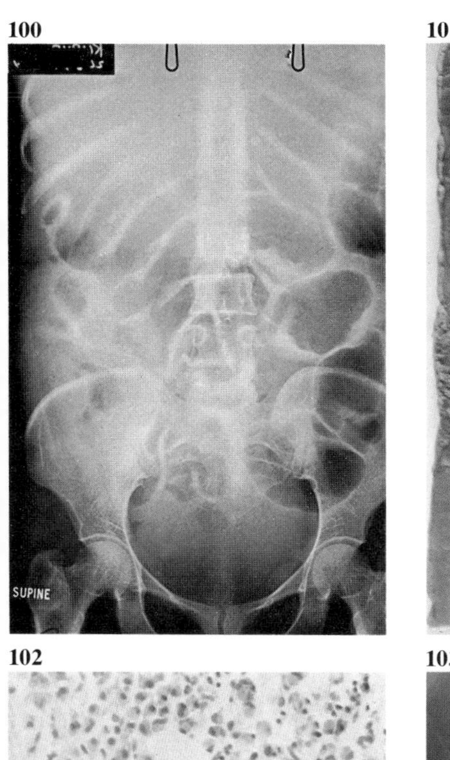

101

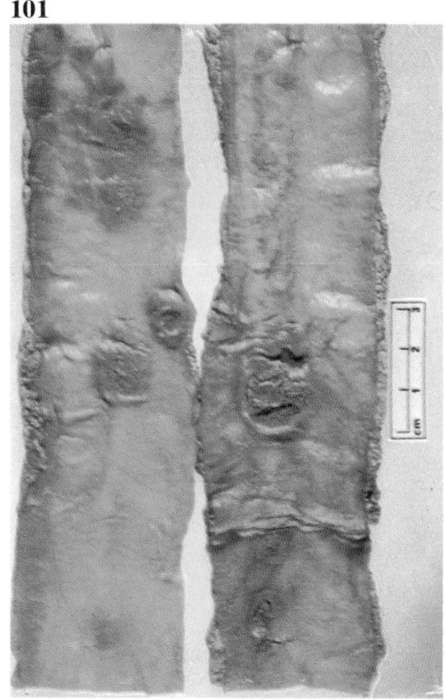

102

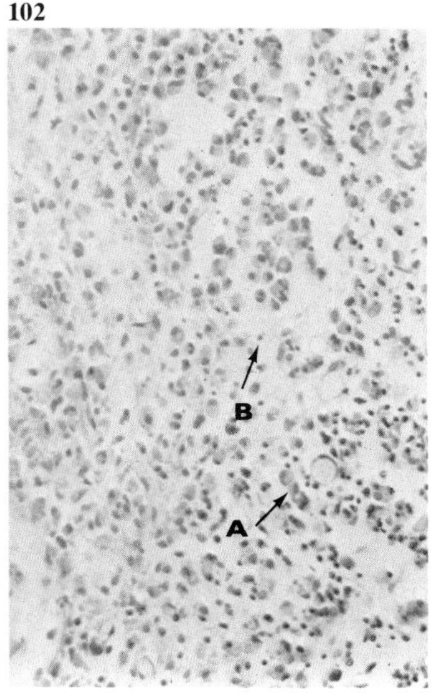

103

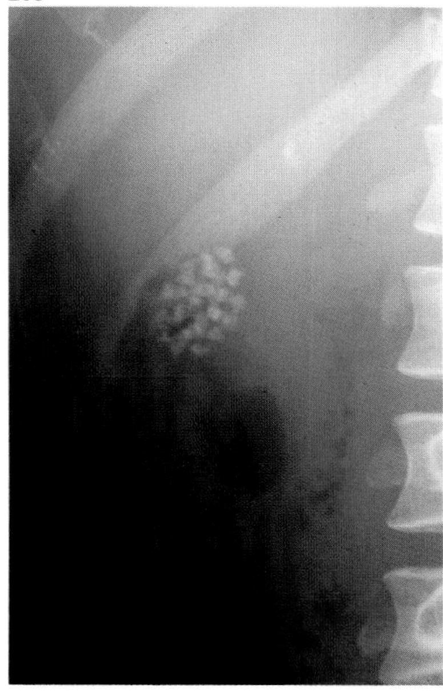

104 Chart — response to treatment with chloramphenicol. The temperature falls slowly by lysis over a period of three or four days.

105 Chart — combined treatment with chloramphenicol and corticosteroid. In gravely ill typhoid patients a combination of chloramphenicol and corticosteroids may produce a sudden drop in temperature with dramatic improvement in the general condition. With high dosage the combination may produce a precipitate fall in temperature to a subnormal level accompanied by circulatory disturbance, but with moderate dosage this problem is seldom encountered. The risk of aggravating or precipitating haemorrhage and perforation appears to be theoretical.

104

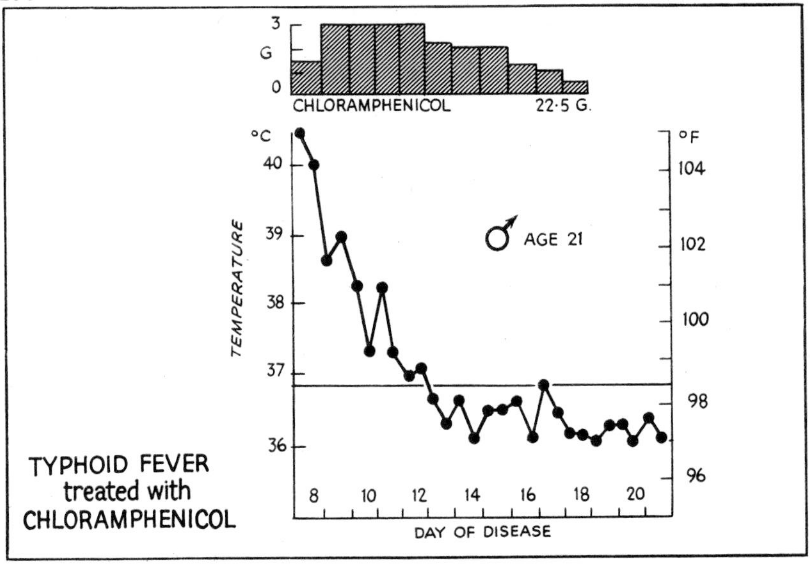

TYPHOID FEVER treated with CHLORAMPHENICOL

105

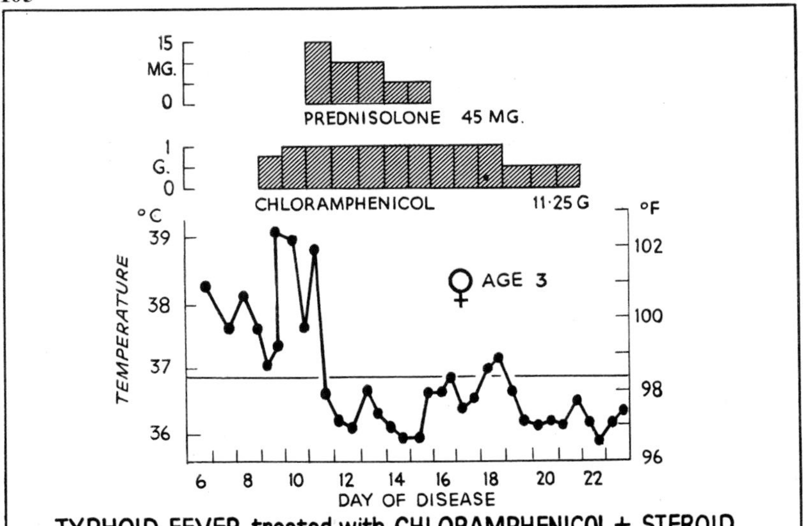

TYPHOID FEVER treated with CHLORAMPHENICOL + STEROID

106 Chart — relapse and treatment. The rate of relapse in untreated typhoid fever varies from 5 to 15%. In cases treated with chloramphenicol for less than 14 days the rate of relapse is greatly increased and may exceed 50%. When chloramphenicol is given for longer periods less than 10% of patients relapse. Relapses usually occur 7 to 10 days after the temperature has returned to normal but are often delayed in patients treated with chloramphenicol and have even been recorded after three weeks of normal temperature. Relapses are generally milder and shorter than the original attack but may be fatal. The illness follows a similar pattern to the primary attack, and rose spots may reappear.

107 Typhoid spine. X-ray of lumbar spine — anteroposterior view. Osteomyelitis and arthritis are rare complications of typhoid fever. Periostitis may occur in late convalescence and usually affects the tibia or ribs. Abscesses may form and discharge pus containing *Salmonella typhi.*

Osteomyelitis of the spine may follow an attack of typhoid. In some instances it is caused directly by the typhoid bacillus, but in others secondary infection with the tubercle bacillus is responsible. The anteroposterior view shows involvement of L4 and L5.

106

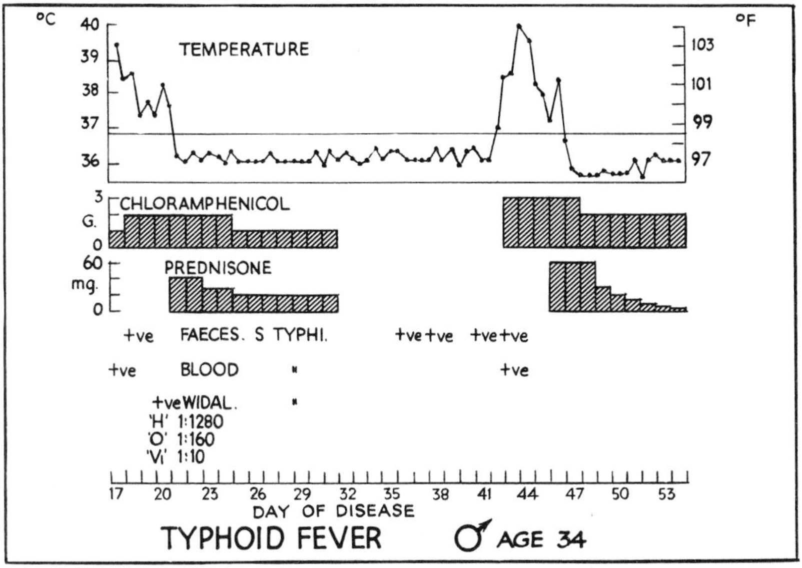

°C 40 39 38 37 36

TEMPERATURE

°F 103 101 99 97

3 G. 0 CHLORAMPHENICOL

60 mg. 0 PREDNISONE

+ve FAECES. S TYPHI. +ve +ve +ve +ve

+ve BLOOD * +ve

+ve WIDAL. *
'H' 1:1280
'O' 1:160
'Vi' 1:10

17 20 23 26 29 32 35 38 41 44 47 50 53
DAY OF DISEASE

TYPHOID FEVER ♂ AGE 34

107

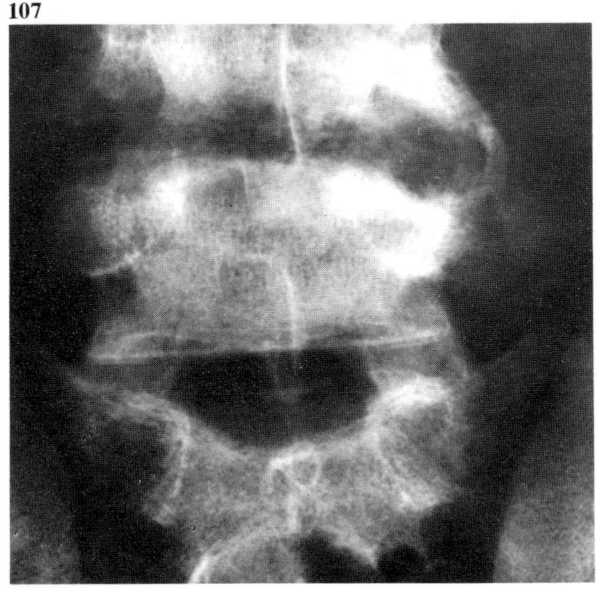

108

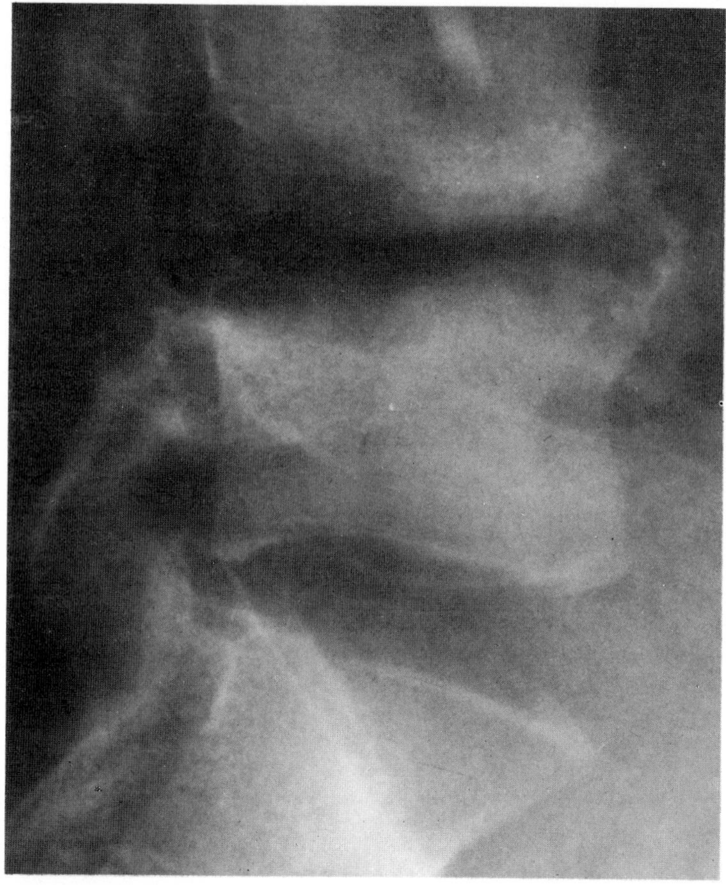

108 Typhoid spine. X-ray of lumbar vertebra — lateral view. This view of the spine shows areas of decalcification and irregular deposition of new bone in the fifth lumbar vertebra of a patient with a typhoid infection.

109

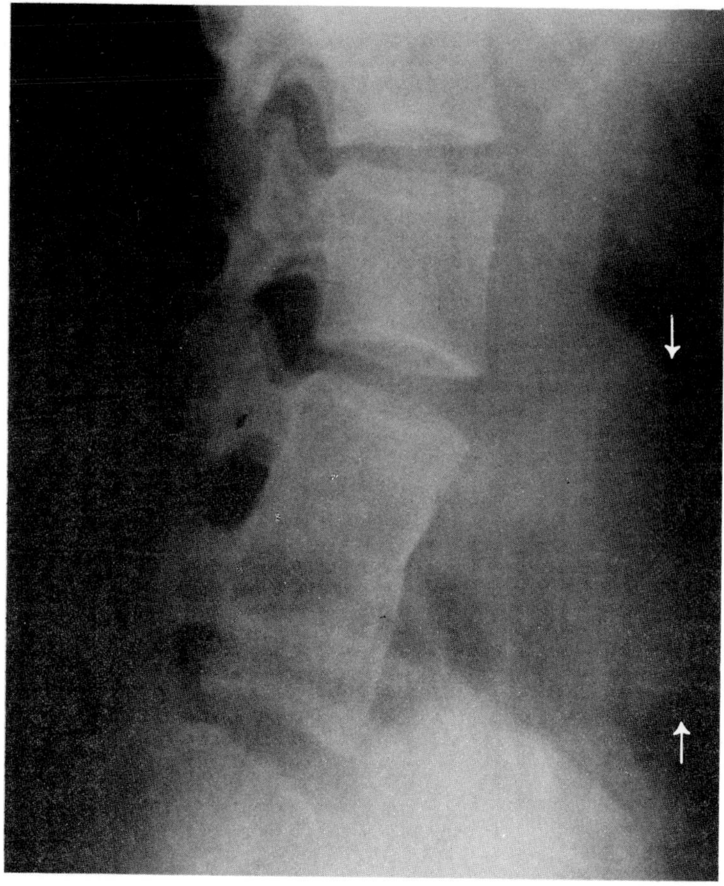

109 Osteomyelitis of spine, and psoas abscess in paratyphoid B. Infection with paratyphoid B is more likely to cause a suppurative lesion, such as osteomyelitis, than paratyphoid A. The lateral view of the lumbar spine shows a large psoas abscess, which originated from a paratyphoid infection of L4 and L5. The vertebral bodies are fused. Although the attack of paratyphoid occurred many years previously, the organism was cultured from the pus drained at operation. (The arrows indicate the abscess.)

110 Sickle-cell anaemia with paratyphoid osteomyelitis. Patients with sickle-cell disease are especially prone to salmonella infections of bone. Salmonella osteomyelitis usually occurs in children. It commonly affects long bones and may affect more than one.

The radiograph shows characteristic changes of osteomyelitis in a young child with paratyphoid B infection of the radius and ulna. Note the patchy decalcification and the periosteal reaction.

111 Sickle-cell disease with osteomyelitis complicating food poisoning. X-ray of tibia. Osteomyelitis may complicate salmonella food poisoning in patients with sickle-cell disease. The diagnosis is not easy but the possibility should always be considered when a patient with sickle-cell anaemia has persistent fever and localised pain during or after an attack of salmonella food poisoning. Blood cultures may show systemic invasion by a salmonella, but three weeks or longer may elapse before radiographic changes can be detected.

110

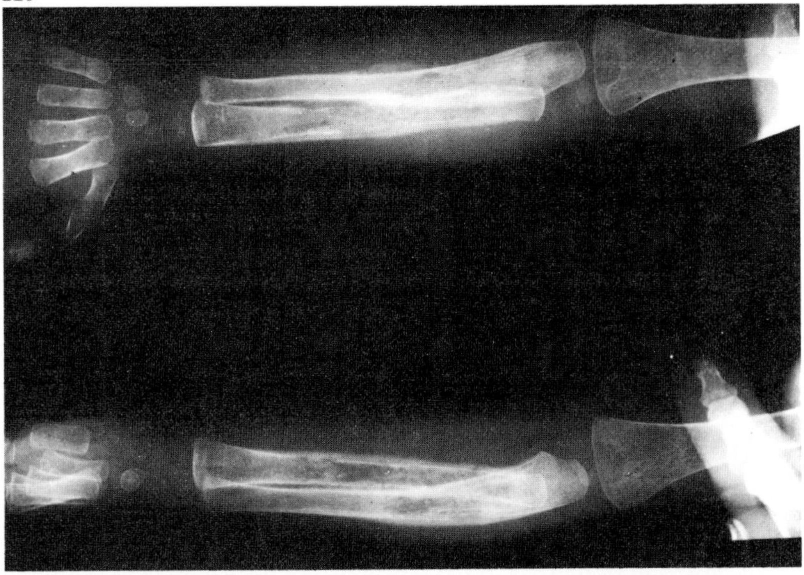

111

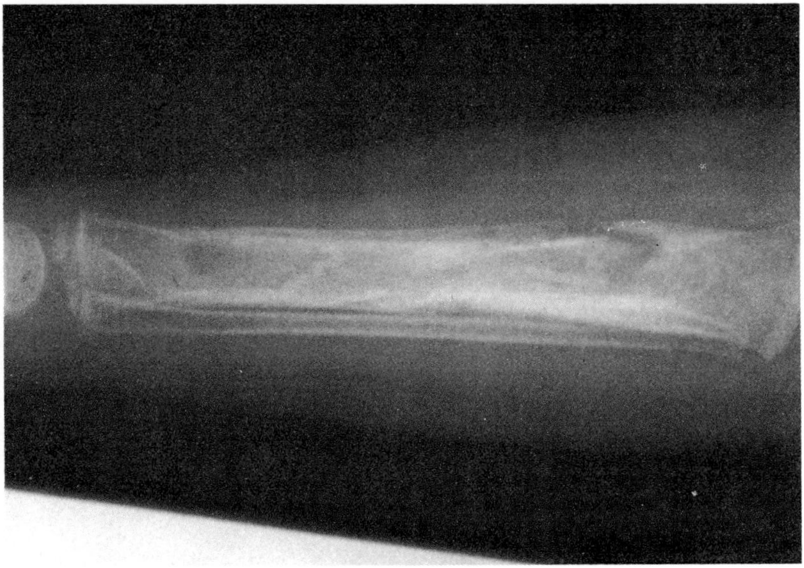

Gastroenteritis

Gastroenteritis may affect any age group, but the disease is most severe in young children, amongst whom most deaths occur. In many cases it is not possible to isolate a recognisable bacterial pathogen or demonstrate a virus to which there is an antibody response. Some outbreaks are associated with enteropathogenic strains of *Escherichia coli.* This type of gastroenteritis is particularly common in children under two years of age and spreads very readily in institutions. Campylobacters, vibrio-like microaerophilic Gram-negative bacteria, are another very common cause of gastroenteritis affecting all age groups.

112 Electron micrograph of rotaviruses. A number of different viruses have been detected by electron microscopy from faeces of patients with gastroenteritis. Perhaps the commonest of these has been rotavirus, a double-stranded RNA virus with a characteristic wheel-like appearance on electron microscopy. Rotavirus gastroenteritis is particularly common in children between the ages of six months and two years, but may affect older children and adults. Gastroenteritis varies greatly according to the aetiology of the infection and the age of the patient. In infants and young children vomiting and diarrhoea rapidly lead to dehydration and imbalance of electrolytes; consequently gastroenteritis is a serious disease with an appreciable mortality. In older children and adults the illness may be incapacitating but seldom fatal.

Clinical features

113 Dehydration — mild (white child). In mild dehydration there may be loss of up to 5% of body weight. The baby is irritable and cries miserably. As a result of vasoconstriction the skin is pale, but the lips remain a vivid pink because of haemoconcentration.

114 Dehydration — mild (black child). The clinical features are very similar, but the colour of the lips does not contrast so sharply with the dark skin.

112

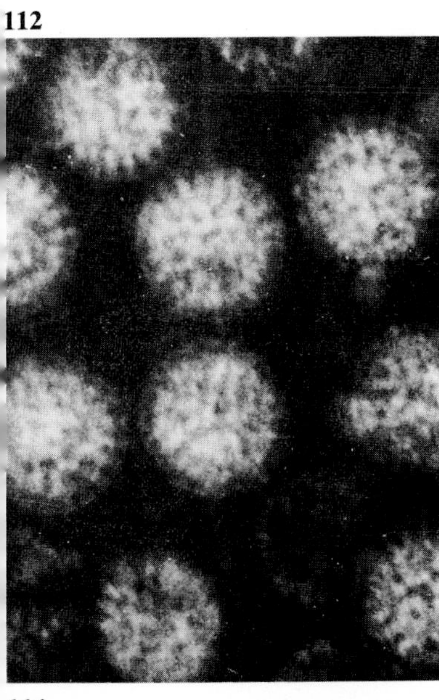

113

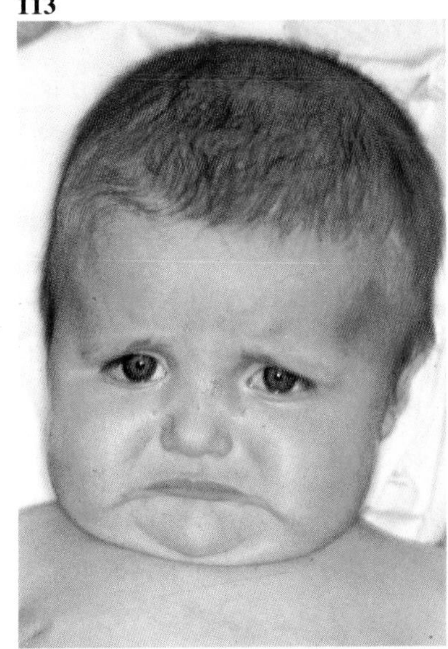

114

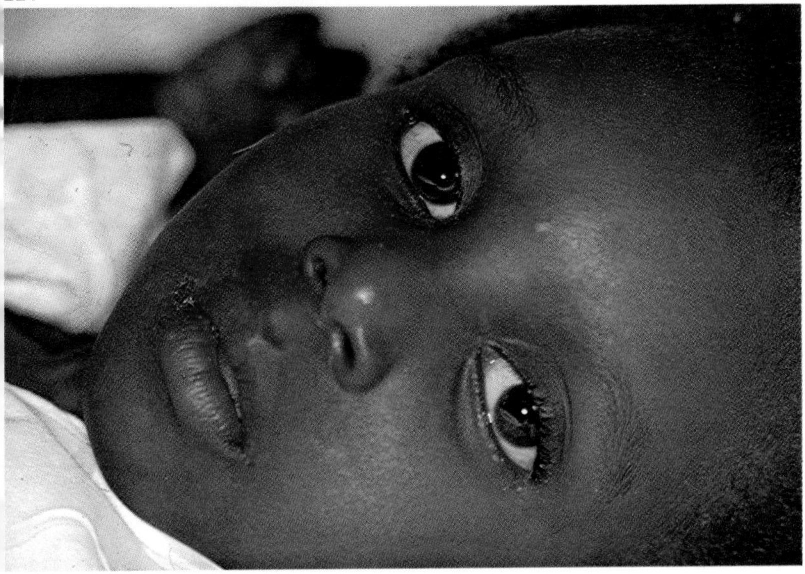

115 Dehydration — moderate (Indian child). In moderate dehydration up to 10% of body weight may be lost. Pallor is still a striking feature, but irritability gives way to listlessness as dehydration increases. Water is lost from the retro-orbital pad of fat, and the eyes become sunken. The fontanelle is depressed, and the mouth parched.

116 Dehydration — moderate (Indian child). The skin loses its turgor and elasticity. Normally when a fold of skin is pinched and then released, it subsides immediately but in dehydration it settles very slowly. This phenomenon can be seen clearly on the anterior abdominal wall of this child. Note the wrinkled skin.

15

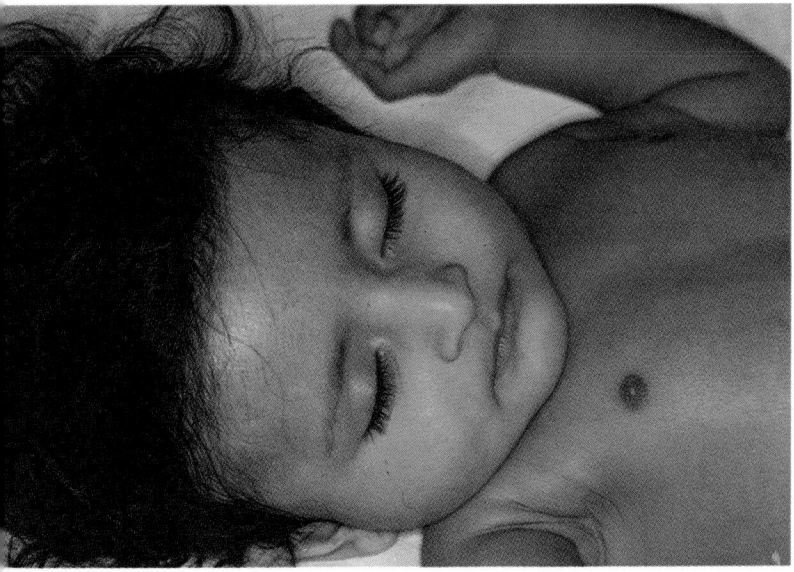

16

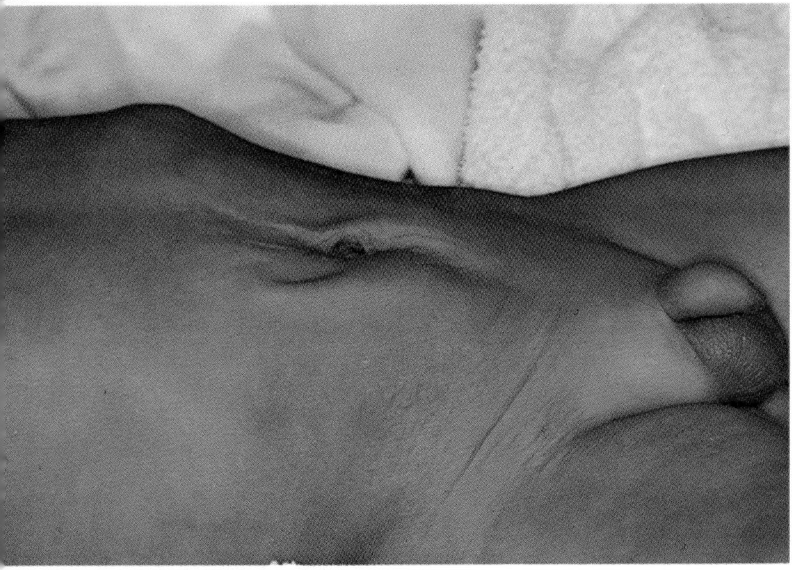

117 and 118 Dehydration — severe (white child). In extreme dehydration, when 10 to 15% of body weight has been lost, peripheral circulatory failure supervenes. The child is limp and apathetic. The extremities feel icy-cold, and the peripheral pulses are absent. Drowsiness gives way to coma. Finally, the child lies as if dead with eyeballs rolled upwards, and sclerae showing white between the half-closed eyelids. Oliguria is invariably present, and the blood urea concentration rises rapidly. Bleeding may occur into the gastrointestinal tract. Acidosis is usually present. The mortality in such severely dehydrated patients is 50%.

117

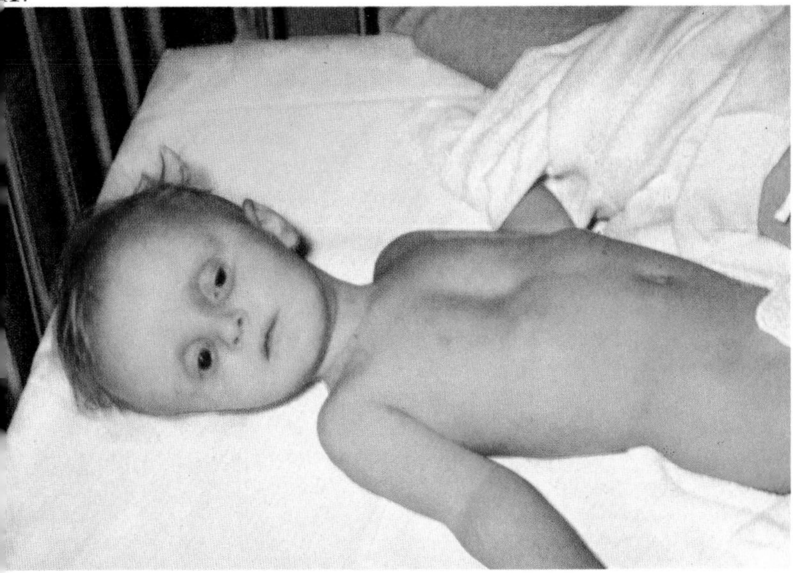

118

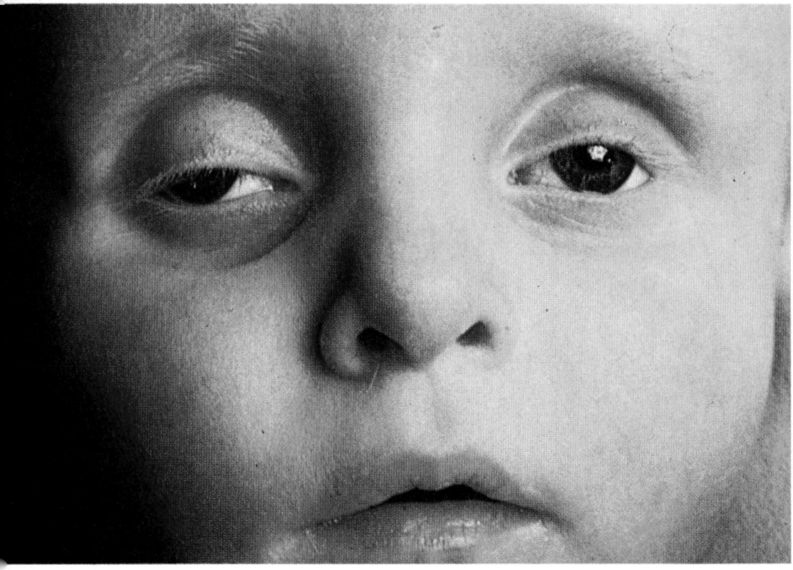

119 Hypernatraemia — conjunctival congestion. Hypernatraemic dehydration may be suspected clinically when a dehydrated child is exceptionally irritable or has neck stiffness. Convulsions are common in this group, especially when the dehydration is corrected rapidly with hypotonic infusions. Permanent brain damage or death may result. Conjunctival congestion is a common finding in these patients. The diagnosis should be confirmed by measuring the serum electrolyte concentrations.

120 Marasmus following attack of gastroenteritis in an Indian baby. In severe gastroenteritis the infant may become intolerant to all types of oral feeding and enter a chronic state of dehydration and wasting from malnutrition. Despite intravenous feeding mortality remains high, varying from 10 to 50% in different outbreaks. Temporary lactose intolerance is not uncommon after severe gastroenteritis. In such patients the reintroduction of milk into the diet exacerbates diarrhoea.

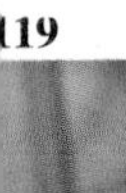

119

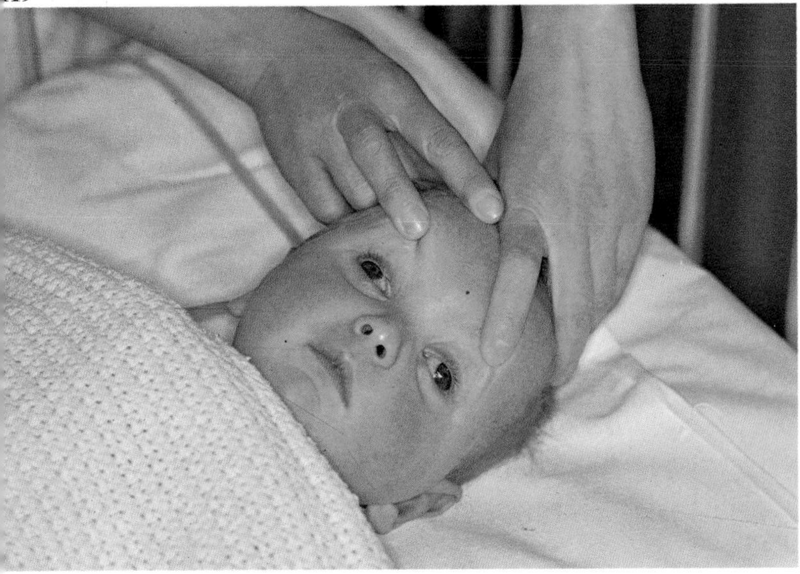

120

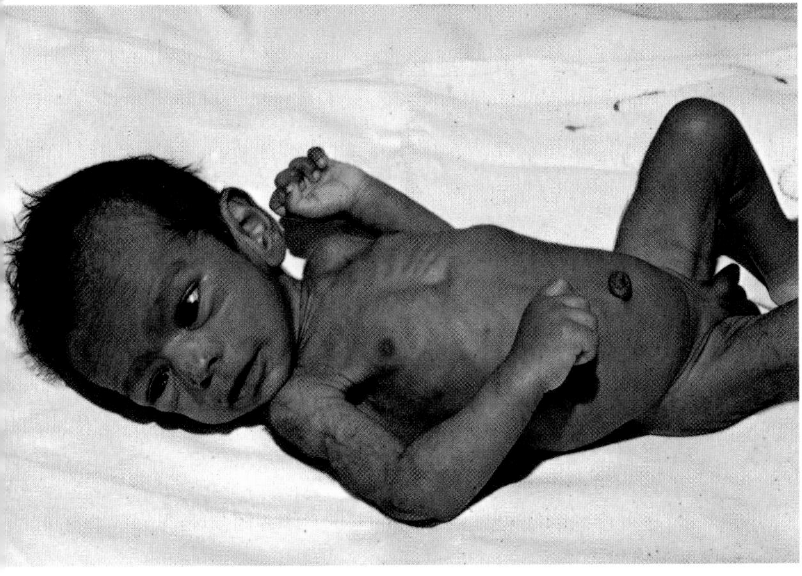

Diphtheria

Corynebacterium diphtheriae, the causative organism of diphtheria, produces a powerful exotoxin that is absorbed from the site of infection on the surface of the body and carried to the heart and nervous system, where it causes severe damage. Human cases or carriers are the sole source of infection, which is spread by close contact at school or at home, the organism being transferred by droplets or by contaminated articles. The clinical manifestations vary with the extent and site of the local lesion and the degree of damage to susceptible structures by exotoxin.

Organism

121 ***Corynebacterium diphtheriae mitis*** **(Albert's stain of smear).** *C. diphtheriae* is a slender, non-motile, non-sporing, Gram-positive bacillus, measuring 3 to 5 μm in length. It can be classified into three types, mitis, intermedius, and gravis, according to a) the appearance of the colonies on blood-tellurite media, b) biochemical reactions, and c) staining characteristics.

The staining reaction by Albert's method is uneven, and metachromatic granules are often present. These may be bipolar or scattered irregularly throughout the protoplasm; pleomorphism is common. In contrast, diphtheroid bacilli are much more regular in appearance. The morphological appearances, however, cannot be relied upon to distinguish one type of diphtheria bacillus from another, or diphtheria bacilli from diphtheroids. Cultural and biochemical characteristics must be taken into account.

122 ***Corynebacterium diphtheriae gravis*****. Smear from culture.** The arrangement of diphtheria bacilli is distinctive. They may be found singly or in groups. In groups the organisms tend to be arranged at angles to each other, probably as a result of incomplete separation at the moment of division. They look like the letters L or V, and the combinations bear a resemblance to Chinese or cuneiform writing.

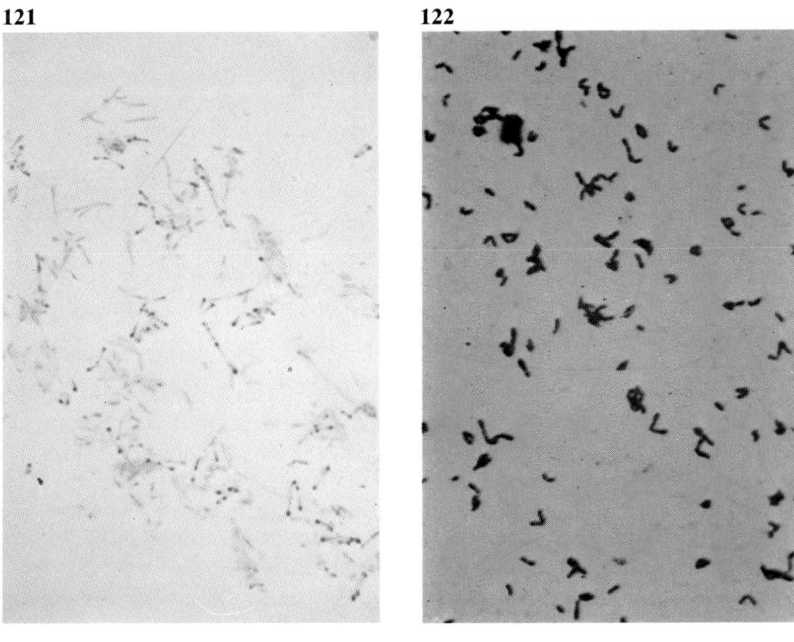
121

122

123 Colonies of *C. diphtheriae gravis* on McLeod's medium (x 4·4). On McLeod's chocolate tellurite agar the three types produce characteristic colonies. Mitis colonies are black, shiny, and dome-shaped; intermedius has pointed, pinhead-sized colonies; gravis has dull matt colonies with a central dome and a crenated edge like a daisy head.

Corynebacterium diphtheriae ferments glucose but not sucrose. The gravis form alone ferments starch.

The diphtheria bacillus may be divided serologically into many subtypes and classified by bacteriophage into at least 19 types. Some strains of mitis are avirulent but may be converted to produce exotoxin under the influence of bacteriophage.

124 Elek plate. Toxigenic strains may be identified by a gel-diffusion test. A strip of filter paper, impregnated with antitoxin, is set in culture medium and diphtheria bacilli streaked on the surface at right angles to the paper. Toxin from the diphtheria bacilli diffuses sideways from the streak, and antitoxin diffuses from the filter paper. A thin white line of precipitate marks the interface where antitoxin combines with toxin. This method is not as reliable as in vivo tests for virulence.

In the Elek plate illustrated the outer two organisms are non-toxigenic, the inner two are known to be toxigenic strains, and the central organism is being tested against these controls. A reaction of identity can be seen between the lines produced by the suspect strain and the two toxigenic strains. There is no reaction from the outer non-toxigenic organisms.

125 Virulence tests in rabbit. Rabbits and guineapigs are highly susceptible to diphtheria toxin and may be used to test strains for virulence. The minimal lethal dose is determined by injecting various dilutions of toxin subcutaneously, and the minimal reacting dose is established by intradermal inoculation. Gravis and intermedius strains are nearly always virulent, whereas mitis strains are often avirulent.

Two days after inoculation a few positive reactions are shown on a rabbit's skin, but most are negative.

123

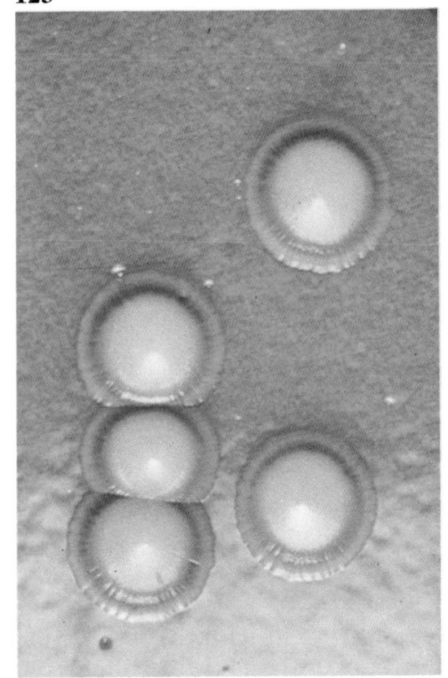

124

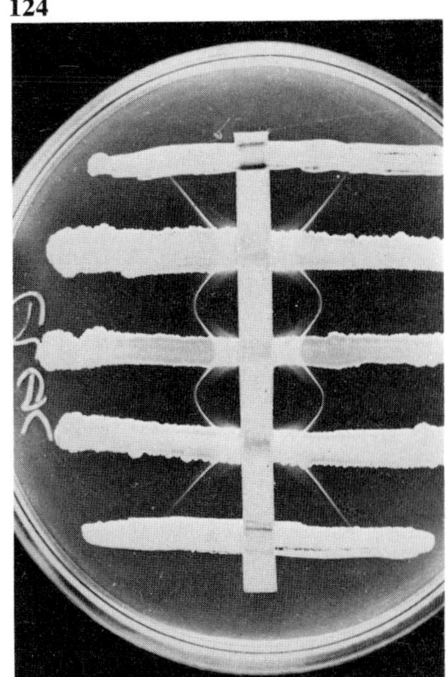

125

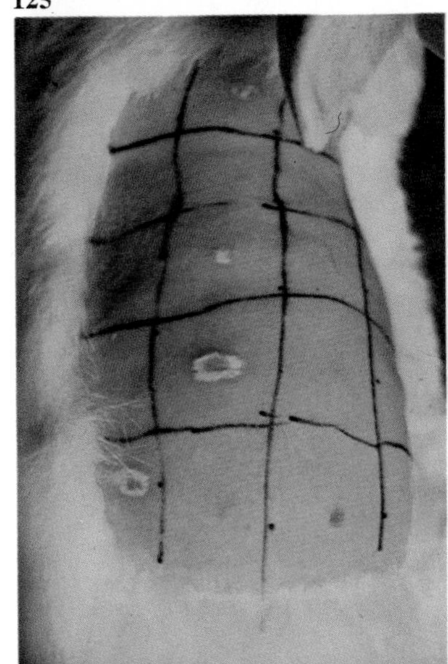

Clinical features

126 Nasal diphtheria. The possibility of diphtheria or a foreign body should always be considered when a child has a unilateral blood-stained discharge from the nose. In anterior nasal diphtheria the skin round the nostril or on the upper lip may be excoriated and membrane or crusting visible inside the nose.

Absorption of toxin is slight so there is no threat to life, but large numbers of diphtheria bacilli are shed and these patients are dangerous to others.

127 'Bull-neck' of diphtheria. Extensive diphtheria of the throat is always accompanied by marked swelling of the neck resulting from enlargement of lymph nodes and oedema of surrounding tissues. The swelling feels solid, and it is difficult to palpate the underlying lymph nodes. There is little pain.

128 Distinguishing between mumps and 'bull-neck' diphtheria. Failure to examine the throat of a child with 'bull-neck' diphtheria may lead to a mistaken and tragic diagnosis of mumps. The child with serious diphtheria looks pale, limp, and toxic, whereas the child with mumps looks comparatively well. Moreover, the swelling of mumps lies superior to that of diphtheria and usually fills the hollow behind the angle of the mandible. Careful inspection of the throat settles the diagnosis.

126

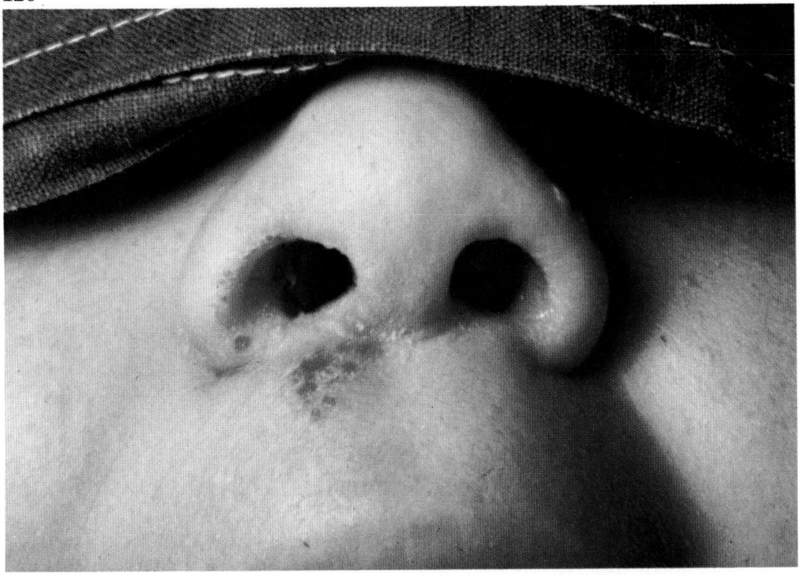

127

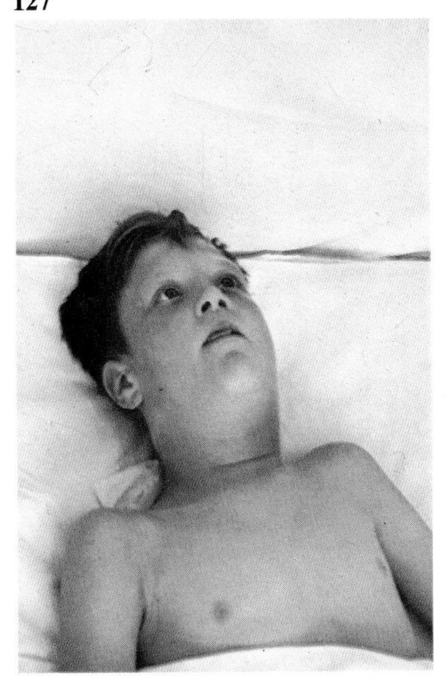

128

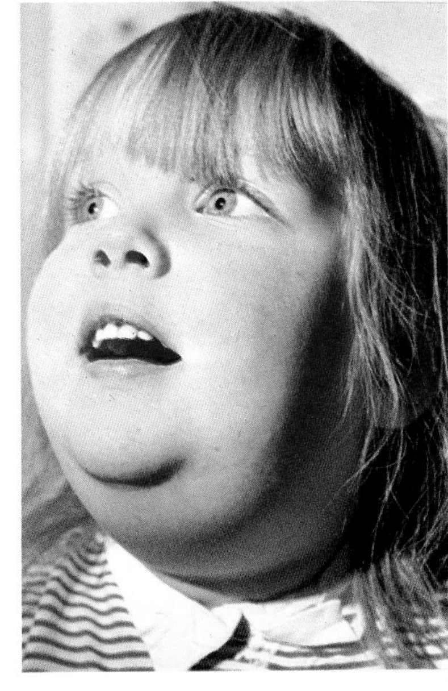

129 Tonsillar diphtheria. Membrane is confined to the tonsils, where absorption of toxin is moderate. It starts as a small patch on one tonsil and usually spreads to both. The membrane is ivory-white or greyish-yellow in colour. The edge is wrinkled but sharply demarcated, and bordered by a narrow band of inflammation. The child is listless and off-colour but may not complain of a sore throat, and the cause of the illness may be overlooked. Pyrexia is slight or absent.

130 Severe pharyngeal diphtheria. In severe diphtheria the membrane may be thin and transparent especially at the spreading edge. The older parts of the membrane are usually greyish-yellow, but if there has been bleeding into the membrane the colour may alter to green or black. The membrane is firmly adherent and forcible removal causes slight bleeding. The underlying mucosa is not ulcerated and membrane forms again after 24 hours. The fauces are oedematous.

131 Spread of membrane in pharyngeal diphtheria. Membrane spreads rapidly from the tonsils across the soft palate to the uvula and over the pharyngeal wall into the nasopharynx. Toxin is readily absorbed, and general symptoms are severe with waxy pallor, extreme lassitude, and drowsiness progressing to stupor. The patient's temperature may be subnormal, and death quickly ensues from circulatory failure.

129

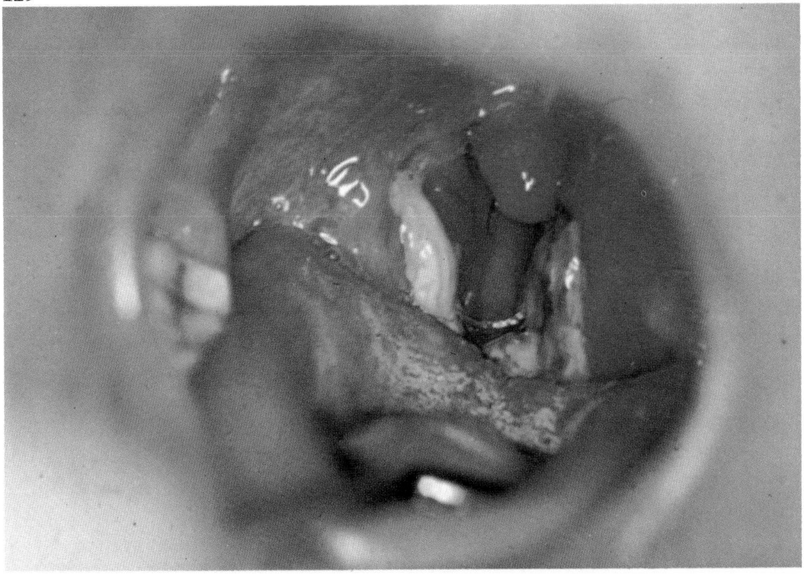

130

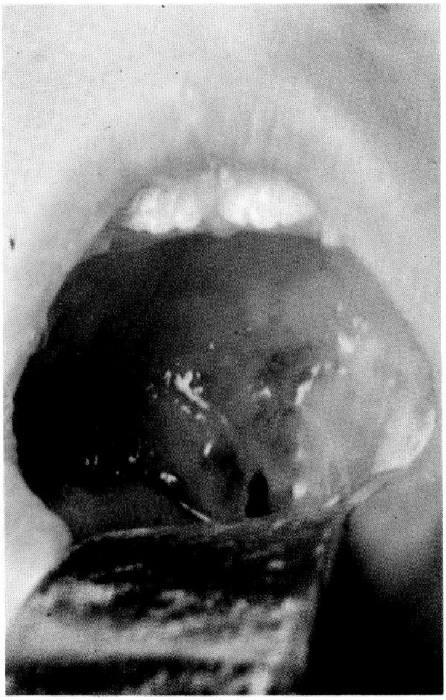

131

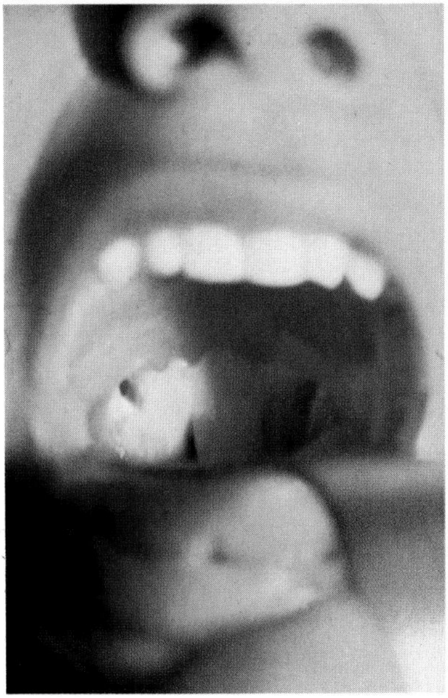

132 Anginose variety of infectious mononucleosis. The anginose form of infectious mononucleosis is of similar appearance to diphtheria, but the exudate usually retains a striking white hue and does not spread further than the tonsils. Despite the alarming exudate on the tonsils, the patient's general condition remains good. Generalised enlargement of lymph nodes and splenomegaly indicate the correct clinical diagnosis, which is confirmed by finding characteristic mononuclear cells in the blood and a positive Paul–Bunnell test or one of its simplified variants.

133 Laryngeal diphtheria. Diphtheria of the larynx may be primary or secondary to pharyngeal diphtheria. Toxic absorption is slight, and the illness is dominated by respiratory obstruction caused by the membrane. As breathing becomes more difficult the accessory muscles are brought into play, and the soft parts of the chest wall and supraclavicular fossae are sucked inwards. The child becomes restless and frightened as he struggles for breath. Eventually the violent muscular effort can no longer be sustained, the child falls back exhausted, and death swiftly follows.

Diagnosis of laryngeal diphtheria is easy when membrane is visible in the pharynx but otherwise presents difficulty. Viral forms of laryngitis are associated with catarrhal signs in other parts of the respiratory tract and generally have a more abrupt onset than diphtheria.

134 Histological changes in diphtheritic tracheobronchitis. Diphtheria bacilli, multiplying on the respiratory mucosa, provoke an inflammatory response. The superficial tissues become infiltrated by leucocytes and fibrin-rich fluid exudes from the engorged vessels. The epithelial cells die and are enmeshed with the bacteria in a coagulum of protein to form a membrane. In the lower respiratory tract, where the ciliated epithelium is loosely attached, the membrane is easily dislodged and may be coughed out at tracheotomy or impacted in the larynx. (A = membrane, B = submucosa infiltrated by leucocytes, C = cartilage ring.)

132

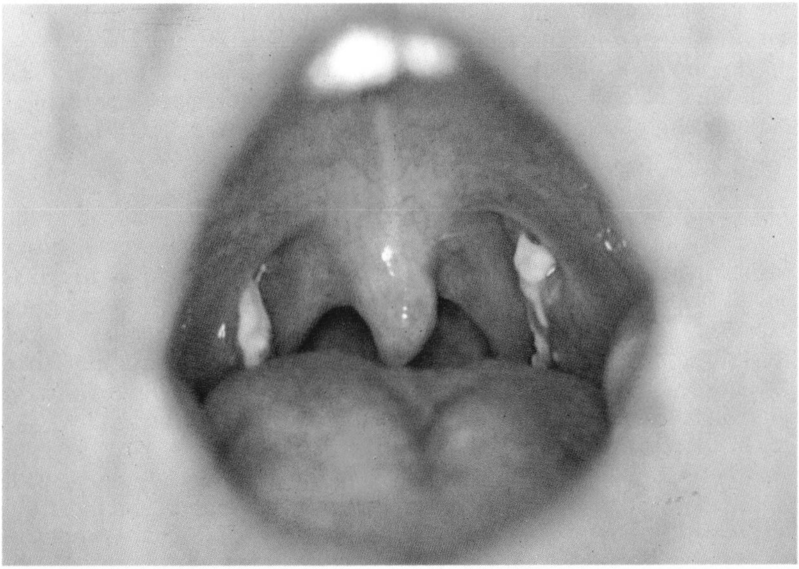

133

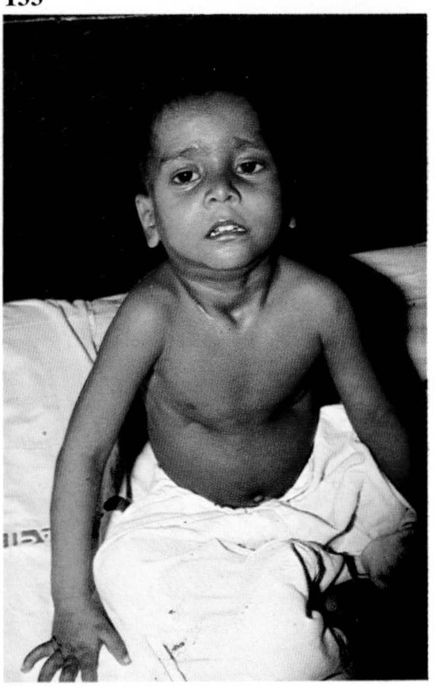

134

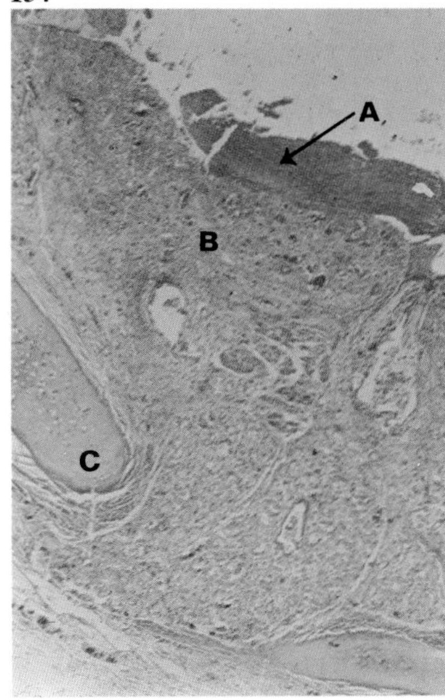

135 Histology of the heart in diphtheria. Diphtheria toxin appears to act primarily on cardiac muscle cells causing fatty degeneration. These patchy areas of damaged myocardium soon become surrounded and infiltrated by leucocytes, many of which are macrophages. In surviving patients fibroblastic repair results in microscopical scars but these do not seem to impair cardiac function.

136 Electrocardiographic changes in diphtheria. Toxic damage to the heart manifests clinically about the eighth to tenth day but may appear earlier in severe cases. The first signs are tachycardia and an irregular pulse. Inversion of T waves or alterations in the ST segment are to be expected in the early stage, and complete heart block may ensue. Restlessness, pallor, vomiting, precordial pain and oliguria are grave prognostic signs. Death commonly occurs about the fifteenth day; survival beyond this stage makes the outlook more hopeful.

This electrocardiogram shows severe changes in a fatal case of diphtheria caused by a mitis stain. Nodal bradycardia is present with ventricular ectopic escape, depression of the ST segment, and inversion of T waves.

135

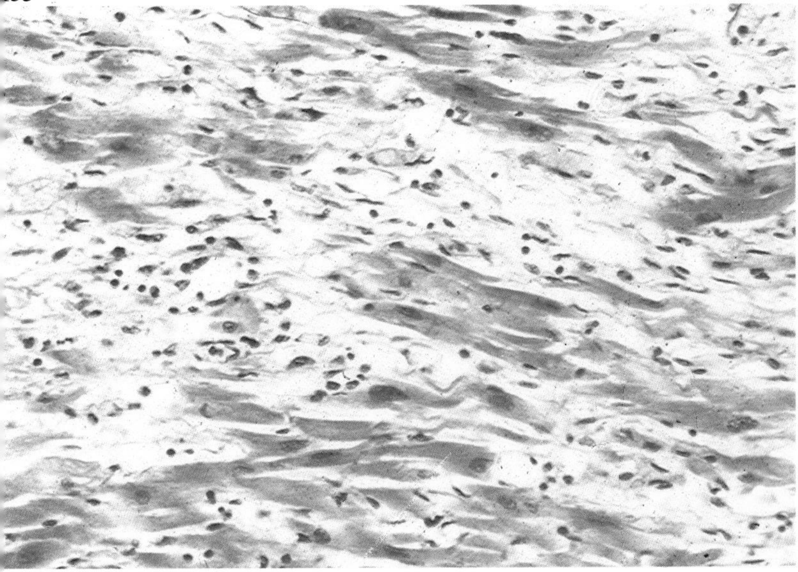

136

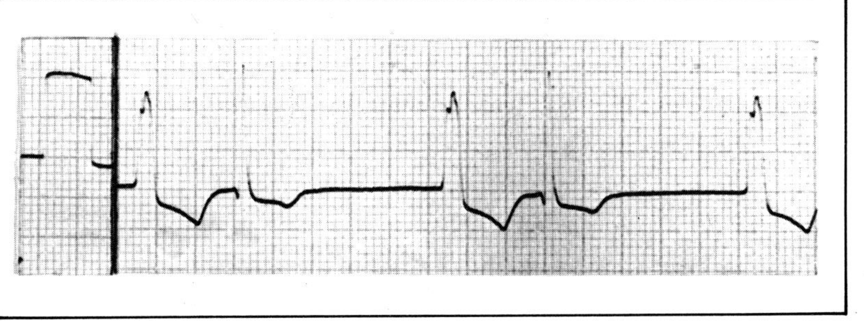

Vincent's infection

137 Vincent's organisms. Dilute carbol fuchsin. A spirochaete and fusiform bacillus are found in large numbers in certain mouth lesions and in ulcerative or necrotic lesions elsewhere. The spirochaete, *Borrelia vincentii*, measures 7 to 18 μm in length and has three to eight loose, open coils. It is actively motile and is an obligate anaerobe. The associated bacillus, *Fusobacterium fusiforme*, is cigar-shaped and measures 5 to 14 μm. It is non-motile and a strict anaerobe. Both organisms are easily detected in smears, stained by dilute carbol fuchsin, but are difficult to culture.

138 Vincent's angina. Vincent's organisms may be found in small numbers on healthy gums. They do not usually act as primary pathogens but as secondary invaders when superficial tissues have been damaged or are defective as a result of trauma, other infections, malnutrition, agranulocytosis or leukaemia. In temperate climates infection is confined to the buccal cavity or respiratory tract, but in tropical climates the organisms may be found in skin ulcers (see **356**).

In Vincent's angina membranous ulcers may be present on the tonsils or pharynx. Halitosis is a feature, but general disturbance is slight. Infection may spread to adjacent areas of the palate.

139 Acute ulcerative gingivitis. When the gums are involved there is destruction of the interdental papillae, leaving shallow concave ulcers with white necrotic margins. Vincent's infection may cause widespread destruction with extensive ulceration. The regional lymph nodes are enlarged.

137

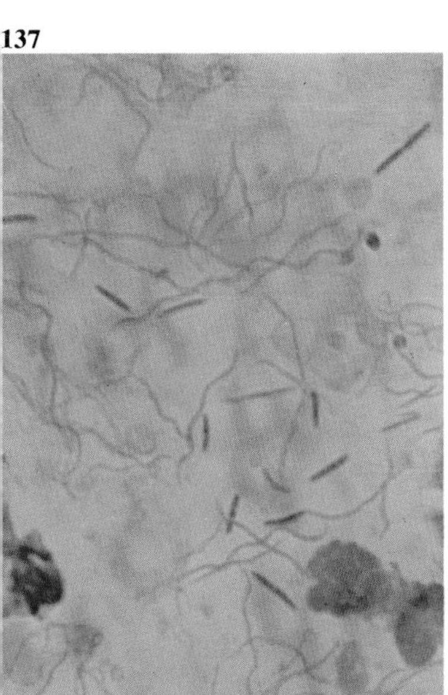

138

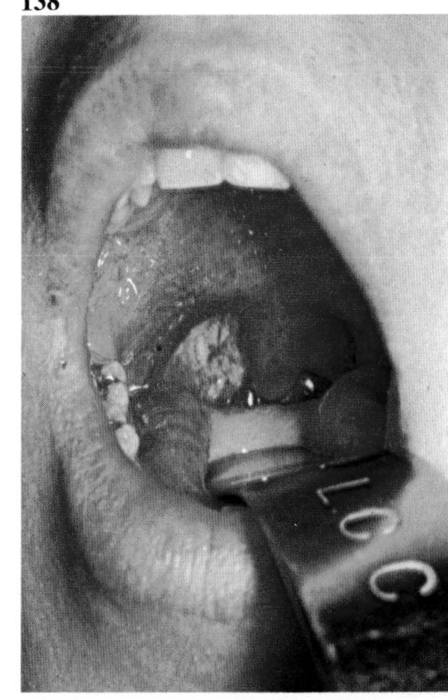

139

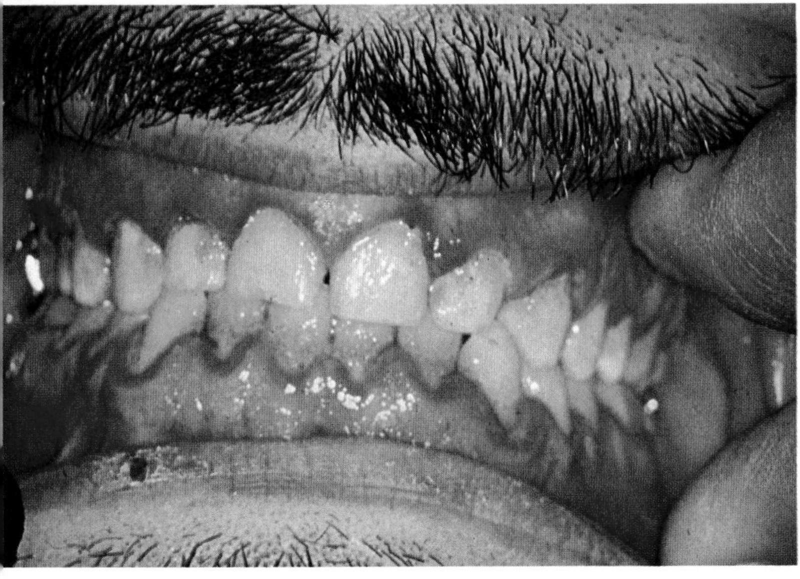

Thrush

140 ***Candida albicans*.** When conditions are favourable the fungus appears as spherical or oval yeast cells, called blastospores, which reproduce by budding. When conditions are less favourable it grows as a pseudomycelium of non-branching, filamentous cells, which divide by constriction. Further yeast cells are formed by budding at these division sites; both forms are thin-walled. Some yeast cells become larger, develop thick walls, and enter a resting phase. These resting cells are termed chlamydospores. *C. albicans* is Gram positive.

141 ***Candida albicans*. Gram stain of smear from 48 hour growth on blood agar at 37°C.** *Candida albicans* is a yeast-like fungus found in man, animals and birds. It is a common surface commensal in man and is present in the mouth and faeces of 20 to 30% of healthy people. Superficial infection of skin or mucous membranes occurs in debilitated patients or when there has been local disturbance as a result of infection or antibiotic treatment. Deep-seated infections and chronic superficial infections may complicate disorders of immunity.

142 **Oral thrush.** Thrush infection of the mouth may occur in infants as a result of cross-infection from the mother or from other infants, especially in bottle-fed babies. In adults, infection is usually endogenous and is found in dehydrated or debilitated patients, or when the bacterial flora of the buccal cavity has been disturbed by antibiotic therapy. The raw inflamed mucous membrane is covered with patches of creamy-white exudate.

140

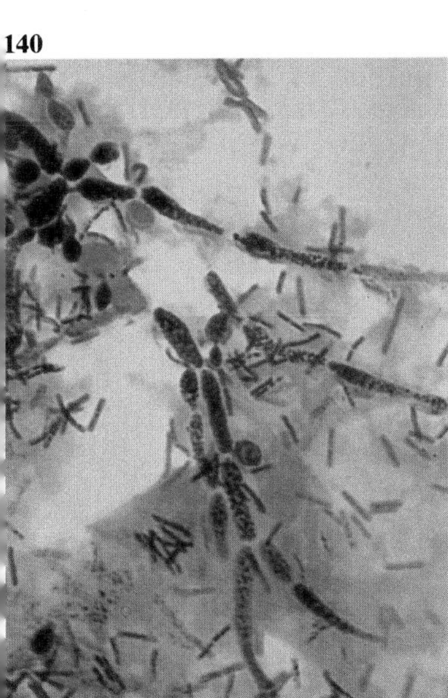

141

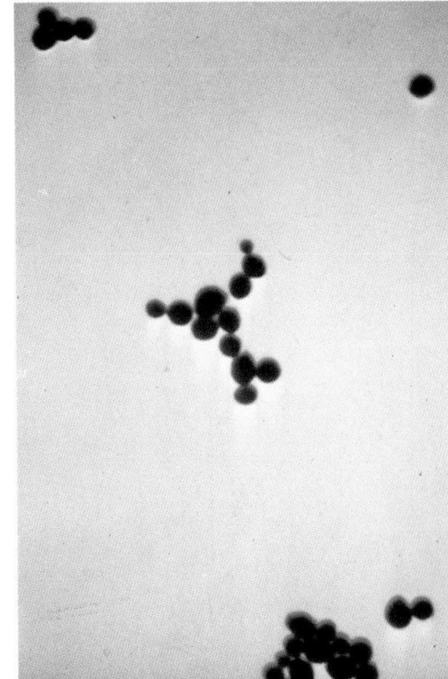

142

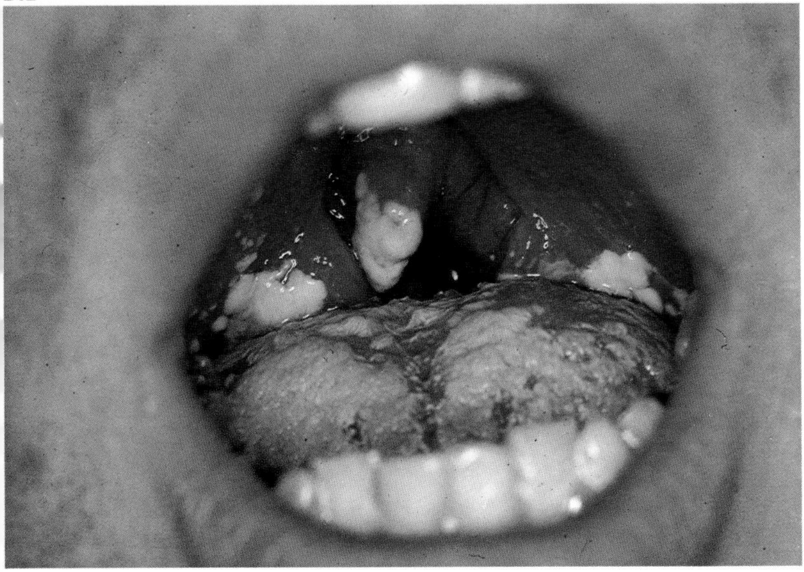

143 Chronic oral thrush. Chronic infection of the mouth may be associated with immunodeficiency, such as the acquired immune deficiency syndrome (AIDS). Firm, diffuse, white plaques or numerous white papules with intervening erythema may be found in the buccal cavity and persist for months or even years depending on the nature of the underlying deficiency.

144 Vulvovaginitis. Nappy rash in babies may be caused by candida and is particularly common in those with diarrhoea or those receiving antibiotic treatment. The rash starts round the anus and spreads over the perineum affecting skin in contact with the nappy. There is a well-defined area of redness with raised edges. Satellite lesions may begin as small pustules that rupture to leave small raw patches. The skin is macerated. In an ammoniacal rash the skin folds tend to be spared.

Genital thrush may prove troublesome in women using oral contraceptives or during pregnancy. Redness of the vagina and labia may be accompanied by severe pruritus and scanty or thick white discharge.

143

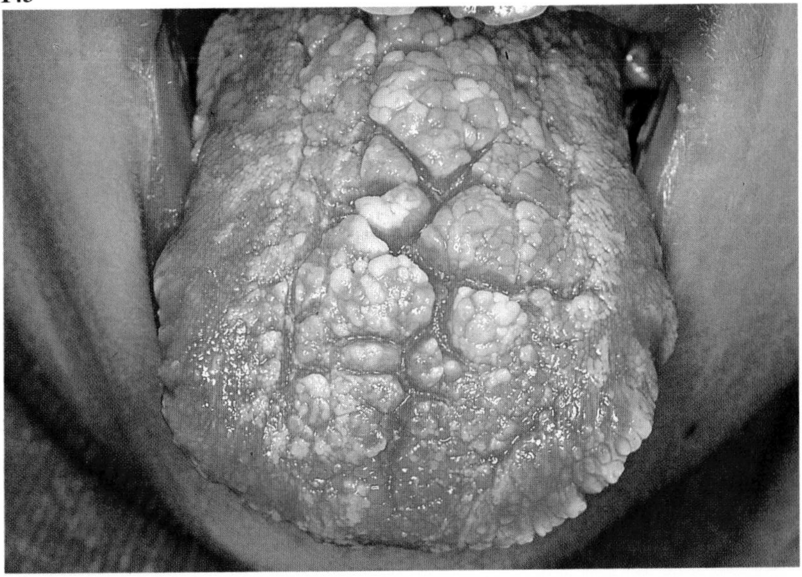

144

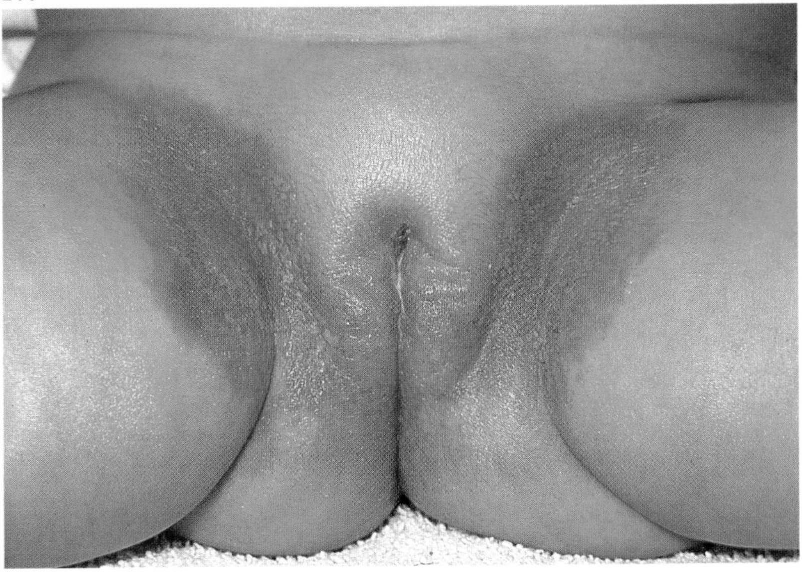

145 Balanitis. Poor hygiene may result in severe irritation of the foreskin and glans with blistering and patches of thrush.

146 Paronychia. Candida infection may spread from the nail fold under the adjacent nail causing deformity and even loss of the nail. It is especially common in those whose hands are frequently immersed in water, and in patients with diabetes or endocrine disorders. Nail infection as a manifestation of chronic mucocutaneous candidiasis may occur in patients with immunological defects. In this child the infection was caused by persistent thumb-sucking.

145

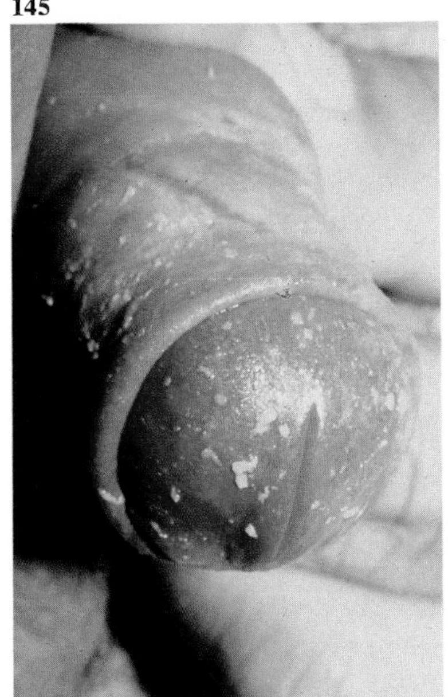

146

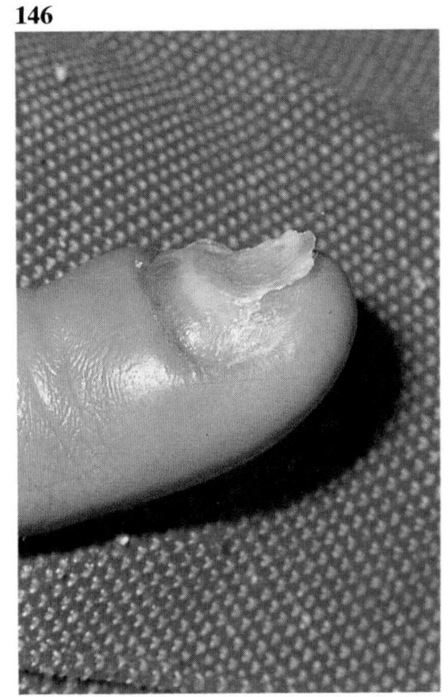

Leprosy

Leprosy is caused by *Mycobacterium leprae*, and man is the only natural host. The disease is found mainly in the tropics and subtropics. Close and continuous household contact is necessary for spread, and infection is usually derived from the nasal discharges of an infectious patient. Most infected people do not develop the disease; in those who do, the pattern of disease exhibits a spectrum from the tuberculoid, showing notable delayed hypersensitivity, to the lepromatous, in which there is virtually no cellular reaction by the host.

147 Organism — *M. leprae*. This is a slender acid-fast bacillus, which has not been cultured on media or in tissue culture, but grows exceedingly slowly in the footpads of mice and armadillos. It replicates with a doubling time of about 13 days, and is an obligate intracellular parasite found in macrophages. The large number of organisms in this section of skin suggests that the patient had lepromatous leprosy.

148 Histology. The Schwann cells of peripheral nerves, being phagocytic, may contain bacteria. When there is a host response a granuloma is formed, consisting of epithelioid cells and giant cells surrounded by lymphocytes. As a result, the nerve may be compressed and damaged. Depending on the individual nerve this may result in motor or sensory disturbance or both.

149 Lepromin reaction at four weeks. The lepromin reaction is a skin reaction observed after the intradermal injection of an extract of leprosy bacilli. It is of delayed hypersensitivity type but differs from the tuberculin reaction in that it is seen after several weeks rather than 48 hours. It is strongly positive in patients with tuberculoid leprosy and negative in those towards and at the lepromatous end of the spectrum.

147

148

149

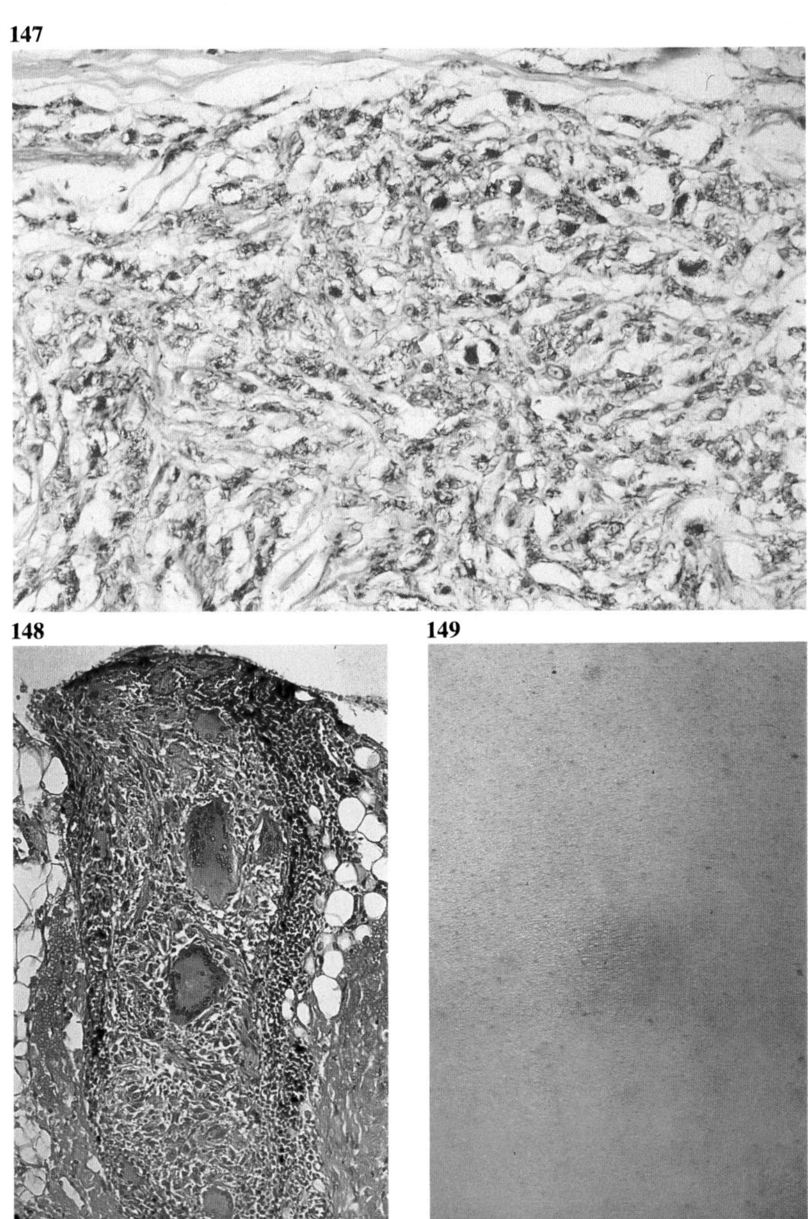

150 Appearance of face. The leonine facies is characteristic of lepromatous leprosy. The skin is thickened and ridged, the nose widened, and the ear lobes also thickened. Bacilli are readily found in large numbers in skin smears and also in the nodules shown here.

151 Erythema nodosum leprosum (ENL). Patients with lepromatous leprosy often suffer from ENL. The eruption is painful and consists of multiple reddened cutaneous nodules. It may be accompanied by constitutional upset, proteinuria, and orchitis. The incidence and severity of attacks vary greatly between patients, and may be precipitated by a variety of circumstances, including emotional factors. The underlying pathology is thought to be a vasculitis secondary to immune complex deposition.

152 'Upgrading' reaction. Patients whose disease is not at the two extremes of the spectrum may move their position in the spectrum according to their response to the organisms. Here, a patient towards the lepromatous end is showing more response than previously and is moving away from the lepromatous end in an upgrading reaction. Clinically, this is seen as areas of erythema. Although this reaction may be considered as protective in nature, the increased cellular response may result in nerve compression and an increase in neurological findings.

150

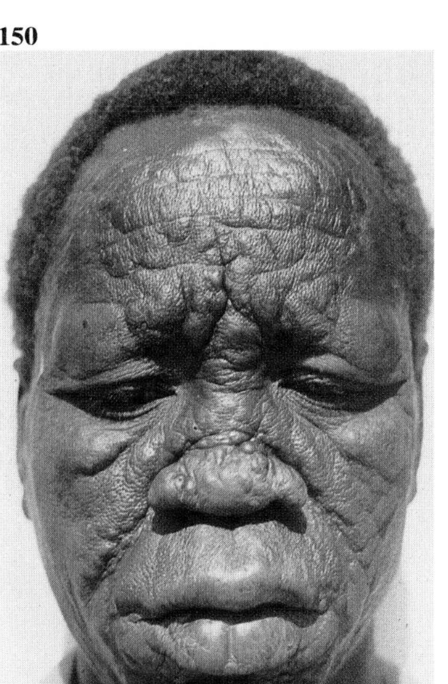

151

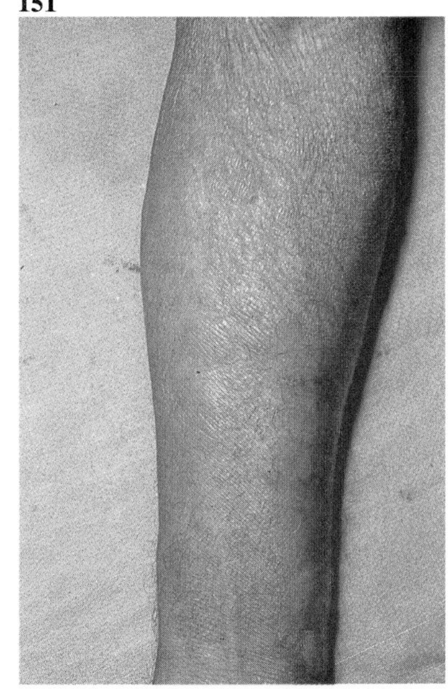

152

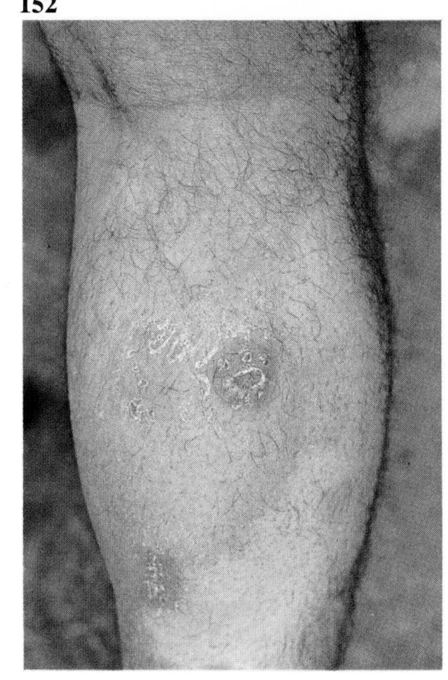

153 Tuberculoid leprosy. This patient is categorised towards the tuberculoid end of the immunological spectrum. Skin lesions are relatively few, asymmetrical, raised, anaesthetic, and do not sweat. Organisms are very scanty. Histologically the lesion is a granuloma; the lepromin test is strongly positive.

154 Nerve infection. In some patients the disease is purely neural and no skin lesions are seen. In this patient the radial nerve is affected causing wrist drop and anaesthesia of the thumb.

153

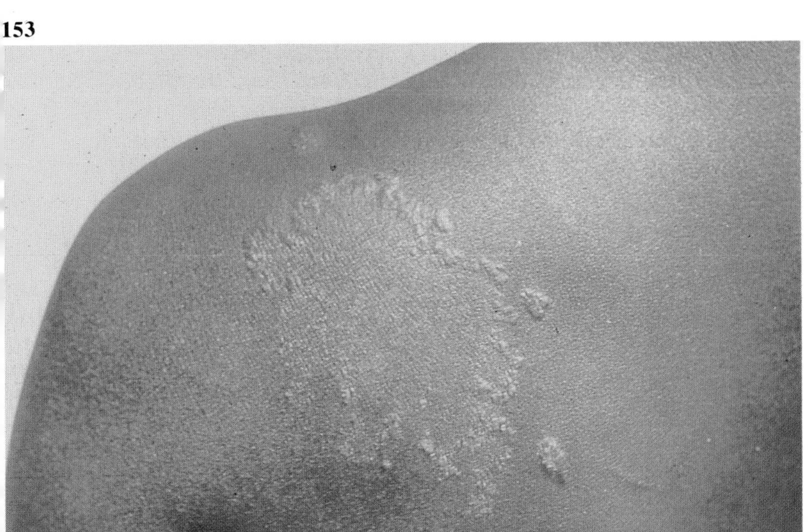

154

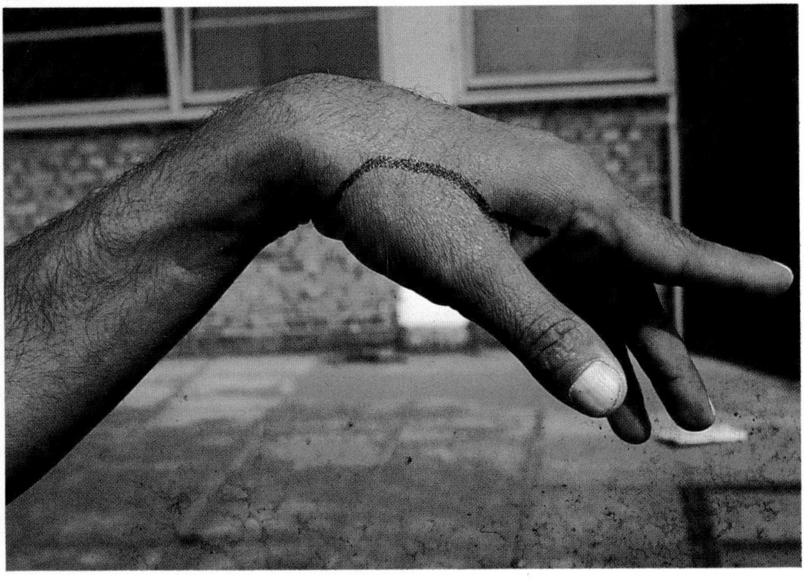

155 Claw hand. Claw hand is a characteristic feature of leprosy, especially in those patients categorised in the middle of the spectrum with borderline disease. The ulnar nerve is affected; patients are unable to flex the metacarpophalangeal joints, and there is prominent wasting of the thenar and hypothenar eminences. The deformity may be aggravated by subsequent contractures. Sensory loss is present in the ulnar distribution.

156 Ulcers. Ulcers of the feet are common in leprosy. They may be perforating ulcers of the sole, similar to those seen in diabetes, or round the ankle, as seen here. Because of anaesthesia the foot is vulnerable to damage from prolonged pressure, burns, or general injuries. The ulcers are slow to heal and tend to break down; they may be associated with considerable loss of tissue, scarring, and deformity.

55

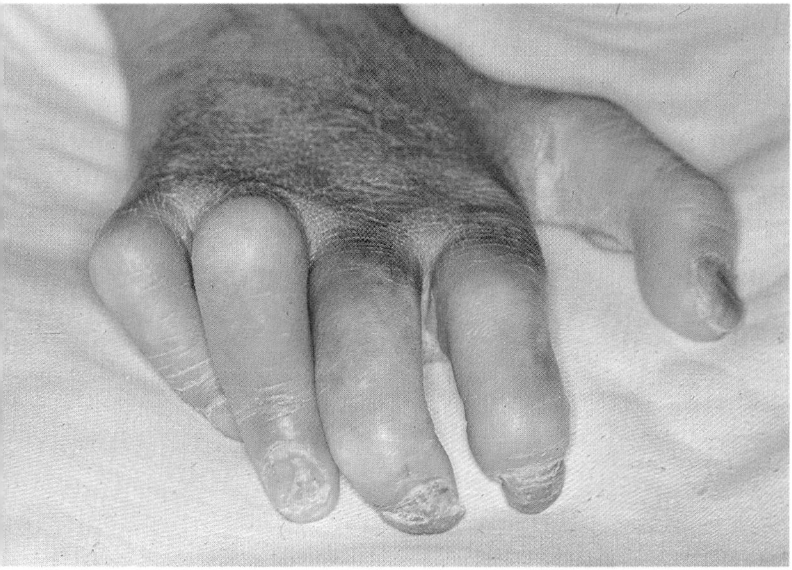

156

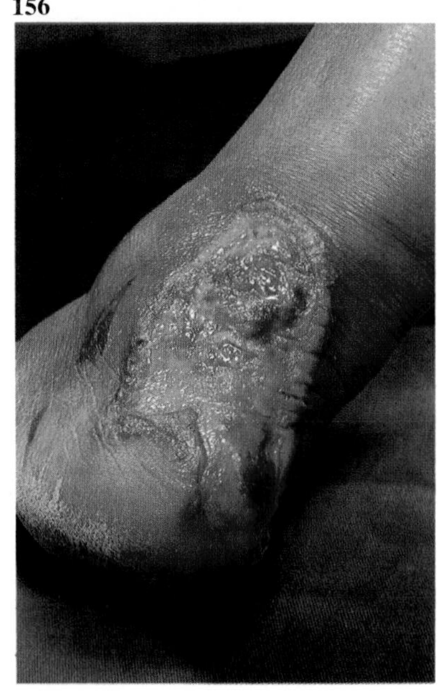

Tetanus

157 ***Clostridium tetani*** **(negative stain with nigrosin).** The tetanus organism is ubiquitous, being present in soil and dust, though the degree of contamination varies from district to district. It is often found in the intestinal tract of animals and sometimes in man. *Clostridium tetani* is a Gram-positive rod measuring 2·5 μm in length and is a strict anaerobe. It forms spherical terminal spores, highly resistant to heat and disinfectants.

The vegetative bacillus produces a powerful exotoxin with a special affinity for nervous tissue. The organism usually gains access through a wound and multiplies locally in the damaged tissues, producing exotoxin. This is absorbed and conveyed to the nervous system, where it disturbs the regulation of reflex arcs and abolishes reciprocal innervation. Consequently afferent stimuli produce an exaggerated response.

158 Trismus. The first evidence of tetanus is usually difficulty in opening the mouth because of increased tone in the masseters. At this early stage mumps may be suspected, but hypertonus can generally be detected elsewhere, and there is no evidence of salivary gland involvement.

Pain and stiffness in the neck and back may simulate meningitis, but the correct diagnosis soon becomes apparent as the disease advances.

57

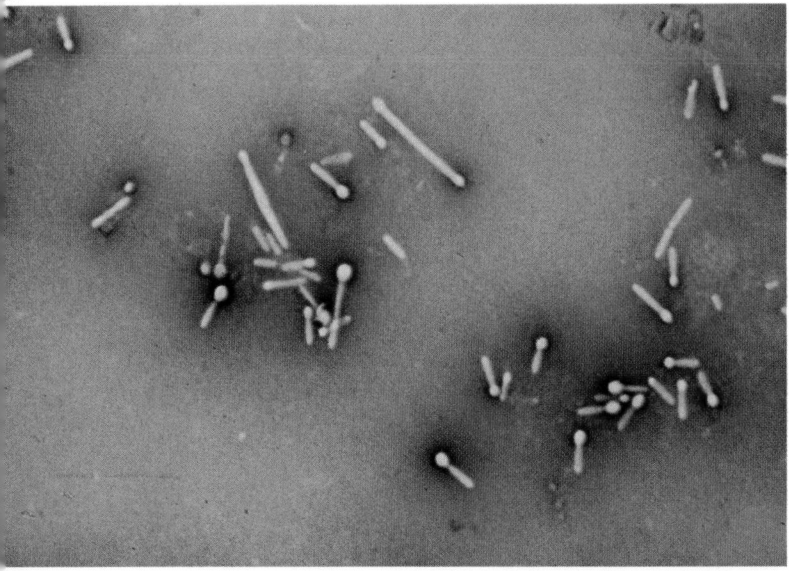

58

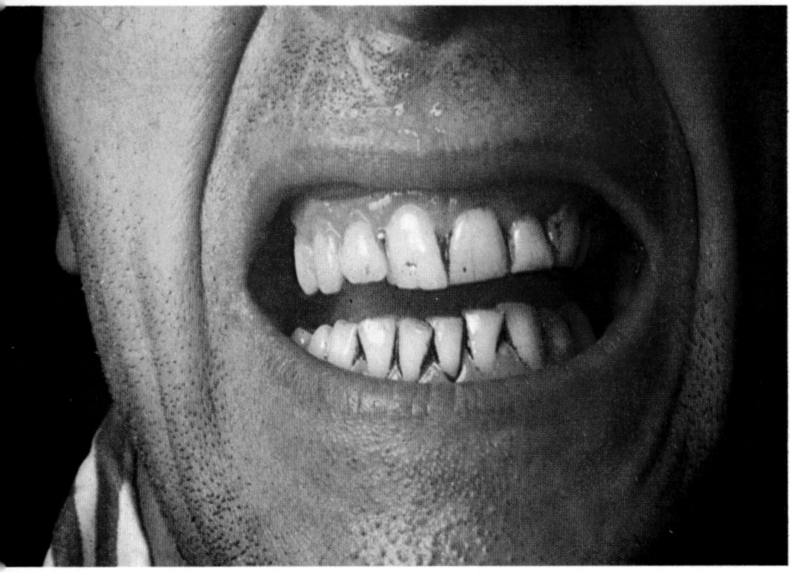

159 Risus sardonicus. Spasm of the facial muscles causes retraction o the angles of mouth to expose the clenched teeth in a characteristi snarling grin.

160 Opisthotonus in a child. Tetanus toxin causes overactivity of moto nerve cells resulting in muscle rigidity and spasm. Tonic rigidity i present in every case and persists throughout the illness. When th spinal muscles are severely affected opisthotonus results. In mild attack the disease may be arrested at the stage of rigidity, and spasms do no develop.

If the disease advances spasms appear and become progressivel more frequent and severe. With the onset of a convulsion the whol body is suddenly thrown into a violent spasm by the sustained contrac tion of all somatic muscles. The jaws are tightly clenched, the bacl arched, and the limbs are usually extended. Each paroxysm may b accompanied by muscle cramp so severe that the patient lies in dread o the next attack. Patients remain fully conscious throughout their terrify ing ordeal.

161 Tetanus neonatorum. The stump of the umbilical cord may b infected by the use of non-sterile instruments or dressings and this ma lead to neonatal tetanus. Failure to suck is an early sign and this i followed by hypertonus and muscle spasms. Despite treatment mortalit is often greater than 50%.

159

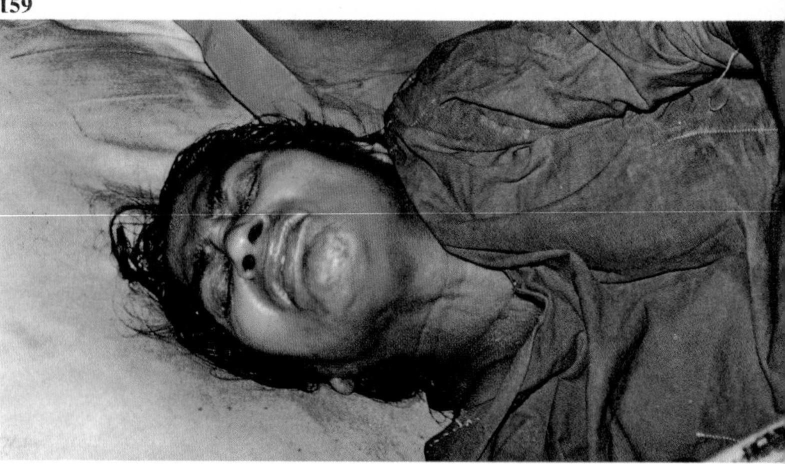

160

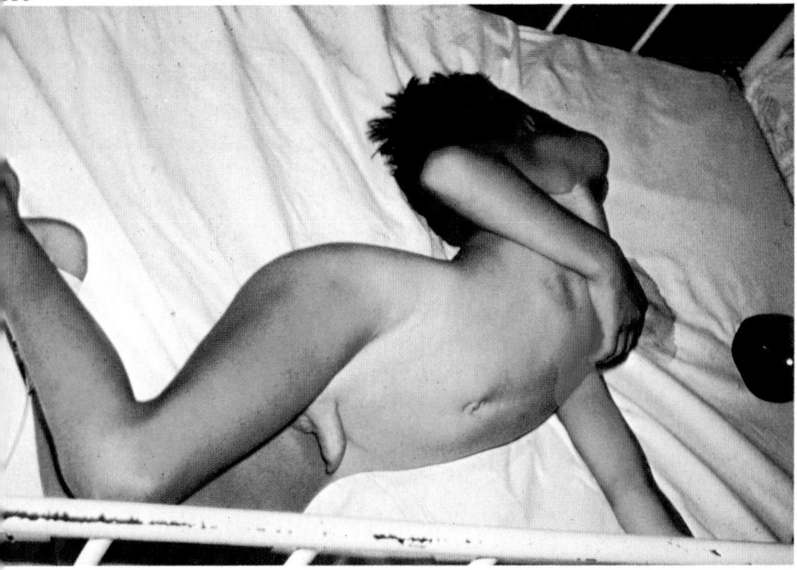

161

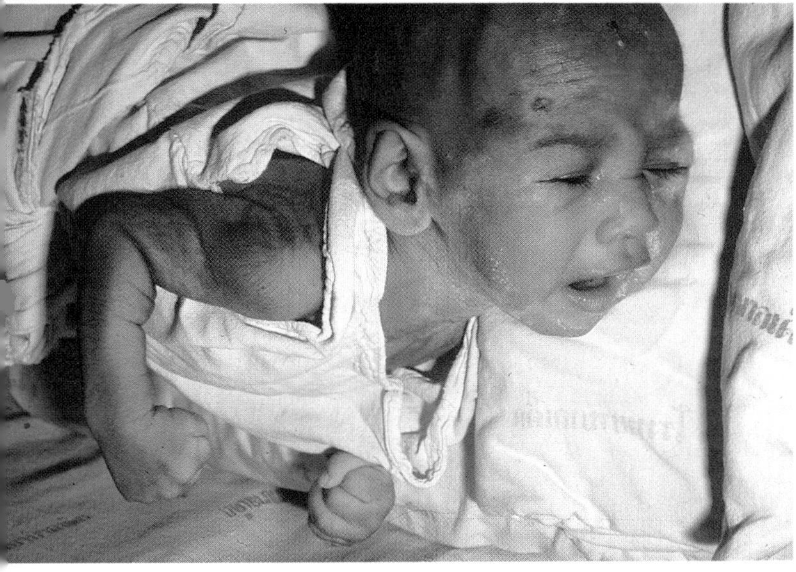

Anthrax

162 Smear from culture of anthrax bacilli. Anthrax is primarily a disease of animals, caused by a bacillus that forms highly resistant spores on exposure to oxygen. In tropical countries, where climatic conditions favour rapid sporulation with heavy contamination of soil, anthrax is mainly spread from infected pasture. In temperate zones sporulation is less rapid, and vegetative bacilli are readily destroyed by soil bacteria; therefore contamination is slight. Under these conditions anthrax is seldom acquired from grazing and is usually derived from imported foodstuffs. Sheep, cattle, horses and goats are very susceptible.

The anthrax bacillus is a non-motile, Gram-positive rod. It measures 4 to 10 μm in length by 1 to 1·5 μm in width and is one of the largest of the pathogenic bacteria. In smears from infected animals the bacilli are encapsulated and lie singly or in short chains, but in cultures on nutrient agar capsules are not formed and the organism is arranged in long strands. When exposed to oxygen it forms spores that are oval in shape with a double-layered outer membrane.

163 Anthrax bacilli in pulmonary capillaries. Gram stain (x 880). Pulmonary anthrax or wool-sorter's disease is a rare condition in man, acquired by inhaling anthrax spores in dust from infected wool or hair. The onset is abrupt and the illness follows a swift course with frequent haemoptyses and acute respiratory distress culminating in death within two or three days.

On postmortem examination there is severe pulmonary oedema with widespread haemorrhagic bronchopneumonia. Large numbers of anthrax bacilli are present and are very conspicuous in Gram-stained preparations because of their large size and deep blue colour.

162

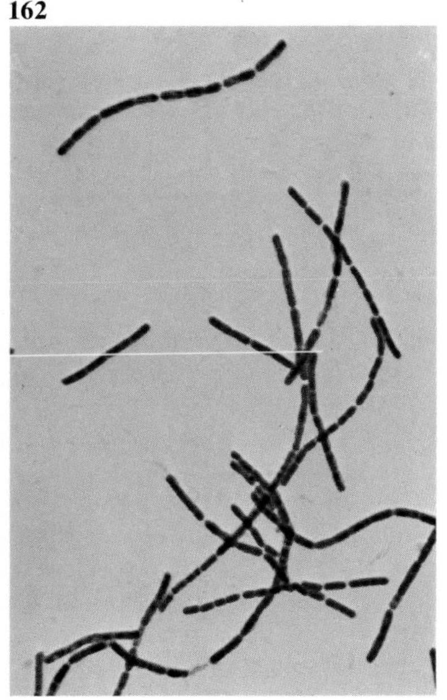

163

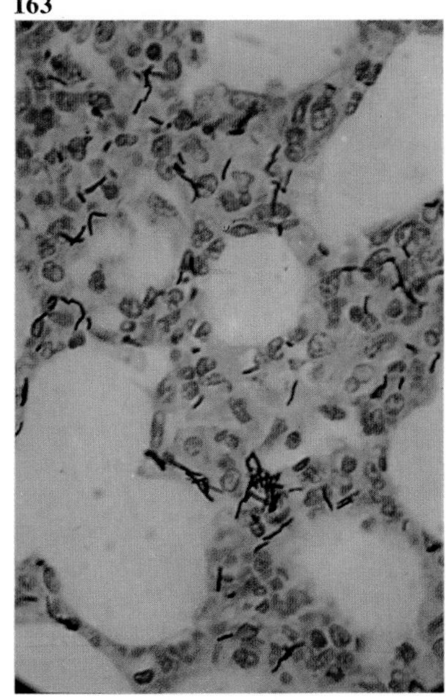

164 Cutaneous anthrax (malignant pustule). Early lesion on neck. The skin is involved in 98% of human infections, and lesions are found most commonly on exposed areas of the body. Cutaneous anthrax is chiefly an occupational disease. Infection may be acquired directly from animals, but it is derived more commonly from hides, wool, hair, raw bonemeal or other animal products.

Anthrax of the neck is an occupational disease of hide porters. An itchy papule develops at the site of entry and is surrounded within a day or two by a ring of haemorrhagic vesicles. Oedema is a striking feature in cutaneous anthrax. It commences round the original lesion and spreads extensively wherever the subcutaneous tissues are lax. The skin may retain its normal colour or become intensely red. Blood cultures may prove positive.

165 Anthrax lesion on neck. As the lesion progresses the central area ulcerates and dries, forming a thick, leathery, dark scab which later extends into the vesicular zone. The crust is firmly attached to the underlying tissues and gradually separates over a period of two or three weeks, leaving a deep ulcer which slowly fills with granulation tissue. The lesion is painless and pus seldom forms, except on rare occasions when there is secondary infection. Before the introduction of antibiotic treatment mortality from anthrax of the neck was much greater than from anthrax of the forehead.

164

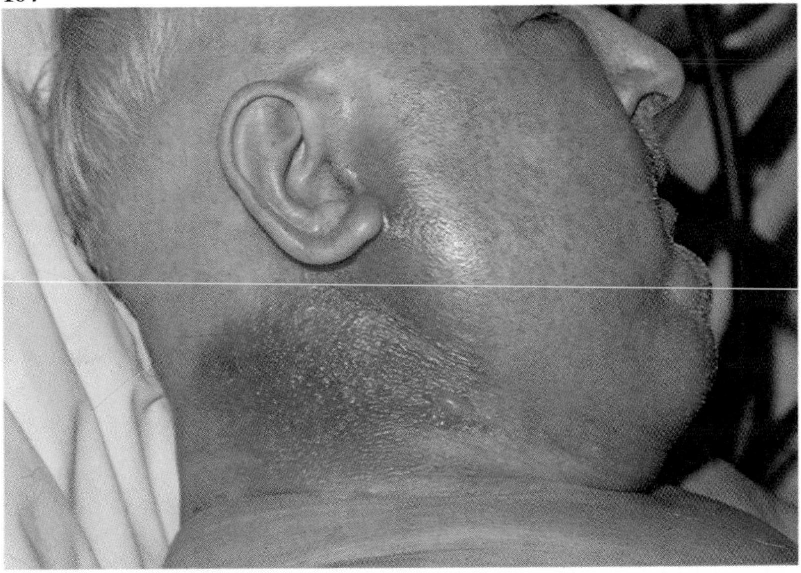

165

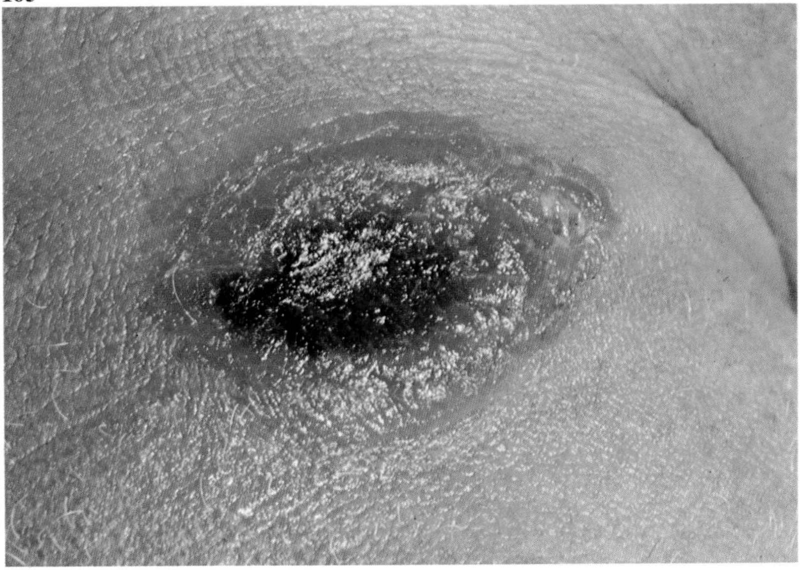

166 Anthrax of forearm. This may occur in butchers handling infected carcases or in gardeners using contaminated bonemeal. Oedema may be slight. This illustration shows the eschar beginning to separate.

167 Anthrax of back. The lower limb and trunk are affected in only 1·9% of cases. The patient opposite worked in a factory manufacturing paint brushes. She developed a large lesion over her left scapula, but there was very little constitutional disturbance. By the time the photograph was taken the vesicles had already ruptured and had been incorporated in the eschar, which was firmly adherent.

166

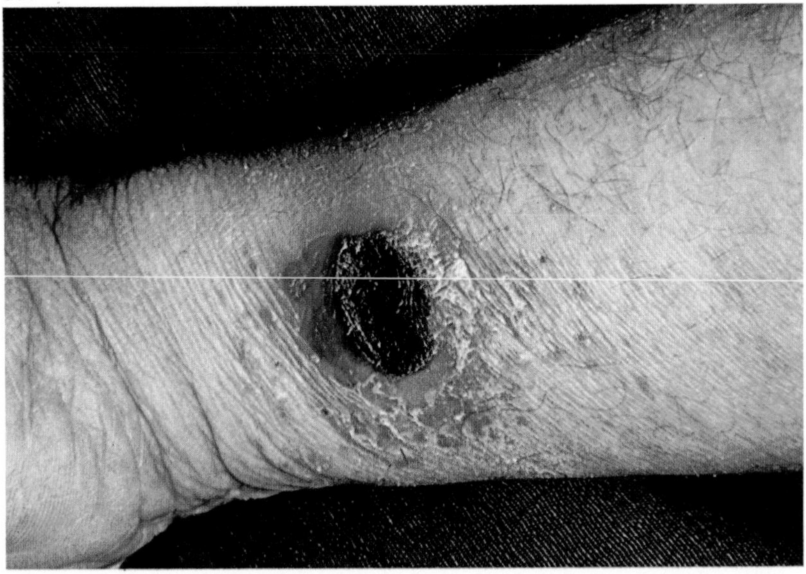

167

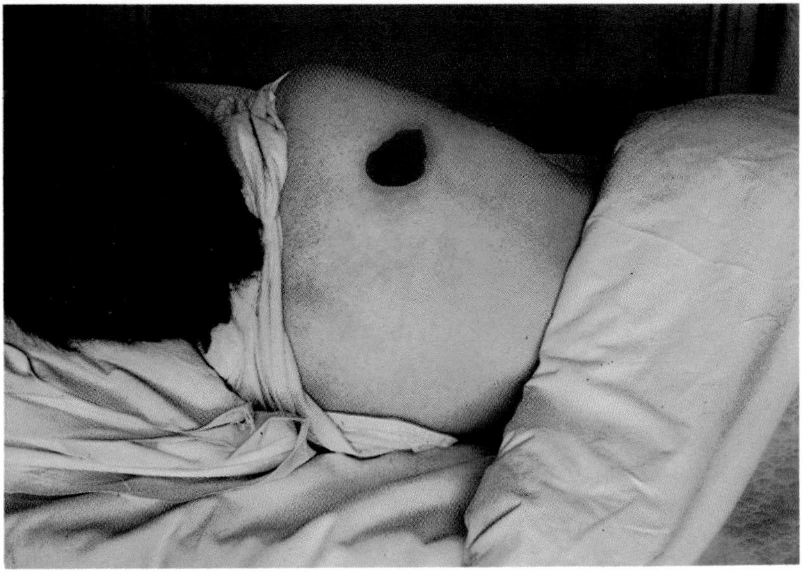

Leptospirosis

168 Smear from culture of *Leptospira icterohaemorrhagiae* (silver impregnation stain). The genus *Leptospira* includes two main species: *L. interrogens* and *L. biflexa*. Both species contain many serotypes (serovars), some of which are pathogenic, and others saprophytic. Parasitic leptospires are indistinguishable from one another morphologically or culturally but can be classified serologically. More than 50 serotypes have already been identified. Leptospires are about 7 to 14 μm long and have a closely coiled body with hooked ends. On electron microscopy the cytoplasm is seen to be wound round a single, straight and stiff axostyle. The organism is actively motile. It is an aerobe, and parasitic strains grow readily on fluid culture medium containing animal serum.

Leptospirosis is a zoonosis affecting rodents, dogs, cats, pigs and cattle. Leptospires may cause little harm to the primary host, where they colonise the renal tubules and are shed in large numbers in the urine. Man and susceptible animals may be infected indirectly by water or articles contaminated by such urine. The organism enters through minor breaches in the skin or mucosa. Farm workers and sewage workers are at special risk.

169 Section of liver showing leptospires (silver impregnation). There is no obvious reaction at the portal of entry, and the organisms quickly enter the bloodstream. When death occurs during the first week of illness leptospires can be found in many tissues but subsequently they are most easily detected in the kidneys. They are best demonstrated by fluorescent antibody technique.

There is a striking contrast between the depth of jaundice in severe cases of leptospirosis and the histological changes in the liver. Damage to the liver cells is much less severe than in viral hepatitis, and the serum transaminase activity is often only slightly increased. Cholestasis is the most prominent feature. In postmortem preparations the parenchymal cells are seen to be separated from each other, and there is a high incidence of mitotic figures.

In this section, stained by Levaditi's silver impregnation method, a large number of leptospires with characteristic closely wound spirals can be seen scattered between the liver cells. (Arrow = leptospire.)

168

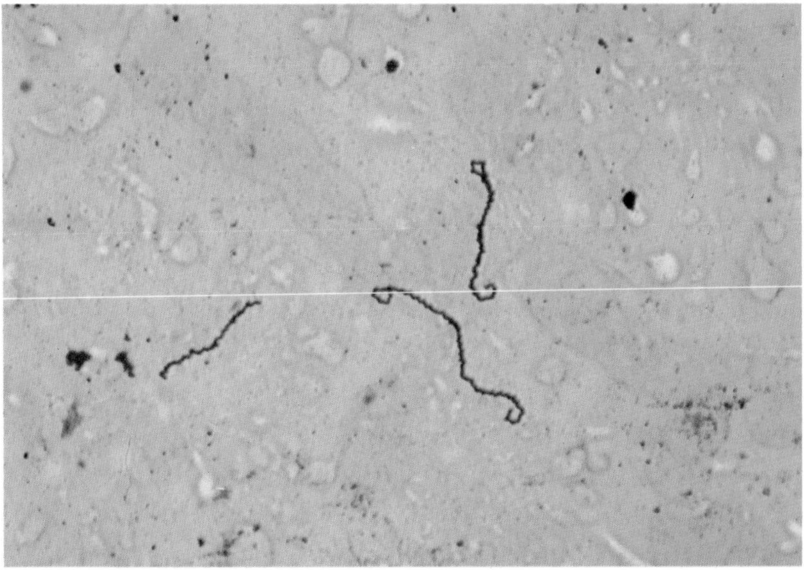

169

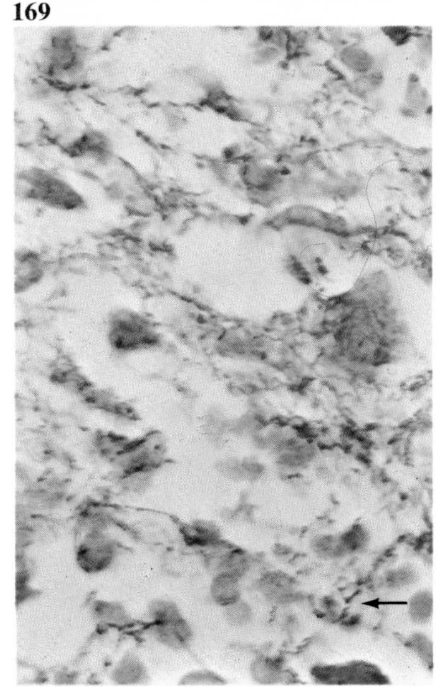

170 Suffusion of conjunctivae. Leptospirosis in man is associated with a wide range of clinical syndromes, including classical Weil's disease, aseptic meningitis, influenza-like illness, and unexplained fever. The onset is abrupt with shivering followed by fever. Headache, myalgia and arthralgia are common features. Conjunctival suffusion is often present and may be accompanied by photophobia. Prostration tends to be severe and disproportionate to the physical signs.

171 Close-up of eye in canicola fever. Human beings usually develop canicola fever through contact with pig or dog urine containing *L. canicola*, although the leptospire is sometimes found in other animals. Severe and intractable headache is an outstanding and distressing symptom. An aseptic form of meningitis is present in 75% of patients. Roughly 20% have jaundice or evidence of renal damage. Nearly 50% have injection of the conjunctivae.

170

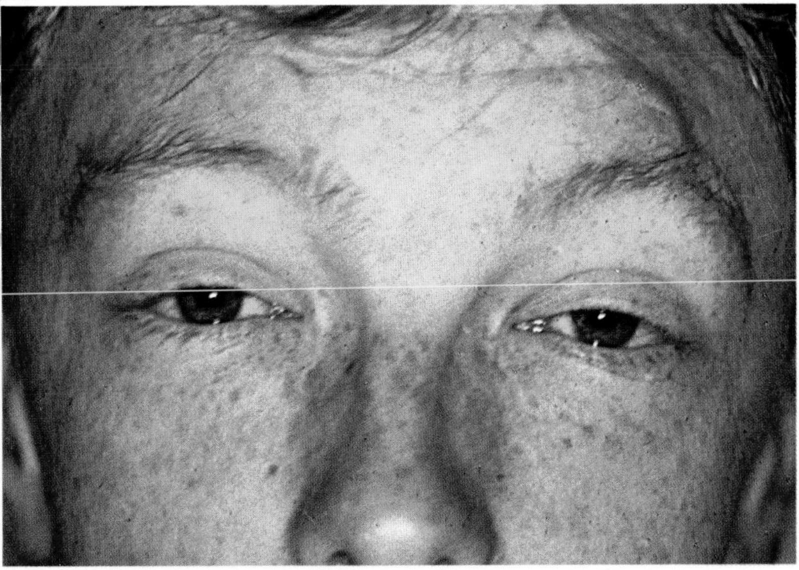

171

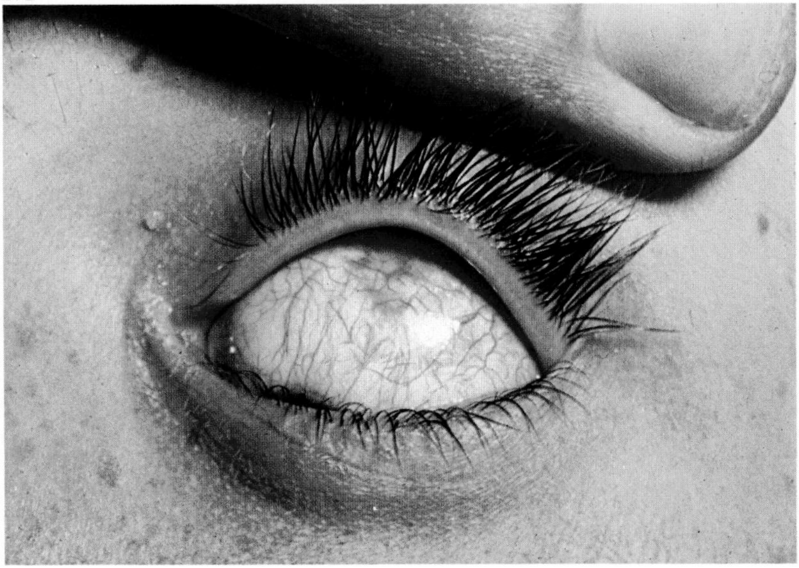

172 Severe Weil's disease. Weil's disease is a severe form of leptospirosis with both hepatic and renal damage. It is commonly caused by *L. icterohaemorrhagiae* derived from rats, but other serotypes have been incriminated. The syndrome is comparatively rare, occurring in roughly 15% of leptospiral infections in man. Even with this most virulent serotype, mild or inapparent infections are not uncommon.

The first week of illness is dominated by fever, headache, severe debility, and muscular pains. Nausea and vomiting may be accompanied by haematemesis, and abdominal pain may be so severe that a surgical emergency is suspected. Jaundice may be the earliest sign but may not develop until the end of the first week. At the same time haemorrhages may appear in the skin and mucous membranes and, if profuse, indicate an unfavourable prognosis. The second week is critical. Jaundice deepens, haemorrhages increase, and renal failure develops. Most deaths take place at this stage from renal failure and some lives may be saved by effective dialysis. During the third week the illness abates, renal function improves, and jaundice lessens. Eventually full renal and hepatic function is restored.

173 Face in Weil's disease. Haemorrhages are common in severely ill patients with jaundice and renal failure. Petechiae or ecchymoses may be found in skin, conjunctivae, or mucous membranes. Epistaxis may be a presenting feature, and there may be profuse bleeding into the bowel during the second week. Mild haemoptysis is not unusual.

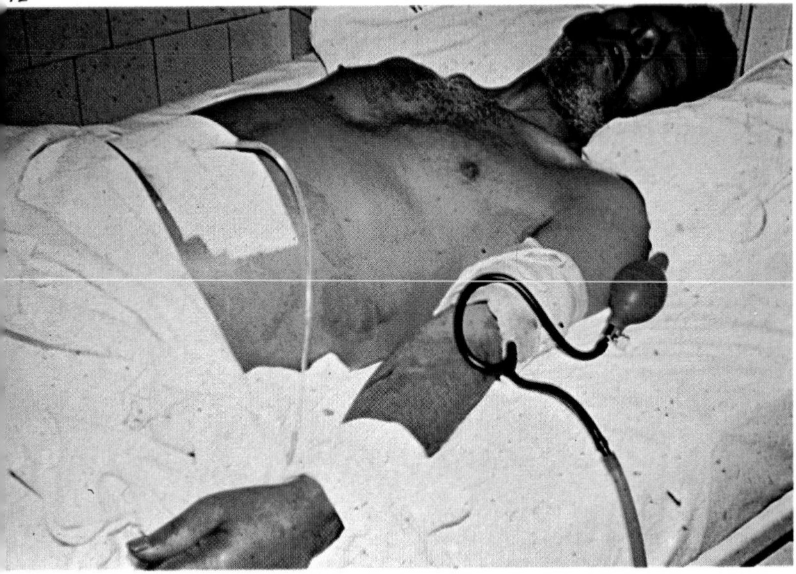

173

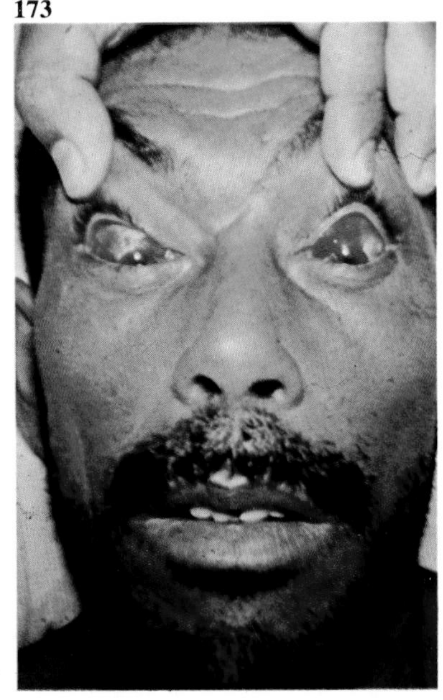

Gonorrhoea

Gonorrhoea is caused by *Neisseria gonorrhoeae*, an infection confined to humans. In adults it is transmitted by sexual contact; in children by non-sexual contact or by fomites. Gonorrhoea in adults may manifest as local infection of the urogenital tract, rectum, conjunctiva or oropharynx, or generalised infection of the skin, joints, meninges, and endocardium. Transmission from the mother during delivery may result in acute conjunctivitis; contamination of flannels and towels may cause acute vulvovaginitis in young girls.

174 Smear of organism (Gram stain). *Neisseria gonorrhoeae* is a Gram-negative bacterium, usually sensitive to human serum and readily ingested by neutrophil polymorphonuclear leucocytes, as seen in this smear stained with Gram stain, where they appear as intracellular diplococci. They have fastidious growth requirements.

175 Urethritis. This is the commonest presentation of gonorrhoea in men. A purulent urethral discharge appears within a few days after exposure and is associated with dysuria. Untreated, this will often last for many weeks before clearing spontaneously. The persistent inflammation predisposes to urethral stricture. Gonococcal urethritis is clinically indistinguishable from non-gonococcal urethritis caused by chlamydia, but can be differentiated by examination of a urethral smear. Painful lymphadenitis is present in 15% of cases. Proctitis may be the presenting feature in homosexuals.

176 Cervicitis. Symptoms are absent in 80% of women infected with the gonococcus. An infected cervix may have a normal appearance with mucoid discharge or may be inflamed with mucopurulent or profuse purulent discharge. The urethra or rectum may be infected from the vaginal discharge. Pelvic spread may result in endometritis, salpingitis or peritonitis.

177 Bartholin's abscess. A more dramatic presentation in women is infection of Bartholin's gland. The lymphadenitis is usually unilateral and may progress to form abscesses. Skene's glands may also be affected.

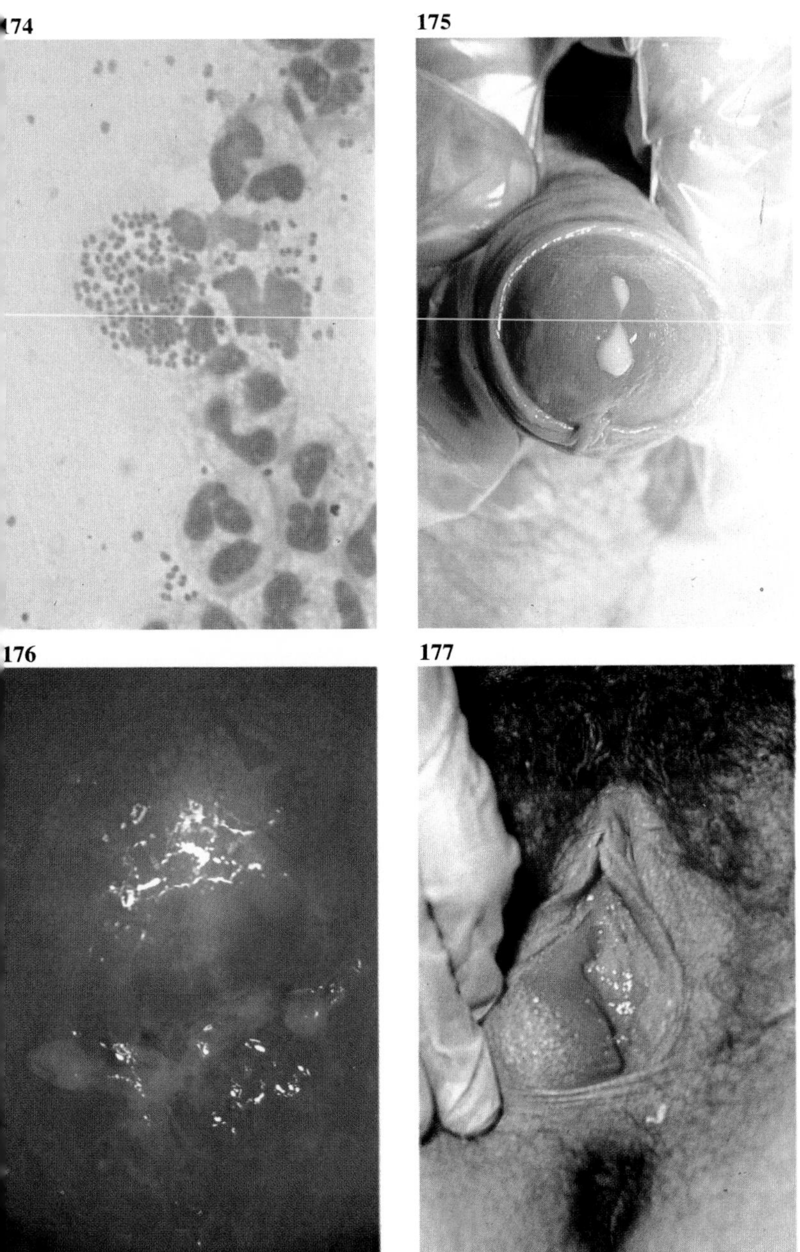
174
175
176
177

178 Gonorrhoea — skin lesions. Disseminated infection is caused by strains of gonococci resistant to serum and accounts for 2% of all gonococcal infection. It is more common in women. Bacteraemia may lead to septic arthritis, tenosynovitis, meningitis, endocarditis or skin lesions. Skin lesions are the most common feature and consist of a sparse rash over the limbs, sparing the face and trunk.

179 Gonorrhoea — skin lesion. The most characteristic lesion is a pustule on an erythematous base. Slight fever is common. Some patients may have no constitutional upset; others may be very ill with a high fever.

180 Gonorrhoea — skin lesion. The skin lesions vary and may consist of macules, papules, pustules, haemorrhagic bullae, or necrotic lesions as shown here. The organism is seldom grown from the skin lesions but may be cultured from blood or purulent joint effusions. Most patients have migratory arthralgia during the first week mainly affecting the large joints. In some cases, this will progress to septic arthritis. Tenosynovitis is found in about 25% of cases.

181 Conjunctivitis. Ophthalmia may result from direct contact with an infected birth canal. It follows two to five days after birth and may cause septicaemia. Transfer of infection from discharges elsewhere may cause conjunctivitis in adults. Young girls living in overcrowded conditions are very susceptible to gonococcal vulvovaginitis spread by moist articles such as flannels or towels. Infection is very seldom spread by fomites to adults.

178

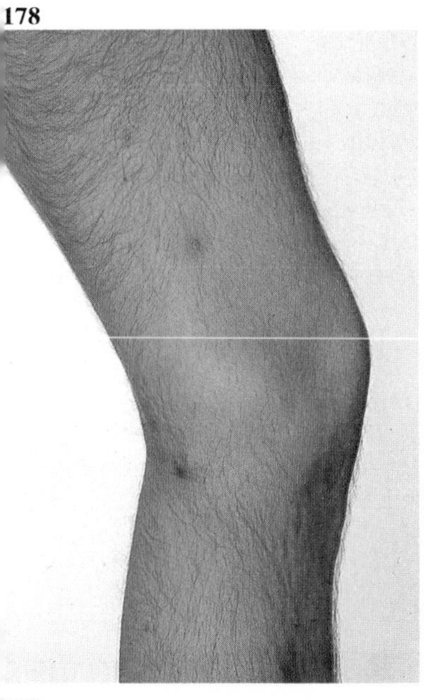

179

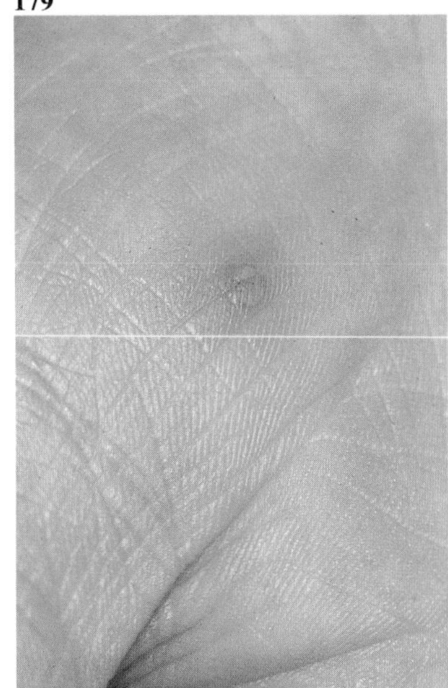

180

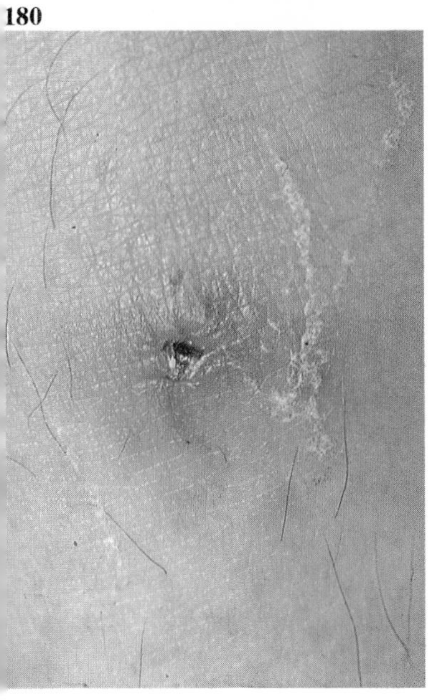

181

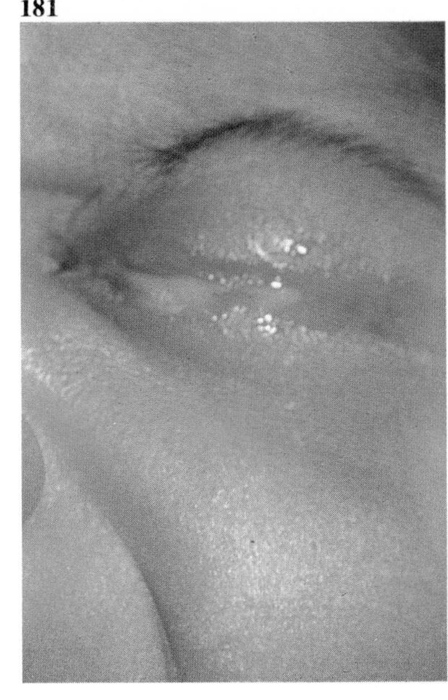

Chlamydial infection

Chlamydia are intracellular parasites, whose genome contains both DNA and RNA. They are considered to be specialised bacteria with a complex form of replication ending in binary fission, and can be divided into two groups sharing a complement-fixing antigen. *Chlamydia trachomatis* (group A) is responsible for genital infections, conjunctivitis at any age and pneumonitis in infancy; *Chlamydia psittaci* (group B) causes ornithosis.

182 Chlamydial infection — conjunctival smear. Conjunctival scrapings from patients with neonatal inclusion conjunctivitis, when stained by Giemsa's method, may show intracytoplasmic basophilic inclusion bodies. The technique is less sensitive in adult inclusion conjunctivitis, and of little or no value in genital infection. Tissue cultures, using pretreated cells, such as McCoy, are more reliable. Humoral antibody may be detected by immunofluorescence, but the results of serological tests must be interpreted with caution.

183 Conjunctivitis in newborn baby. Infection of the eye from the mother's cervix at the time of birth may result in inclusion conjunctivitis of the newborn. A mucopurulent conjunctivitis develops within two weeks of birth and may affect one or both eyes. There are no distinguishing features. The acute stage settles after two weeks or so, but the eye may take several months to return to normal and the disease may progress to mild trachoma.

182

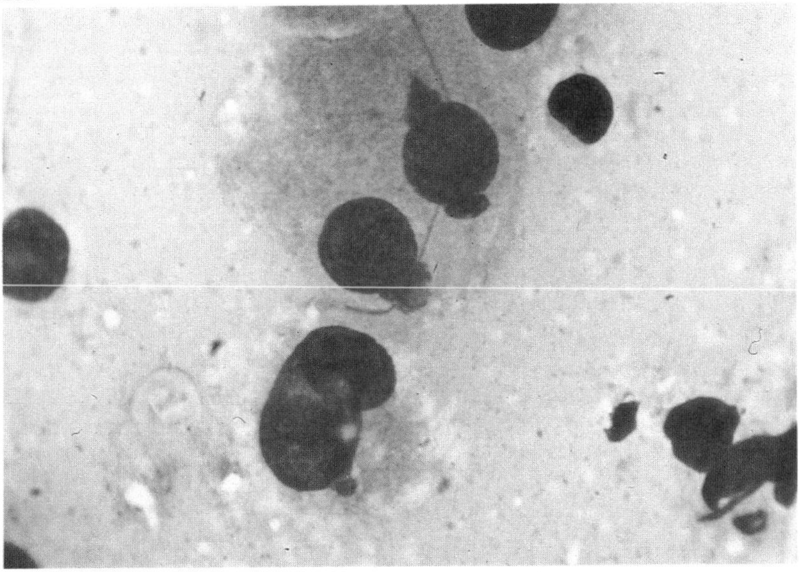

183

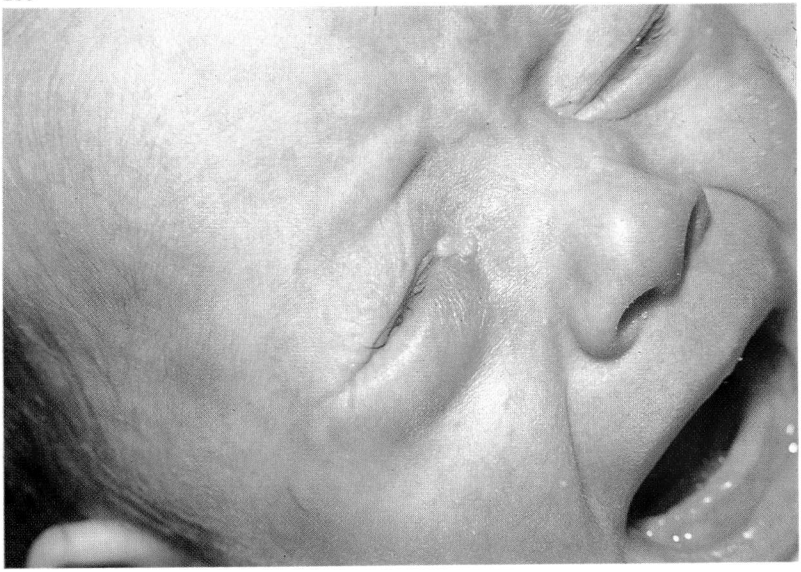

184 Conjunctivitis — adult. Inclusion conjunctivitis in adults also has an acute onset and is accompanied by mucopurulent discharge, conjunctival follicles and superficial punctate keratitis. The follicles are always more prominent in the lower than the upper lid, and appear as rounded swellings, 1 to 2mm in diameter, which are formed by lymphocytic foci in the subepithelial adenoid layer. Healing takes place slowly over a period of one to two years.

185 Trachoma. Trachoma is also caused by TRIC or non-LGV strains of *Chlamydia trachomatis*. The disease is endemic in many parts of the world where people are crowded together under conditions of poor hygiene. Infection is transmitted by conjunctival secretions, which are transferred on fingers or towels and, above all, by flies. The onset is usually subacute and the course is determined by the presence or absence of secondary infection. The conjunctiva is inflamed and follicles appear in the fornices. They spread over the palpebral conjunctiva but rarely on to the bulbar conjunctiva, and may measure up to 5mm in diameter. Trachomatous infiltration may extend deeply into the subepithelial tissues of the palpebral conjunctiva. The cornea is affected at an early stage with a superficial keratitis, which is most marked in the upper part. As the disease progresses the conjunctiva becomes scarred and pannus develops, with cloudiness and vascularization of the cornea.

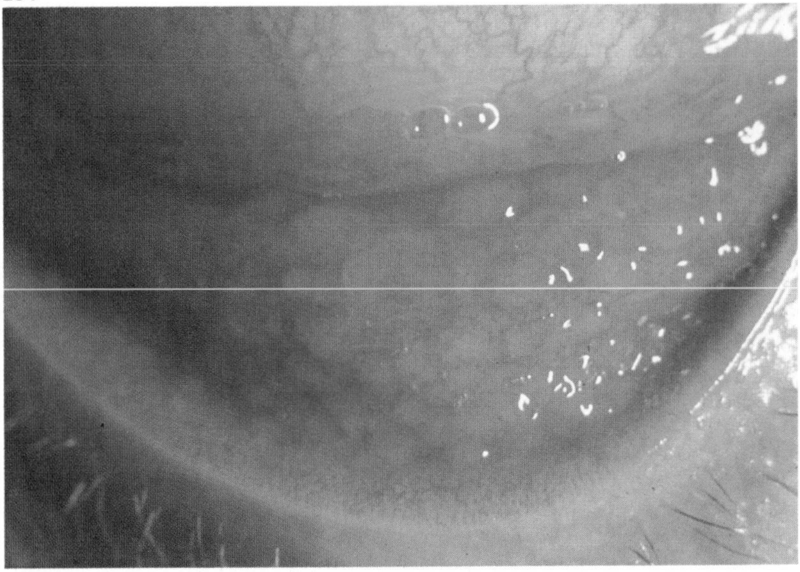

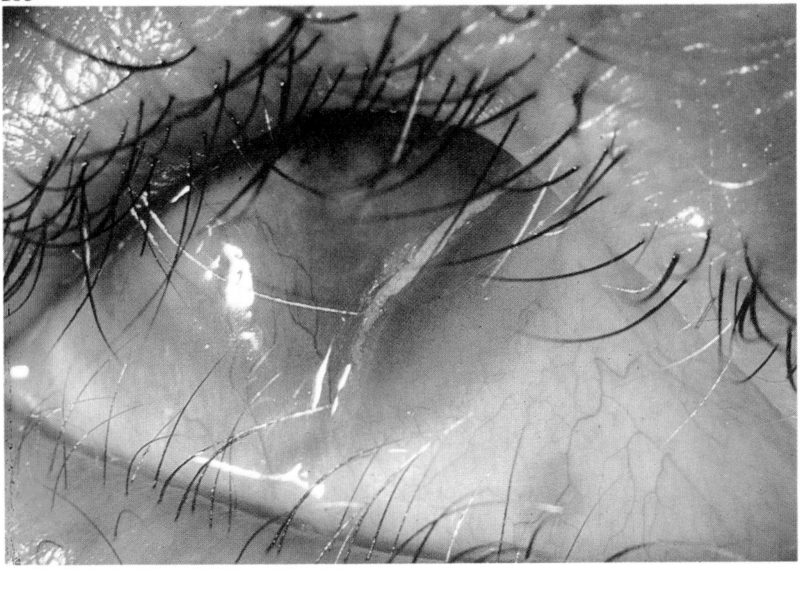

186 Urethritis. *Chlamydia trachomatis* may be isolated from the urethra in up to 5% of symptomless men, 20% of men with gonorrhoea, and 30 to 50% of men with non-specific urethritis. Chlamydial urethritis is clinically indistinguishable from gonococcal, though it tends to be milder. Chlamydial infection is also associated with epididymitis and with Reiter's disease.

187 Cervicitis. Chlamydial infections are common in women: the organism has been detected in up to 5% of healthy women, and up to 60% of women with gonorrhoea. Chlamydial cervicitis is accompanied by mucopurulent discharge from the os and the cervix is reddened and oedematous. Chlamydia is responsible for some cases of salpingitis and proctitis in women. Infection acquired at birth may give rise to inclusion conjunctivitis in the newborn baby, or pneumonitis in the infant.

188 Lymphogranuloma venereum. This sexually transmitted disease is caused by the LGV strain of *Chlamydia trachomatis*. After an incubation period of one to three weeks a primary lesion may be detected on the genitalia in about 10% of patients. This consists of a small papule or vesicle, which may ulcerate, but heals within a few days without leaving a scar.

After two to ten weeks the patient enters the secondary stage, with painful swelling of the regional lymph nodes. This is occasionally accompanied by constitutional disturbance, with fever, headache and arthralgia. As the disease progresses the lymph nodes become matted and attached to the overlying skin, which is reddened. The buboes may suppurate and discharge through sinuses on to the surface of the skin, vagina or bowel.

The disease may resolve after three to four months, or may advance to the third stage, with strictures of the urethra, vagina or rectum. Fistulae or perirectal abscesses may prove troublesome and lymphatic obstruction may result in chronic oedema with enlargement of the penis or vulva.

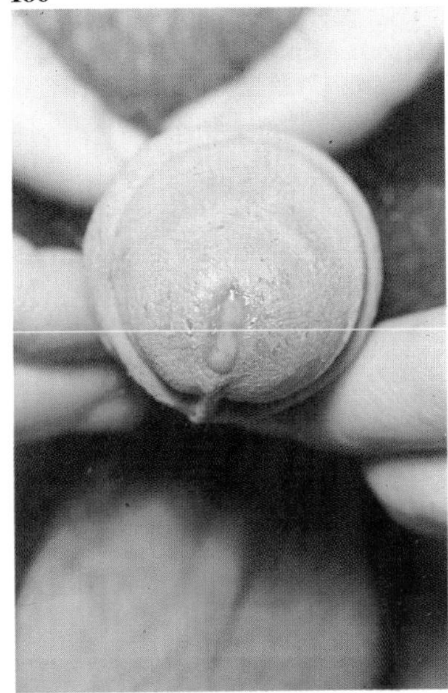

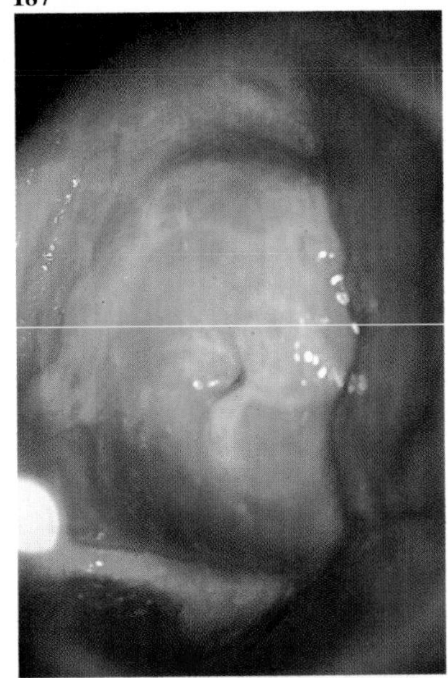

188

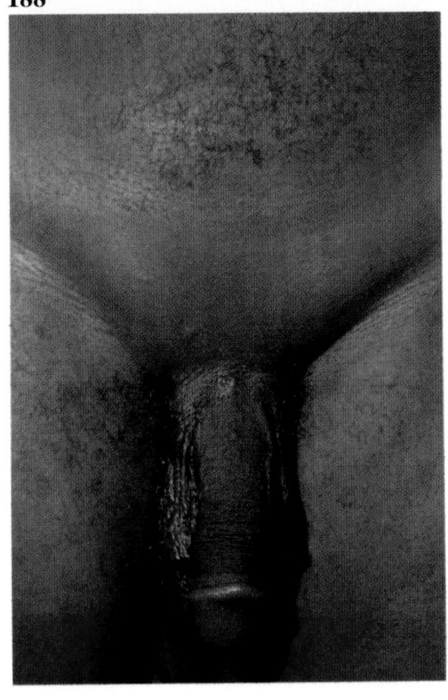

189 Ornithosis. This is a worldwide zoonosis caused by *Chlamydia psittaci*. Infection is common in humans occupationally exposed to psittacine birds in pet shops and aviaries, and other birds in turkey- and duck-processing plants. Infection is rarely transmitted from humans.

Much infection is subclinical or mild, resembling influenza. Severe attacks begin with an influenza-like illness. During the first week the patient has a high fever with relative bradycardia and possible gastrointestinal disturbance with diarrhoea. A dry cough may be present, but there are few chest signs. Evidence of consolidation may appear during the second week, and the extent of the pneumonia or radiological examination is disproportionate to the physical signs. The radiographic appearances are not diagnostic. The erythrocyte sedimentation rate tends to be notably increased, and the diagnosis is confirmed by serological tests. The illness subsides after 7 to 14 days, but convalescence tends to be protracted, and radiological clearance may take several weeks.

189

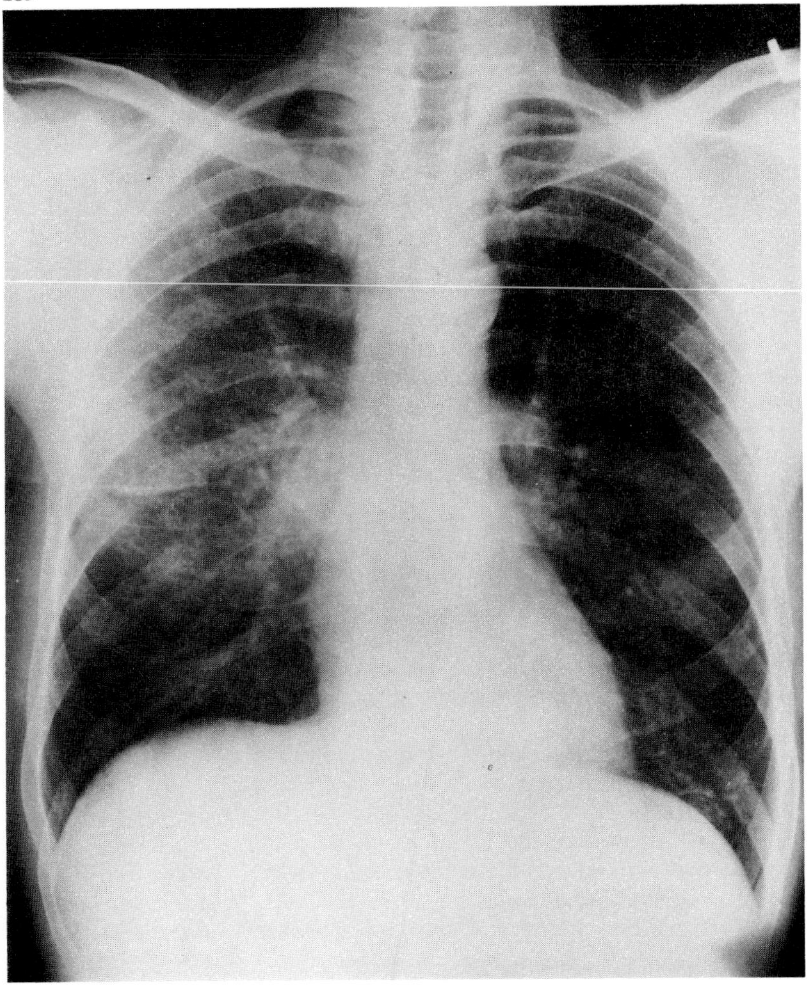

Syphilis

Syphilis is caused by the spirochaete *Treponema pallidum*. Acquired infection is almost entirely transmitted by sexual contact; congenital infection often comes from a mother who has been infected during or shortly before pregnancy. The incidence of syphilis has greatly declined since the introduction of antibiotics.

190 Organism — *Treponema pallidum*. *Treponema pallidum* is a slender spirochaete about 10 μm in length with roughly 10 turns to its spiral. It has an undulating movement and rotates about its long axis. It is sensitive to drying and dies rapidly above 42°C but can survive for some days at 4°C. It cannot be seen by ordinary microscopy but is best seen by dark-field illumination as shown here; it can be stained by silver in tissue sections. It is a human parasite and is indistinguishable morphologically or serologically from treponemes causing yaws, pinta or bejel.

191 Syphilis — chancre in a male. In heterosexual men the primary lesion of syphilis, the chancre, is most commonly found on the glans penis or in the sulcus and less commonly on the penile shaft. The chancre is indurated but is not tender and is often associated with enlarged but painless inguinal lymph nodes. Dark-field preparations are made from serum exuded from the chancre.

192 Syphilis — chancre in a female. Classically, the chancre appears after an incubation period of 21 to 35 days (extremes 9 to 90 days) as a single lesion in 50% of cases. It evolves rapidly from a macule to a papule, which erodes and forms a round, painless ulcer with a clean surface and surrounding hard induration. It heals within three to ten weeks leaving a thin atrophic scar in some cases. Vulval lesions may be readily recognised, but cervical lesions are commonly overlooked.

193 Syphilis — anal chancre. In homosexual men the anus is a major site for the primary lesion. Anal lesions may also be found in women, and mouth lesions occur in both sexes.

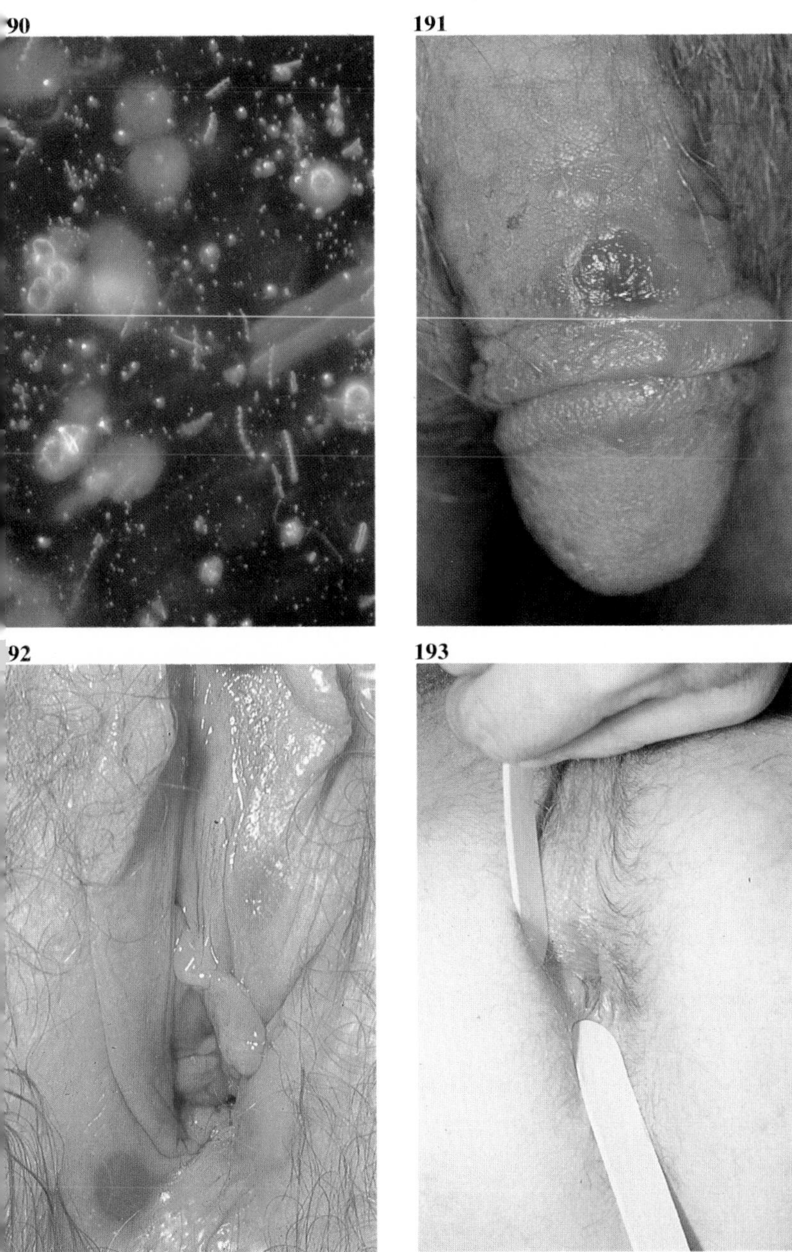
90
191
92
193

194 Syphilis — rash. A rash is the presenting feature in 70% of case and usually appears six to eight weeks after infection, when the primar lesion is declining or has healed. It may be accompanied by genera symptoms of fever, headache, malaise and arthralgia, and associate with mucous patches, lymphadenitis and meningitis. The rash varie greatly in intensity and appearance. It usually appears first on the trunk and proximal parts of the limbs as discrete pinkish macules, which ma evolve into red papules. The lesions do not itch and persist for four t eight weeks.

195 Syphilis — rash. Sometimes the rash may consist of fewer, larger darker red papules.

196 Syphilis — rash. In a few patients the rash may finally becom pustular and form crusts. Lesions of different type may be found on th same patient. Vesicular rashes are not a feature of secondary syphilis.

197 Syphilis — rash. The rash may extend to cover the whole body including the palms and soles. This distribution should suggest possibl secondary syphilis. Involvement of hair follicles may result in patch alopecia.

When the secondary stage subsides the patient enters the stage of laten syphilis. There is no clinical evidence of active disease, but serologica tests remain positive. Some patients with latent syphilis advance to th tertiary stage after an interval of three to ten years or longer.

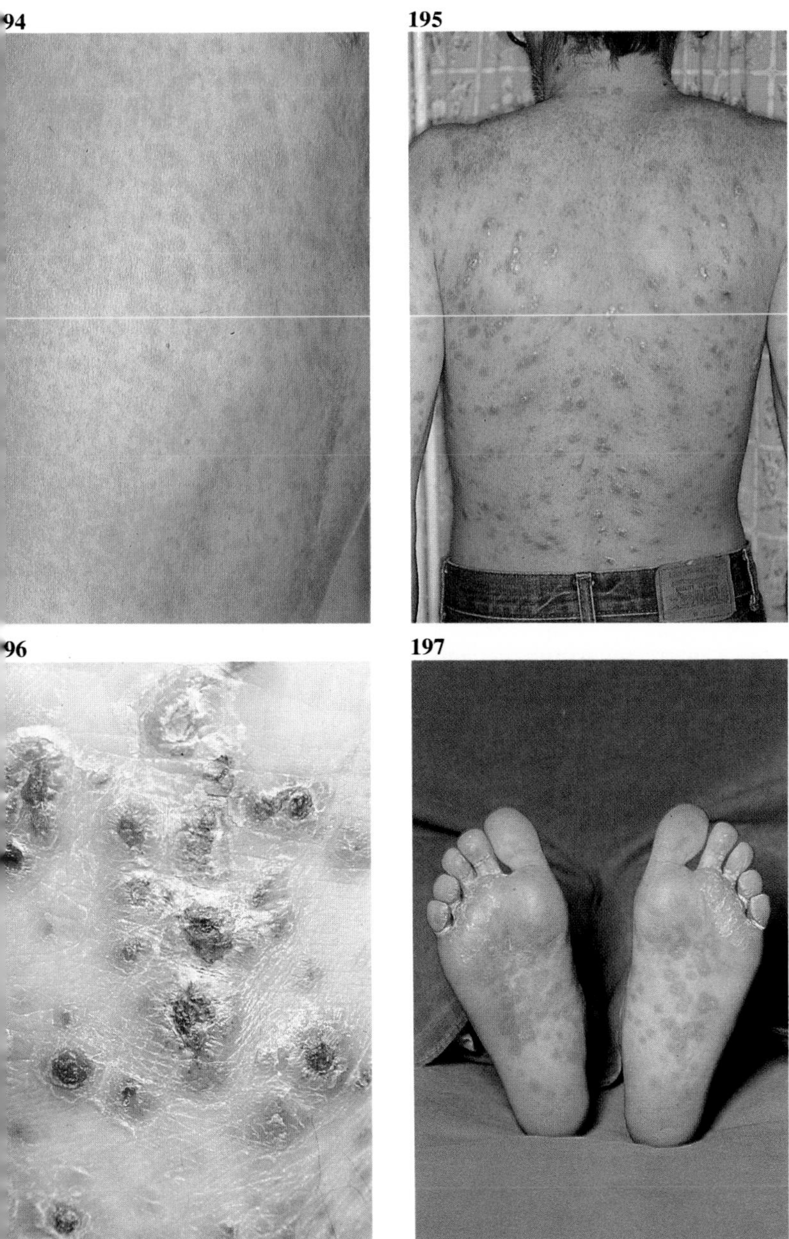

94

195

96

197

198 Syphilis — chest x-ray showing aneurysm. Before the introduction of penicillin for the treatment of syphilis, between 10 and 40% of patients progressed to the tertiary stage. Cardiovascular disease appeared 10 to 30 years after infection and was accompanied by neurosyphilis in about 30% of cases. Vasculitis affecting the vasa vasorum of the aorta results in the loss of elastic tissue and subsequent dilatation of the artery. If the root of the aorta is affected the aortic ring becomes dilated causing aortic incompetence.

199 Syphilis — gumma. The basic lesion of tertiary syphilis is a chronic granuloma, known as a gumma. It tends to be localised, asymmetrical in distribution, and destructive in character. A gumma may affect any part of the body. Sometimes a solitary gumma may appear in the subcutaneous tissues, increasing in size before breaking down to form a gummatous ulcer. Such an ulcer is painless and has a characteristic appearance. It is roughly circular, with sharply defined 'punched out' edges and an indurated base. A slough of necrotic tissue, like a piece of wash-leather, initially occupies the crater and is firmly adherent. Later it separates leaving pale granulations. Spirochaetes cannot be detected in the lesion.

200 Congenital syphilis — early manifestations. Congenital syphilis is now extremely rare in developed countries. The clinical course is very variable and in many cases there may be no obvious clinical signs. One of the earliest features may be a mucopurulent nasal discharge, which may persist for many months and is known as the 'snuffles'. Skin eruptions are common during the first two years of life, and there may be evidence of damage to many structures, including mucous membranes, bones and teeth.

The rash is most commonly maculopapular and may be followed by extensive sloughing of the epithelium on the palms and soles, and around the mouth and anus. Pemphigoid lesions may be found in congenital syphilis but seldom in acquired syphilis. The skin lesions are teeming with treponema.

These early lesions heal and are followed by a latent period before the late features appear. These include damage to teeth, bones, eyes and auditory nerve as well as gummata and neurosyphilis.

98

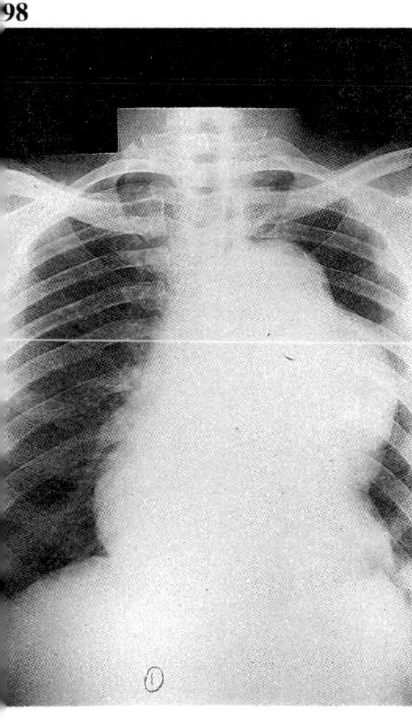

199

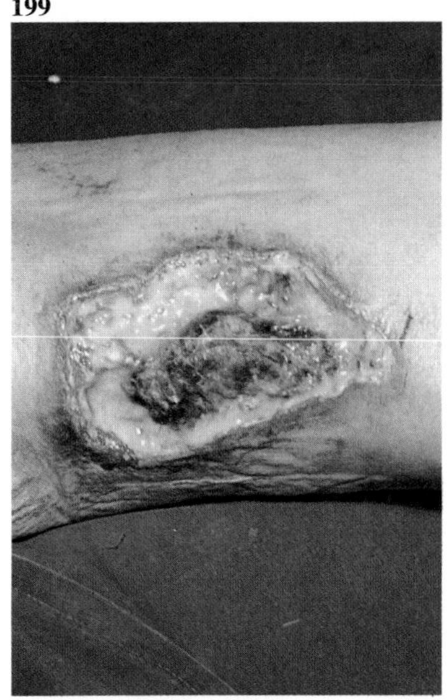

200

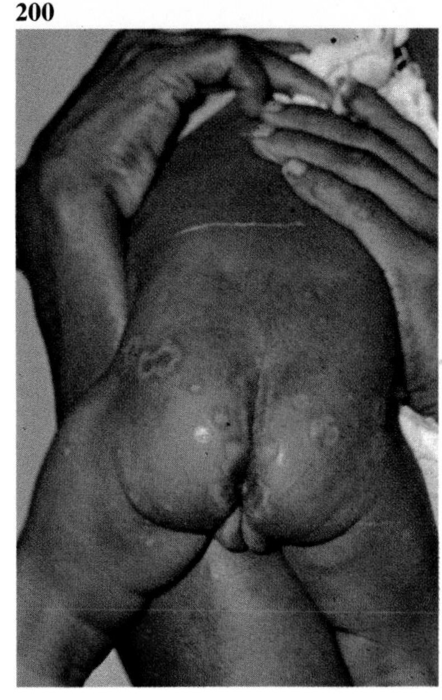

201

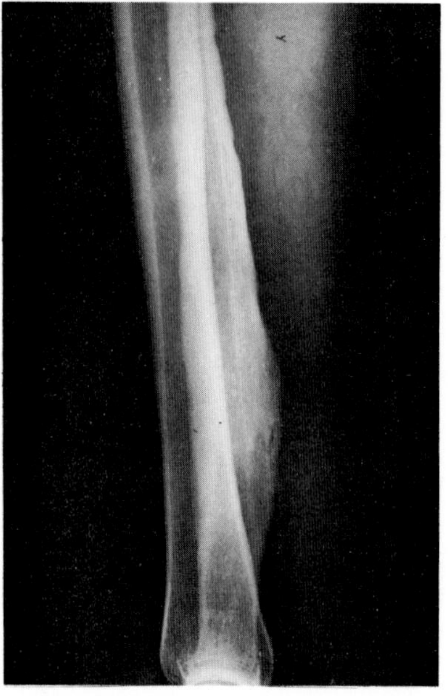

201 Radiograph of tibia and fibula in late form of syphilitic periostitis
Widespread bone disease is very common in young children with congenital syphilis and may present as osteochondritis, periostitis, or osteitis and osteomyelitis, particularly affecting the long bones and the skull. This early disease may be detected at any time from birth to the age of three to four years and usually resolves spontaneously.

Bone disease may reappear between the ages of five to 15 years. This late form is usually very resistant to treatment and may persist indefinitely. The radiological appearances in syphilitic, tuberculous and chronic pyogenic bone disease are very similar, and other factors must be taken into consideration when making a diagnosis. In the juvenile form of syphilitic periostitis or osteitis new bone may be deposited in lamellated layers parallel to the shaft or else on the convexity of the shaft. The tibia is commonly affected, and thickening of the anterior aspect of the proximal half of the bone may produce the appearance of sabre shin of tibia.

hancroid

hancroid is a sexually transmitted disease caused by the Gram-negative occobacillus *Haemophilus ducreyi.* As with a number of sexually ansmitted diseases, it is more commonly recognised in men than omen. The infection is worldwide in distribution and is especially ommon where social, economic, and hygienic conditions are poor.

Lesions are usually confined to the genitalia and perianal region, with econdary lesions in the inguinal lymph nodes. The initial lesion is a ender papule, which becomes pustular and then erodes to form a non-ndurated and painful ulcer. This may coalesce with other lesions, and econdary infection may result in further destruction.

02 Genital lesions in chancroid. Here the penile lesions are associated ith greatly enlarged inguinal glands. The lymphadenitis is usually uni-ateral. The swelling is painful and may rupture to leave a discharging inus. The penile lesions may be difficult to distinguish from those of ranuloma inguinale (Donovanosis). They may also be confused with he primary lesion of syphilis, but can be differentiated by the presence f pain and absence of induration. The two infections coexist in up to 0% of patients, so the possibility of syphilis should always be considered. he diagnosis of chancroid may be confirmed by finding the organism in mears or by culture.

02

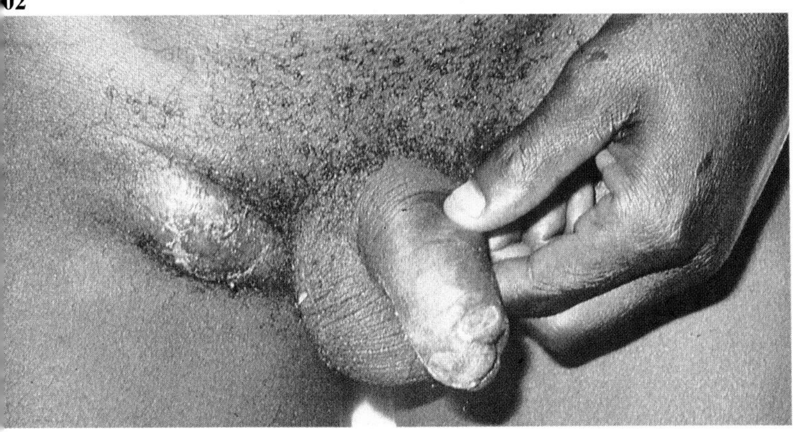

Donovanosis

Donovanosis, granuloma inguinale, and granuloma venereum are names given to the disease produced by *Calymmatobacterium granulomatis,* a Gram-negative encapsulated bacterium, whose relation to other organisms is uncertain. Infection is usually transmitted by sexual contact, but this is not exclusive, as young children may be affected. It is more common in tropical parts of the world.

203 Donovanosis — organism. This is characteristically found in large mononuclear cells and can be demonstrated as deeply staining Donovan bodies in smudge smears made from the lesions. In this smear the preparation was made from the penile lesion. The organism is difficult to culture on artificial media.

204 Donovanosis — lesions. The disease is usually confined to the genitalia, but other sites may be affected. In men the penis is the common site, in women the labia. The primary lesion is an indurated nodule, which becomes ulcerated. Individual lesions may coalesce to form enlarging areas of ulceration, and autoinfection may occur. In this patient from Papua New Guinea spread of infection to the inguinal lymph nodes from the initial penile lesion has resulted in extensive ulceration in the groins. Secondary infection may cause further damage and scarring may lead to deformity.

203

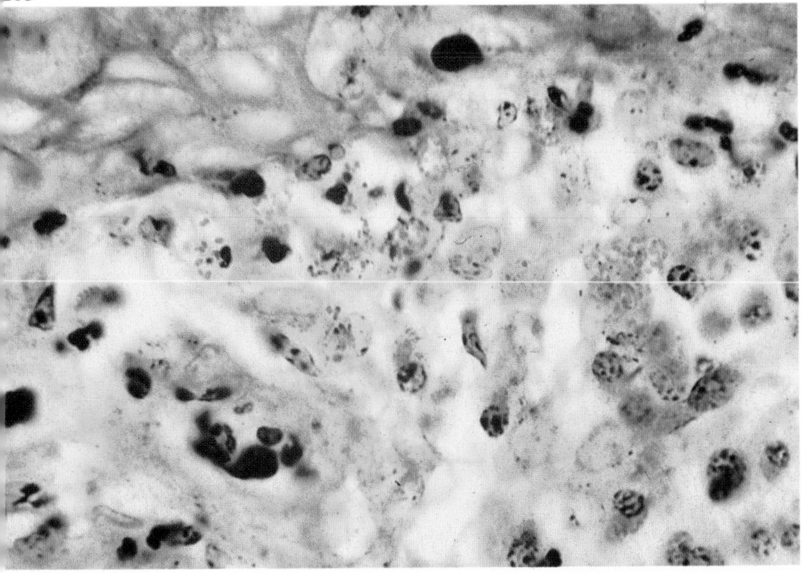

204

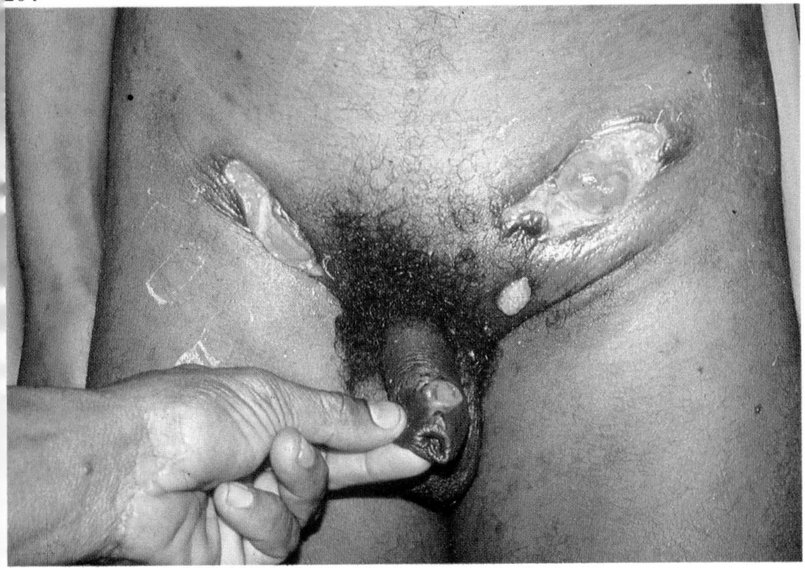

VIRUS INFECTIONS

Herpesvirus group

Members of this group cause important infections in both man and animals. Those associated with disease in man include:

- *Herpesvirus varicellae/zoster* — the cause of chickenpox and herpes zoster.
- Herpes simplex virus.
- *Herpesvirus simiae* — a rare cause of encephalitis in man.
- Cytomegalovirus — benign lymphadenitis and other syndromes.
- Epstein–Barr virus — associated with infectious mononucleosis and neoplastic disease.

The herpesviruses are relatively large, 120 to 180nm, with a central capsid containing DNA and an outer membrane derived from the host cell. They are ether-sensitive. They develop within the nucleus of the host cell and may pass quietly into the cytoplasm and leave the cell without necessarily destroying it. An acidophilic inclusion body surrounded by a halo (Cowdry type A) is characteristically left in the nucleus as a memorial to viral replication. Many viruses in the group show a marked tendency to latency and may become active whenever host immunity is impaired.

Varicella (chickenpox)

Varicella is a highly infectious disease mainly affecting young children, though no age group is exempt. Infection is usually acquired by direct contact with a case during the first few days of illness, when virus is being shed from the respiratory mucosa and skin. The virus is probably transmitted by the airborne route and enters through the respiratory passages. The incubation period varies but commonly lies between 15 and 18 days. In children varicella is generally mild and complications are rare; in adults the illness tends to be more severe with a higher incidence of complications.

The viruses causing chickenpox and herpes zoster appear to be identical and have been designated *Herpesvirus varicellae/zoster*.

Virology and pathology

205 Electron micrograph of *Herpesvirus varicellae/zoster*. On electron microscopy the viruses of varicella, herpes zoster, and herpes simplex are identical. The fully mature particle in the vesicular fluid measures about 150 to 200nm in diameter. There is an electron-dense inner core of DNA enclosed by a shell or capsid. This capsid has an icosahedral structure with an axial symmetry of 5:3:2, and consists of 162 capsomeres, which appear as hollow cylinders with a polygonal cross-section. The outer membrane of the virus is derived from the nuclear membrane of the host cell. Herpesviruses are easily distinguished from poxvirus by electron microscopy.

206 *Herpesvirus varicellae/zoster* in human amnion cells. Chickenpox virus does not grow on the chorioallantois of chick embryos, but can be propagated in a variety of primary cultures of human tissues and in some cultures of monkey tissues. In human amnion culture focal lesions appear in the cell sheet and spread slowly outwards as contiguous cells become infected. Typical intranuclear inclusion bodies are found in the degenerate cells. The supernatant fluid remains free from virus. Chickenpox virus grows readily in human thyroid cells and may be harvested from the supernatant fluid for neutralisation tests. (Arrow = cell with intranuclear inclusion.)

207 Giant cell in human amnion cell culture. Multinucleated giant cells are a characteristic feature in human tissues or in cultures of cells infected with chickenpox virus. The nuclei of these cells contain typical eosinophilic type A inclusions. (Arrow = nucleus with inclusion.)

205

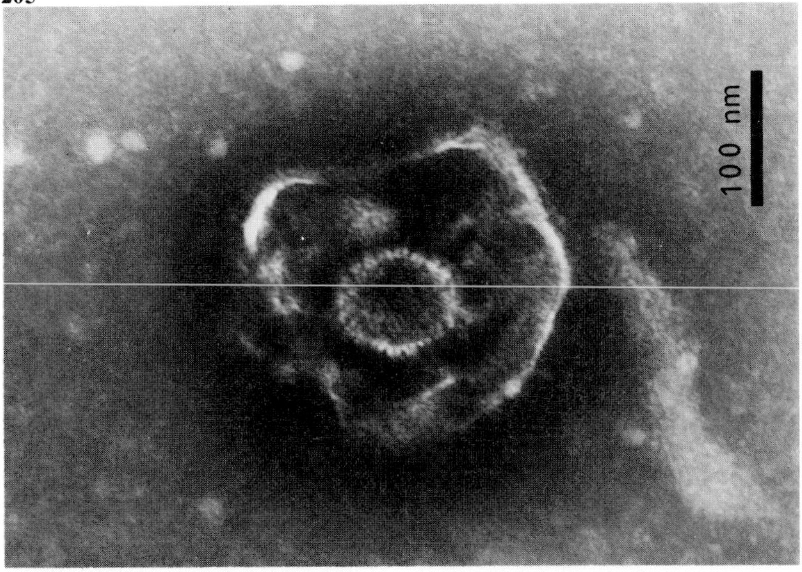

206

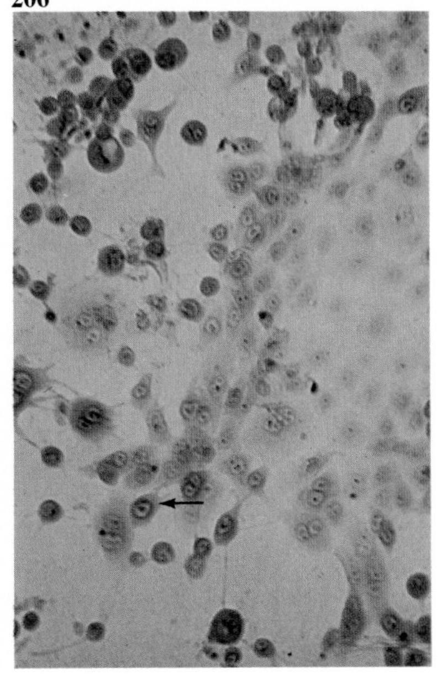

207

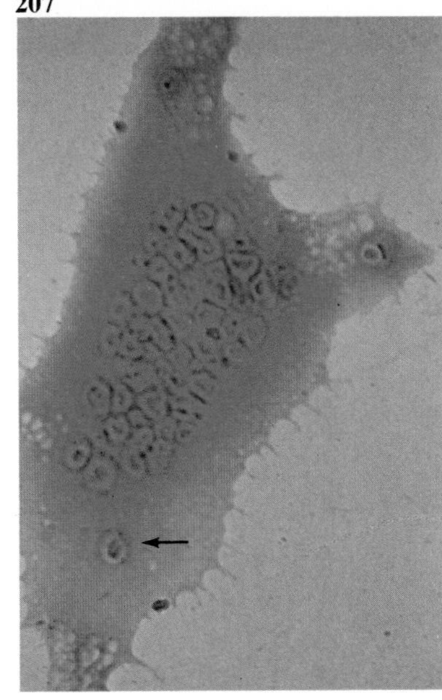

208 Histology of early chickenpox vesicle. The vesicles of varicella, zoster and herpes simplex cannot be distinguished from each other histologically, but may be differentiated from those of poxvirus infections and vaccinia by the presence of multinucleated giant cells.

Vesicles form within the epidermis as a result of cellular degeneration accompanied by intracellular oedema. At first the fluid collects in small pockets, but these eventually merge to form the mature vesicle.

Two types of degeneration are found — 'ballooning' and reticular. 'Ballooning' is peculiar to virus infections but reticular degeneration is also seen in some forms of dermatitis. In 'ballooning' degeneration the epidermal cells swell, lose their intercellular prickles, and become separated from each other. The cytoplasm is intensely eosinophilic. In reticular degeneration the cells swell but remain clear; some may eventually rupture. (A = intra-epidermal vesicle, B = multinucleated giant cell.)

209 Mature vesicle. The small foci seen in **208** have now coalesced to form a large vesicle. There is little cellular reaction in the dermis and the epithelial cells usually survive intact, so scarring seldom follows. An occasional polymorphonuclear cell may be present in the vesicular fluid. (A = intra-epidermal vesicle, B = dermis.)

Clinical features

210 Distribution of rash. A prodromal illness seldom occurs in children, but occasionally the exanthem in adults may be preceded by fever, headache, and sore throat.

Skin lesions are seen first on the body and inner aspects of the thighs but spread quickly to the face, scalp, and proximal parts of the limbs. The distribution of the rash used to be supremely important in differentiating varicella from variola. The rash in chickenpox is heaviest on the trunk and diminishes in intensity towards the periphery. It is prominent on flexor surfaces and extends into the hollows of the body.

208

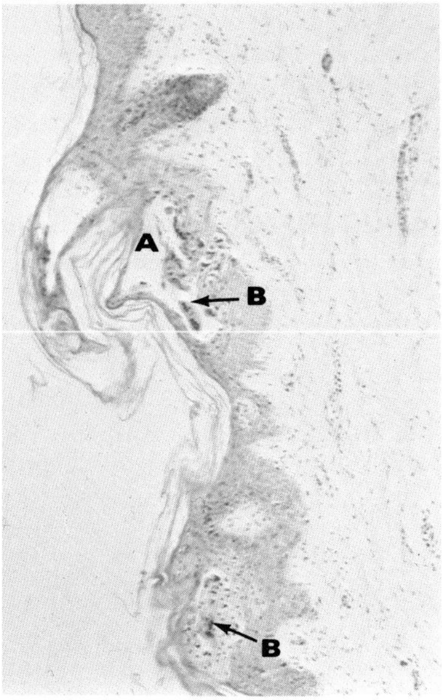

209

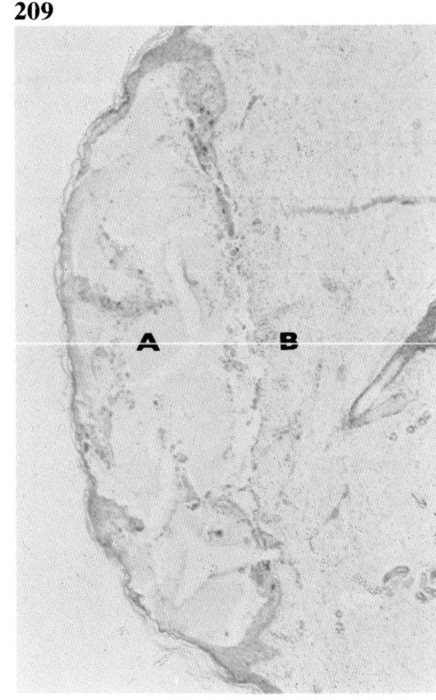

210

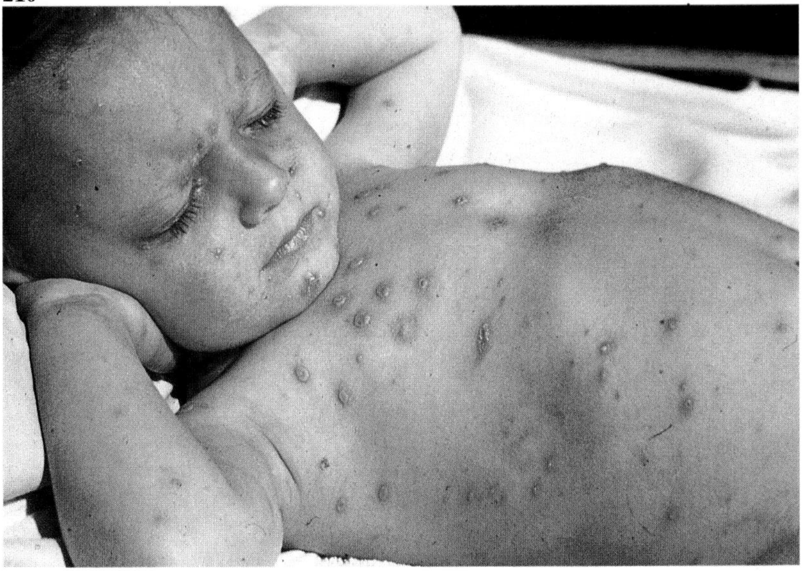

211 Chickenpox rash on dark skin. Detection of a chickenpox rash on heavily pigmented skin is easy: although the individual lesions may appear slightly different, the rash conforms to the rule of centripetal distribution. In this illustration the spots are dense on the arm but gradually diminish on the forearm to become scanty on the hand.

212 Pleomorphic rash. The rash evolves very rapidly through the stages of macule, papule, vesicle, pustule and crust. The first two stages are seldom seen, and the rash has usually reached the vesicular stage before it is discovered. Many lesions abort without undergoing full development.

In chickenpox the lesions emerge in crops at irregular intervals up to a week. As a result, the rash has a pleomorphic character with spots at different stages of development. Pruritus may be very troublesome during the first few days.

211

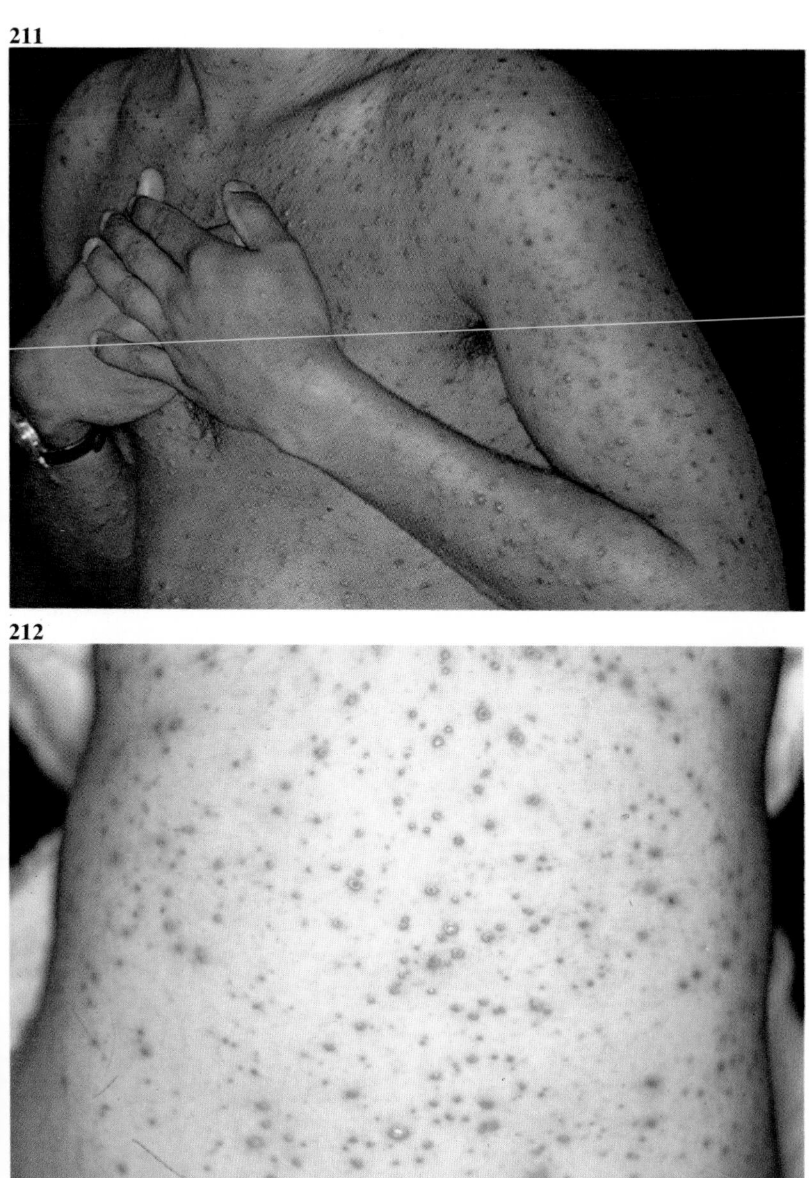

212

213 Close-up of rash on dark skin. In dark-skinned patients it is very common to find a petechial element in the rash and bleeding into the vesicles. The prognosis is not affected by these skin haemorrhages.

214 Close-up of lesions on white skin. Skin lesions vary greatly in size and shape. Fully developed vesicles and pustules are often oval but may be round or even totally irregular. The long axis of the oval lesion tends to follow the natural creases of the skin. Many lesions heal at an early stage. Skin haemorrhages are rare in white patients.

The chickenpox vesicle is unilocular and lies on the surface of the skin like a drop of water. When mature it is often surrounded by an erythematous ring or areola. After two or three days the vesicular fluid becomes cloudy, and a pustule forms with crenated edges.

215 Scarring. Most chickenpox lesions are very superficial, and damaged epidermis is quickly restored, leaving the skin unblemished. Occasionally the damage extends more deeply into the skin, and unsightly scarring results.

216 Close-up of scar. A pitted or foveated scar is the only clinical evidence that a patient has previously had chickenpox. Similar scars may be produced by vaccination against smallpox or by BCG immunisation.

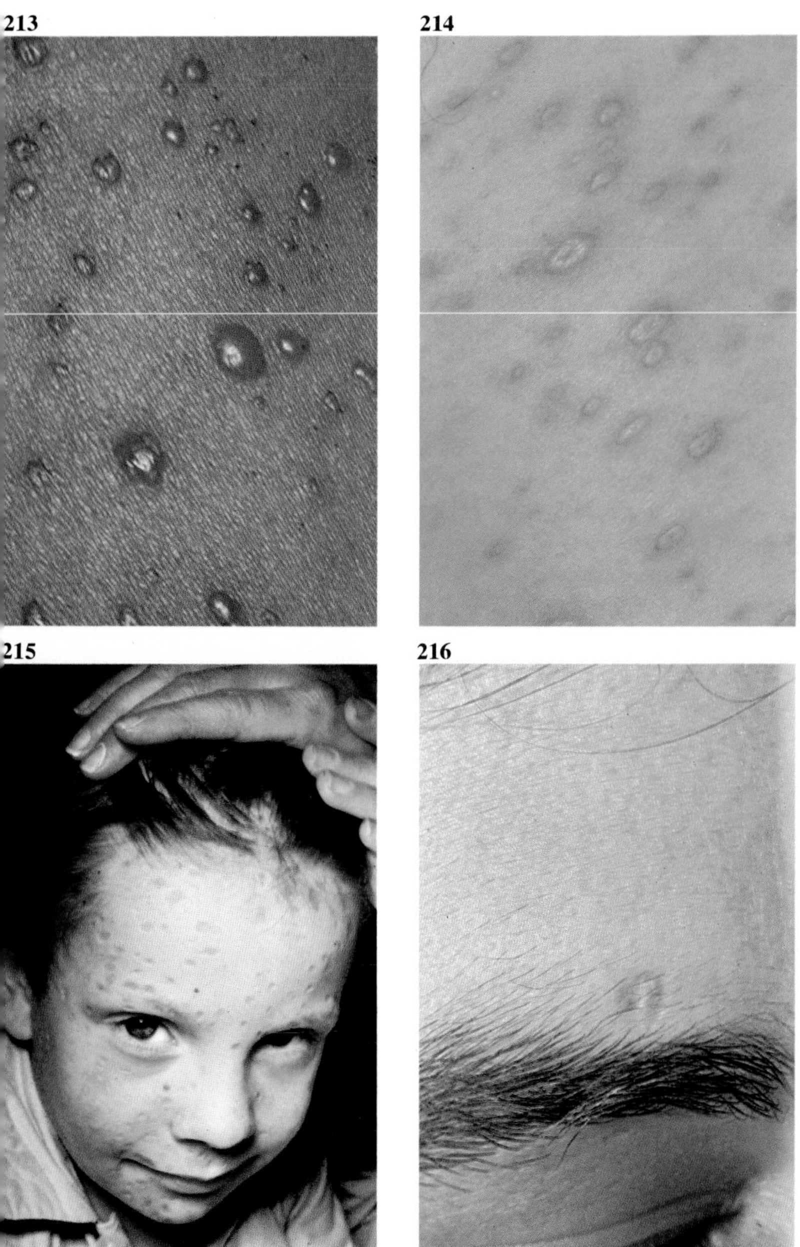
213
214
215
216

217 Petechiae on palate. Fine haemorrhages may be found on the palate in varicella as in many other infections. A vesicle is beginning to form on the palate above the left tonsil.

218 Vesicles on palate. During the first day or two the throat may be painful and inflamed, but no focal lesions are seen. Vesicles may later erupt on the palate and pharynx adding to the discomfort. The thin roof of the vesicle usually ruptures and leaves a shallow ulcer, which heals without scarring.

219 Vesicles on tongue. Vesicles may be found on the mucosa of the mouth and respiratory tract. On the tongue vesicles have a flat top and heal without forming a crust.

220 Vesicle on conjunctiva. Vesicles may be found on the conjunctivae where they pursue a benign course and heal without scarring.

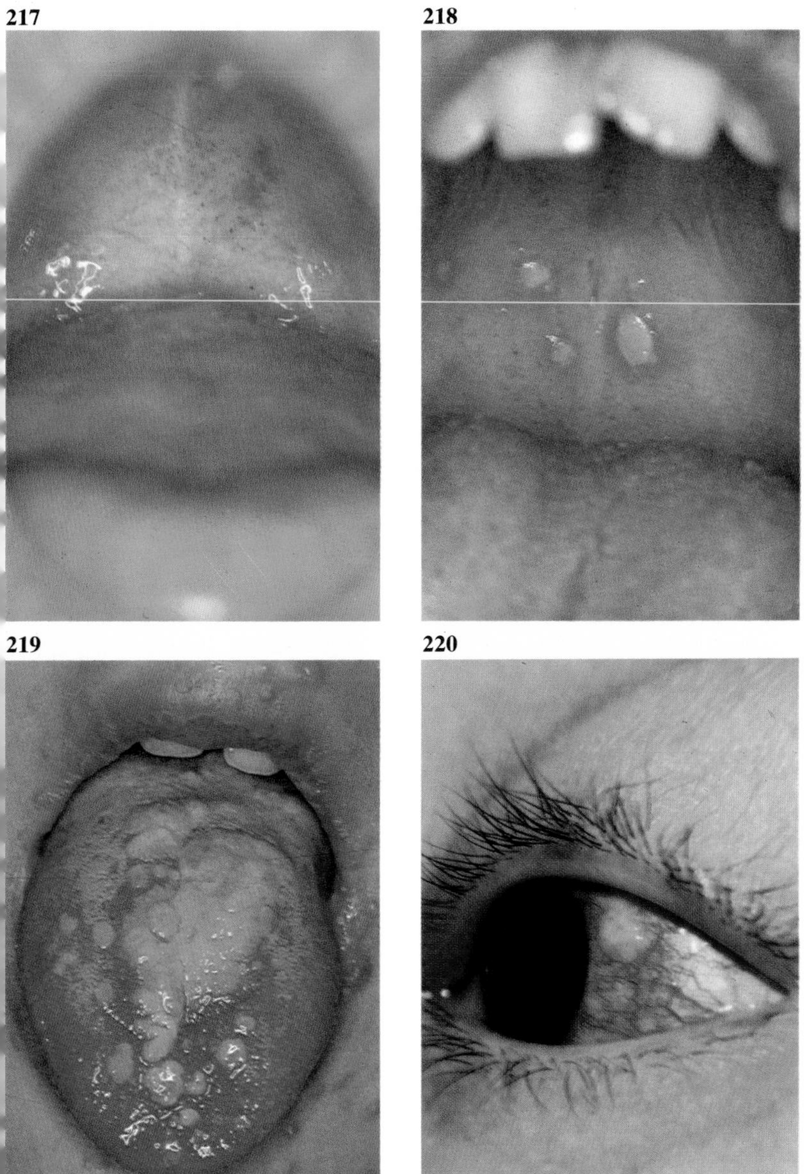
217
218
219
220

Complications

221 Varicella and bullous impetigo. Secondary infection of chickenpox lesions with *Staphylococcus aureus* may give rise to bullous impetigo with widespread infection of the surface of the skin.

222 Gangrene of skin. Invasion of the deeper layers of the skin and subcutaneous tissues by a virulent staphylococcus may result in cellulitis with gangrene and deep ulceration.

Septicaemia may develop with or without evidence of local sepsis, and blood cultures should be performed whenever a patient is unusually ill or the fever unduly prolonged.

223 Varicella and 'surgical' scarlet fever. Local infection of a chickenpox lesion by a haemolytic streptococcus in a patient susceptible to erythrogenic toxin may result in an attack of scarlet fever. The infected lesions can be identified by the surrounding inflammation. Toxin is absorbed from the skin and produces the generalised punctate erythema of scarlet fever.

224 Varicella and 'surgical' scarlet fever — tongue. Although the streptococcus is growing in the skin and not in the throat, the patient nevertheless develops a typical enanthem with a white strawberry tongue (see **27**).

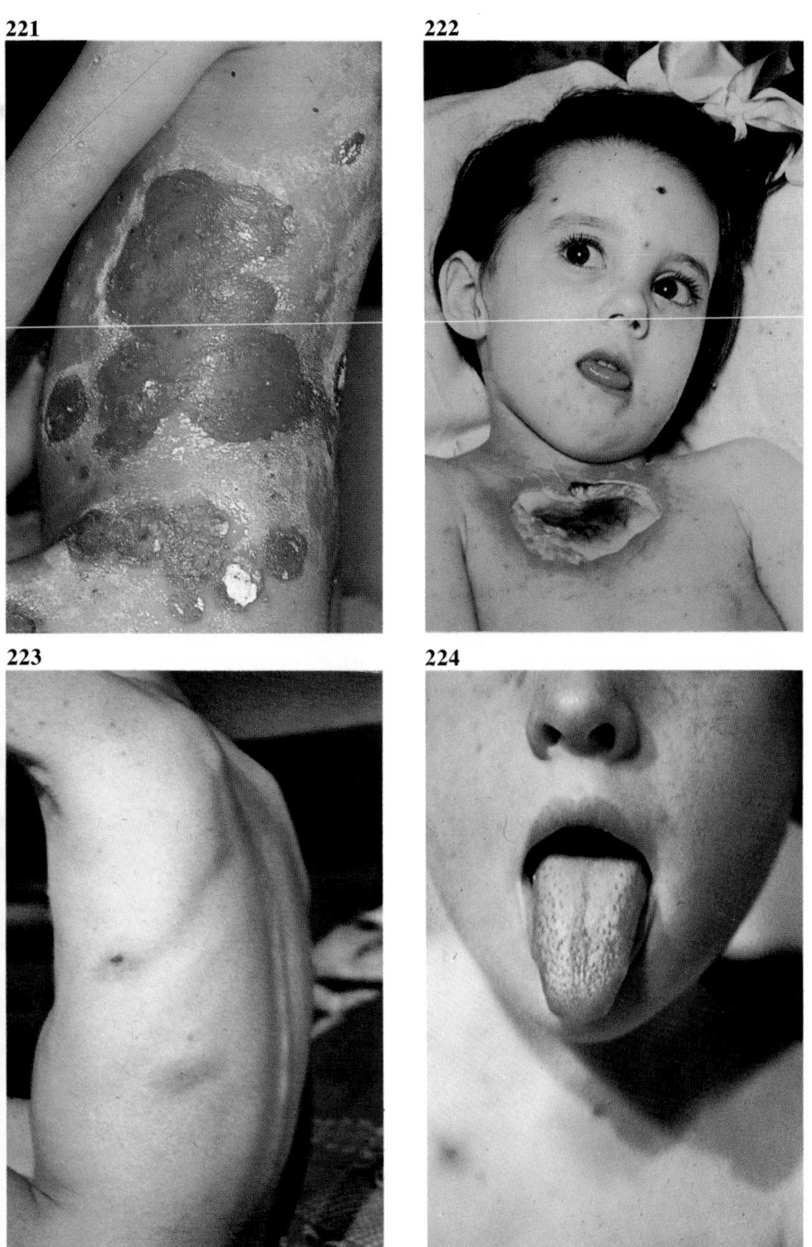

221 222 223 224

225 Chest x-ray of child with staphylococcal pyopneumothorax. Pneumonia complicating chickenpox in children is usually caused by secondary bacterial invasion from the upper respiratory passages, and is predominantly staphylococcal. Abscesses may form in the lungs.

This child's chest x-ray shows gross displacement of the mediastinum caused by pyopneumothorax, which resulted from rupture of a subpleural abscess. Each time the child coughed more air was forced into the pleural cavity through the pulmonary fistula, and continuous suction was necessary to reduce the pressure. Pus aspirated from the chest gave a heavy growth of *Staph. aureus*.

226 Chickenpox pneumonia. Chest x-ray — first week. Chickenpox viral pneumonia is found typically in adult patients and only very exceptionally in children. The condition varies greatly in severity: at one extreme it is so mild that it can be detected only by routine radiography; at the other it presents as a catastrophic illness with severe dyspnoea, cyanosis, haemoptysis and prostration, terminating fatally within 24 to 48 hours.

In a typical case the lungs are affected within two to five days from the onset of the rash. During the first week of the illness the characteristic findings are those of acute inflammatory pulmonary oedema. Dyspnoea and cyanosis are prominent. X-ray examination of the chest at this stage shows widespread soft nodular opacities throughout both lungs, but less noticeable at the apices.

225

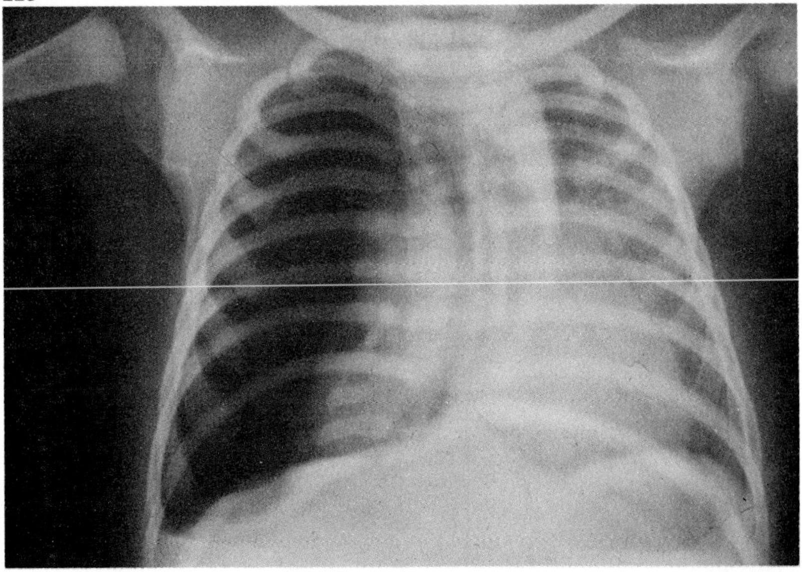

226

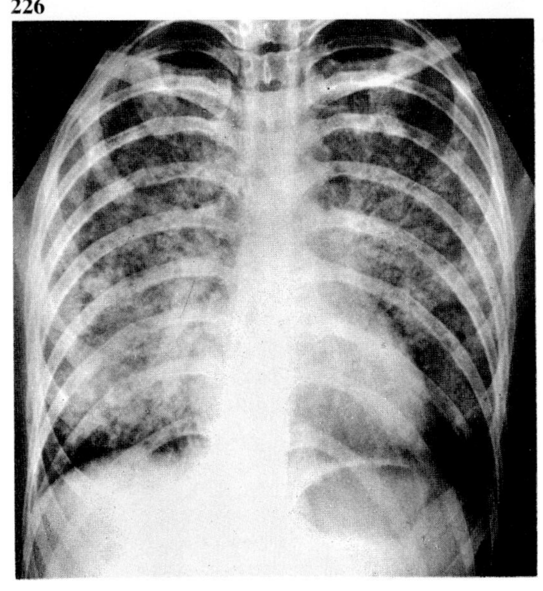

227

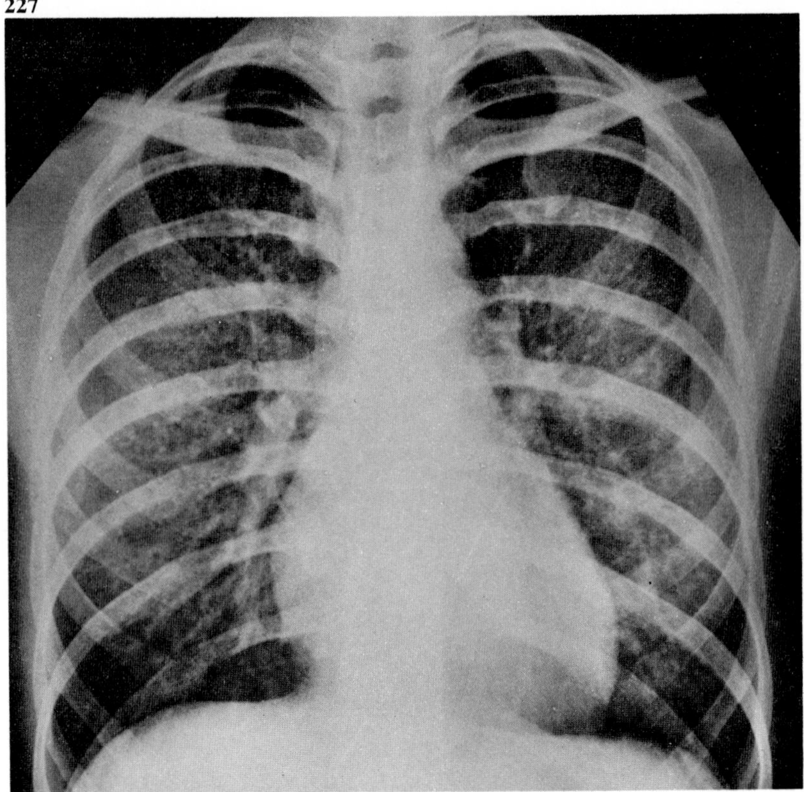

227 Chickenpox pneumonia. Chest x-ray — second week. Mortality is high in pregnant women and in patients with disturbed immunity, who commonly die from respiratory failure during the first week. During the second week the pulmonary oedema abates and the patient begins to improve. The cough lessens, and the abnormal chest signs disappear. Towards the end of the second week the chest radiograph shows changes, as the soft nodular shadowing resolves, leaving a prominent reticular pattern.

228

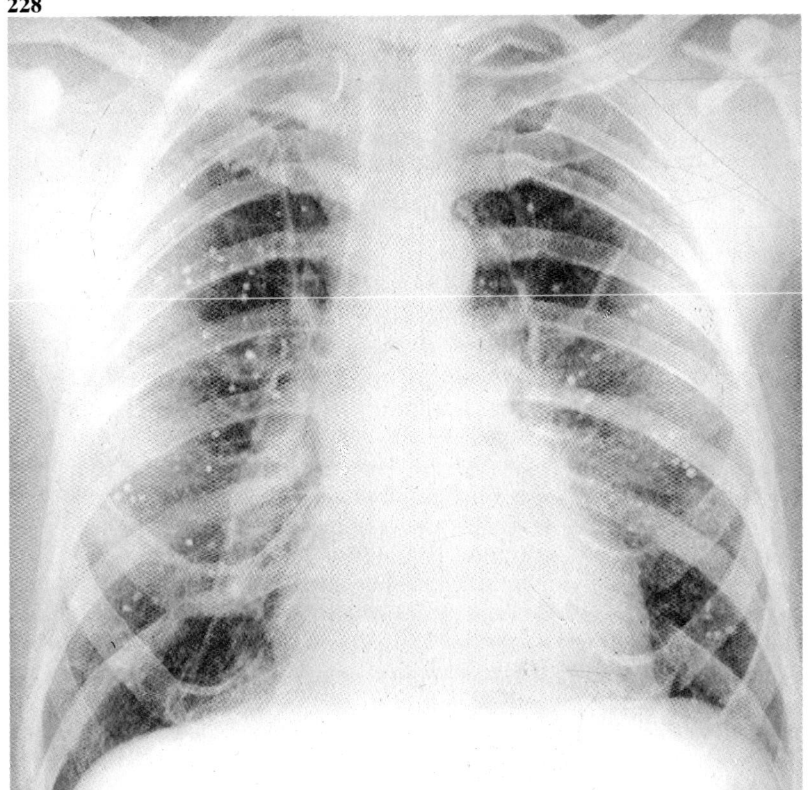

228 Chickenpox pneumonia. Chest x-ray — miliary calcification. After two weeks the patient emerges from the acute stage to face a prolonged period of convalescence. Breathlessness on slight exertion may persist for several weeks or even months, but eventually subsides, and full health is restored. In most patients the coarse reticular pattern gradually fades, though the chest radiograph may reveal abnormalities for many months. Patients found on routine examination to have miliary calcification of the lungs often give a history of severe chickenpox in adult life, and it is believed that calcium salts are deposited in the necrotic foci that are a typical feature of chickenpox pneumonia. Similar appearances may be found as a result of histoplasmosis or miliary tuberculosis.

229 Chickenpox pneumonia — histology of lung. In fatal cases of chickenpox pneumonia the lungs are grossly oedematous, and there are extensive haemorrhages. Histological examination shows widely disseminated interstitial pneumonia with patchy haemorrhagic consolidation.

The illustration shows a 3mm focus of fibrinoid necrosis surrounded by a zone of septal oedema and haemorrhage.

230 Chickenpox pneumonia — alveolar exudate. The alveoli are filled with a protein-rich fluid containing red cells and mononuclear cells. To the left of centre may be seen a degenerate mononuclear cell with a typical intranuclear inclusion. The nuclear membrane is clearly visible, but the cytoplasm is faintly stained. (Arrow = nuclear membrane with inclusion body.)

231 Haemorrhagic chickenpox. Widespread and sometimes fatal bleeding into the skin and mucous membranes may be precipitated by a number of infections, including chickenpox. The extent of the haemorrhages is not necessarily related to the severity of the original illness. In haemorrhagic chickenpox the platelet count is very low, the prothrombin time prolonged, and there may be other evidence of excessive consumption of clotting factors. Intravascular coagulation and endothelial damage by the virus may both contribute to the patient's death. Extensive haemorrhages into the skin or mucous membranes may be accompanied by alarming epistaxis, haematemesis, or haematuria.

232 Concurrent varicella and measles. The importance of the interference phenomenon varies with different virus infections. Sometimes infection with one virus may completely prevent invasion by another. This applies particularly to closely related viruses, such as members of the enterovirus group, but seldom occurs when viruses have notably different characteristics.

In the illustration a chickenpox rash is emerging on the upper limb of a child with a florid measles rash.

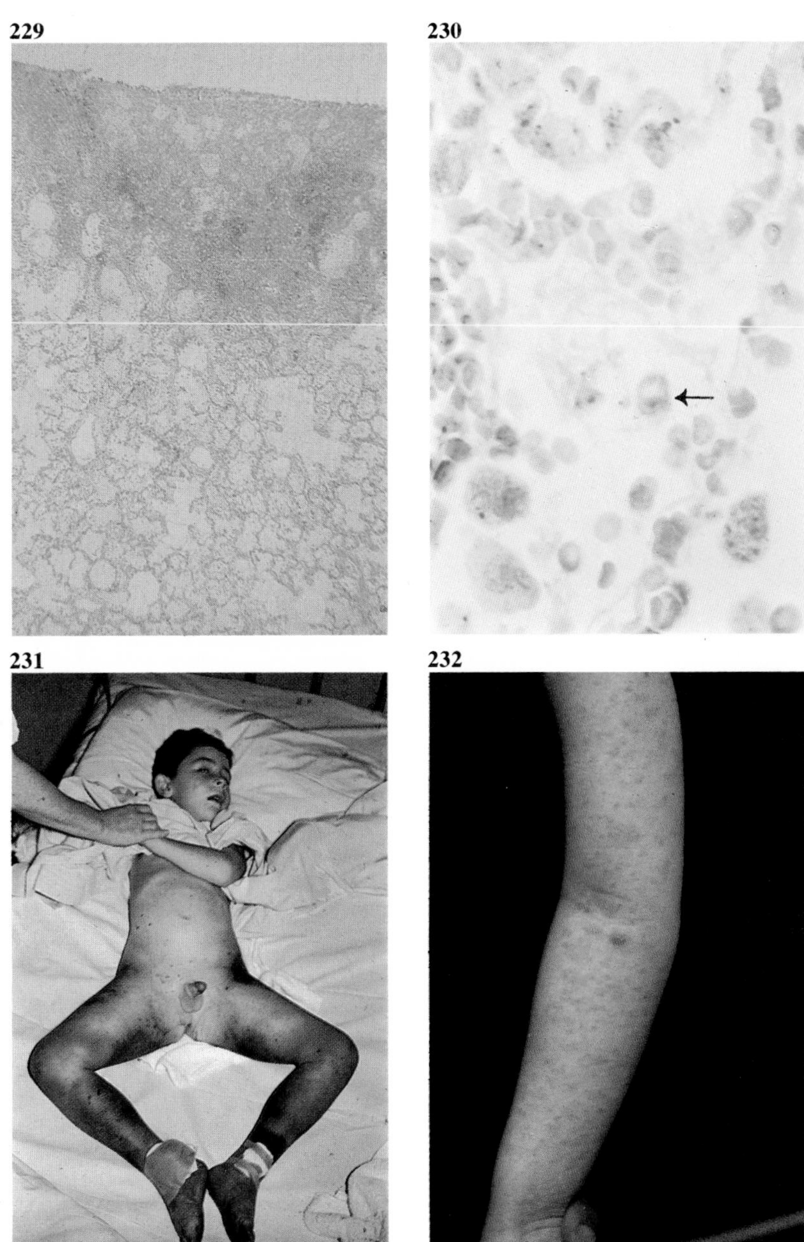
229
230
231
232

Varicella in disturbed immunity

233 Varicella and disturbed immunity. Patients with underlying disease affecting immunity are especially vulnerable to chickenpox, which may follow an exceptionally severe or prolonged course and may terminate in death.

The illustration shows a patient with Hodgkin's disease who contracted chickenpox from her child. Although the rash was not particularly dense, the individual lesions were unusually large and the general disturbance severe. Jaundice developed and 'cropping' continued until the patient died three or four weeks after the onset of her illness.

234 Close-up of lesions in chickenpox associated with defective immunity. The large size of the lesions is striking. The pustular fluid was sterile on culture for bacteria.

Patients who have never had chickenpox and who have defective immunity as a result of disease of the reticuloendothelial system or immunosuppressive treatment, are in grave danger from chickenpox and should not be exposed to this disease or to herpes zoster.

233

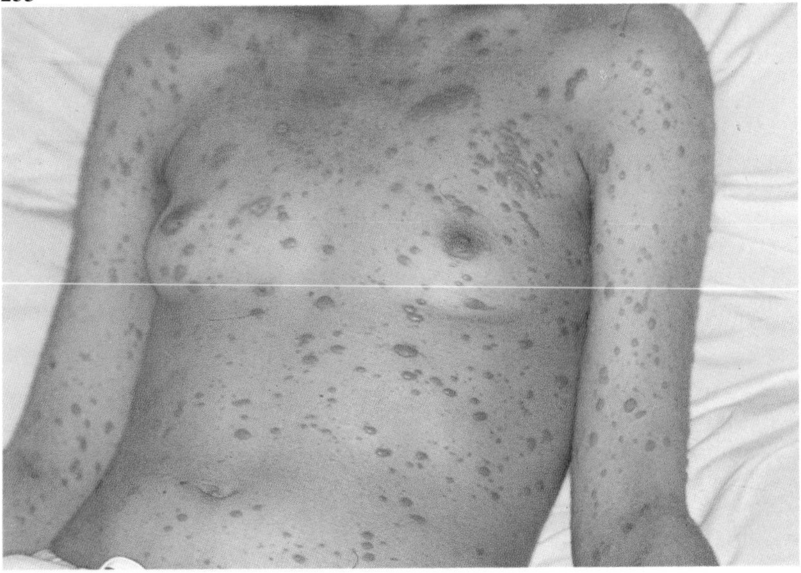

234

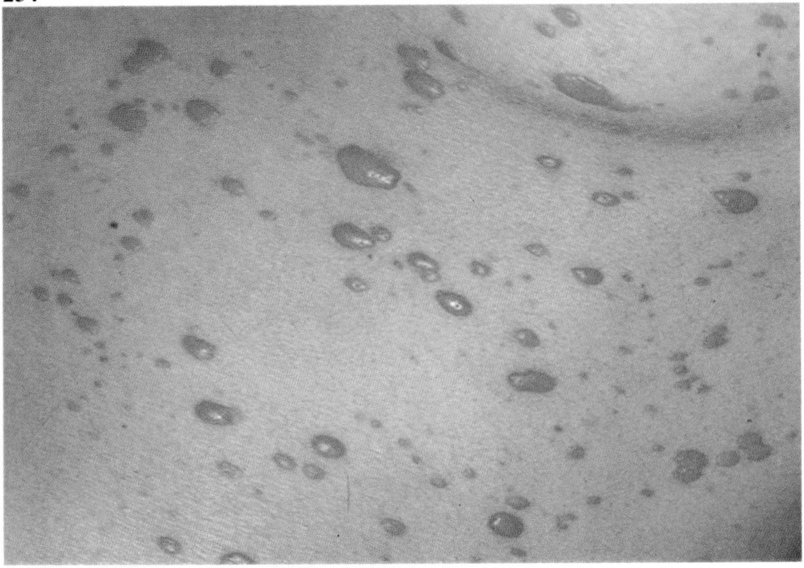

Herpes zoster (shingles)

Pathology

235 Histology of dorsal root ganglion. Herpes zoster is believed to be caused by reactivation of varicella virus lying dormant in cells of a dorsal root ganglion. In the early stages there is an acute inflammatory reaction in the ganglion, or its equivalent in the cranial nerves, which extends into the dorsal root and involves the meninges and spinal cord. Mononuclear cells are conspicuous, but there is a notable absence of polymorphonuclear cells. (A = undegenerate neurones, B = degenerate neurones, C = mononuclear cells.)

236 Histology of peripheral nerve. Virus spreads from the dorsal root ganglion cells along the sensory nerve fibres to the skin, where it enters the epithelial cells. At this stage virus particles may be found in the nuclei and cytoplasm of ganglion cells, in the cytoplasm of perineural cells, in the nuclei and cytoplasm of Schwann cells, and in the nuclei and cytoplasm of cells in the epidermis.

The illustration shows a section of frontal nerve from a patient with trigeminal herpes, who died four days after the onset of the rash. Staining by fluorescent antibody demonstrates viral antigen in two nerve fibre bundles with heavy concentration in the perineurium.

237 Histology of vesicle. The vesicles of herpes zoster and varicella are identical. The vesicle forms in the epidermis as a result of degeneration of the cells, which become swollen and separated, and some rupture. Intercellular oedema is marked and giant cells are a prominent feature. Severe inflammatory reaction in the corium may be followed by scarring.

In this section inflammatory reaction is slight, but many bizarre cells are present. (A = intra-epidermal vesicle, B = multinucleated giant cell, C = dermis.)

235

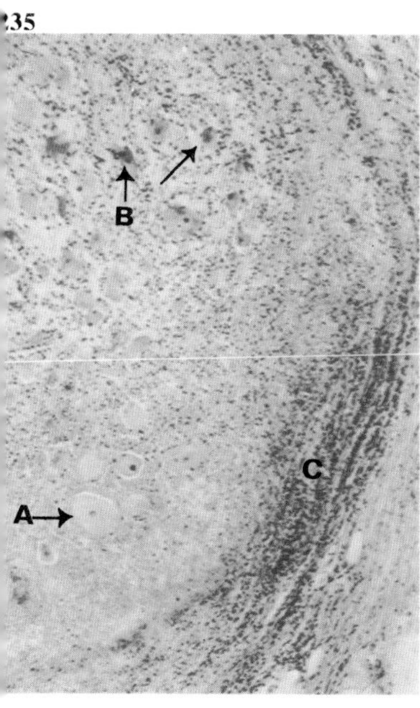

236

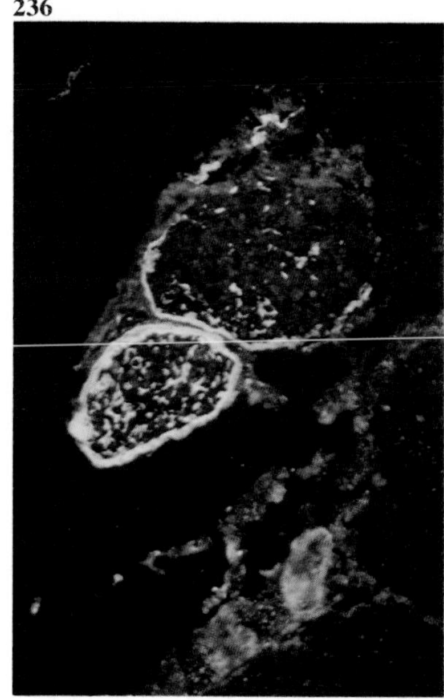

237

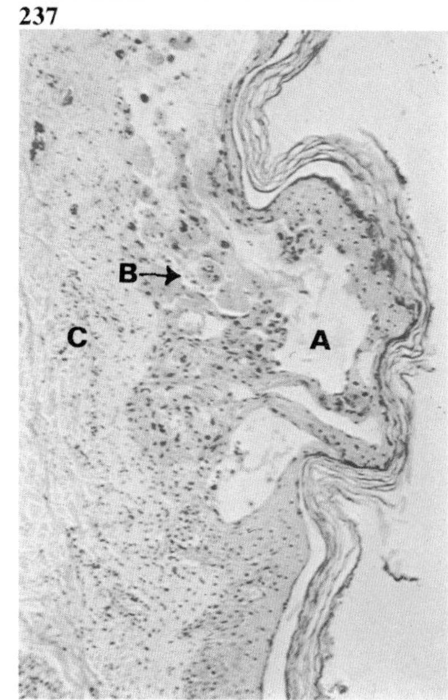

238 Effect of nerve damage on distribution of rash. A patient with hypoaesthesia, a result of section of a cutaneous nerve during a herniotomy 15 months previously, developed an attack of herpes zoster involving the same dermatome. Virus spread readily into the skin where sensation was normal, but round the scar, where the nerve supply had been interrupted, the skin was spared. This would be expected if the virus in herpes zoster gains access to the epidermis along nerve pathways.

Clinical features

239 Evolution of rash — erythema. An attack of herpes zoster begins with pain and hyperaesthesia in the distribution of one or two adjacent sensory nerve roots. Within a few days a rash appears in the same area. At first the skin has a deep red flush, but clusters of vesicles soon emerge. The rash is strictly confined to the midline, but oedema may spread extensively wherever subcutaneous tissues are lax.

238

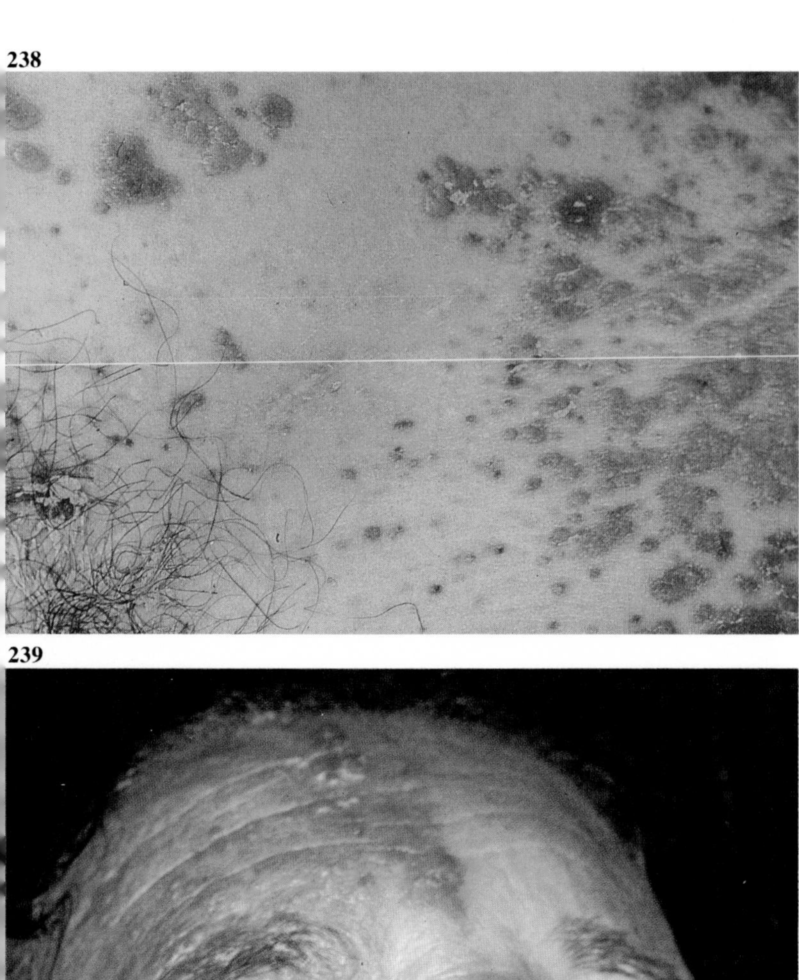

239

240 Evolution of rash — vesicles. The severity of the illness and extent of the rash are extremely variable. Fresh crops of vesicles continue to emerge for several days and may coalesce to form bullae, some of which may be haemorrhagic.

241 Evolution of rash — pustules. After a week or so the vesicles begin to dry up and form scabs but some may go through an intermediate pustular stage. These are usually sterile on bacterial culture.

242 Evolution of rash — crusts. If the rash is heavy, and especially if there is damage to the underlying corium, a thick plate of scabs may form which takes several weeks to separate. Any attempt at forcible removal merely results in the formation of fresh scabs and further harm to the skin. With a rash of average severity the scabs have usually been shed within two or three weeks.

240

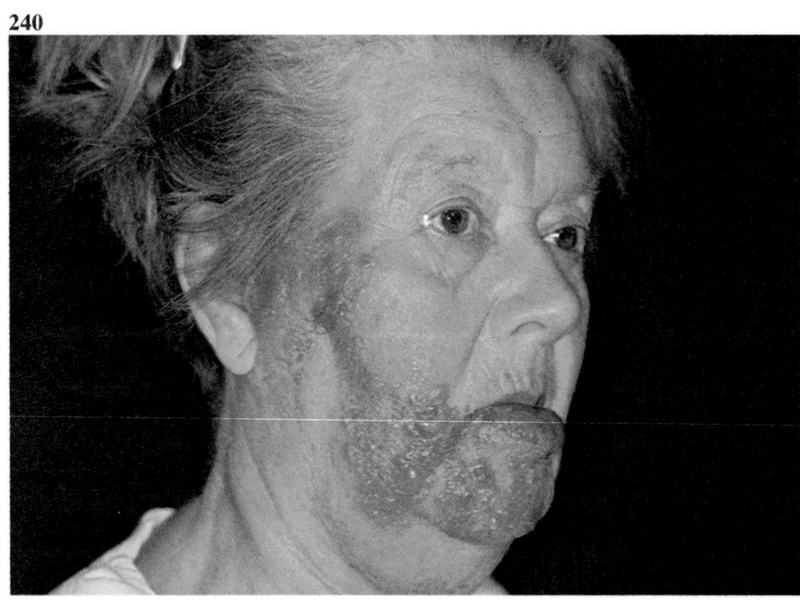

241

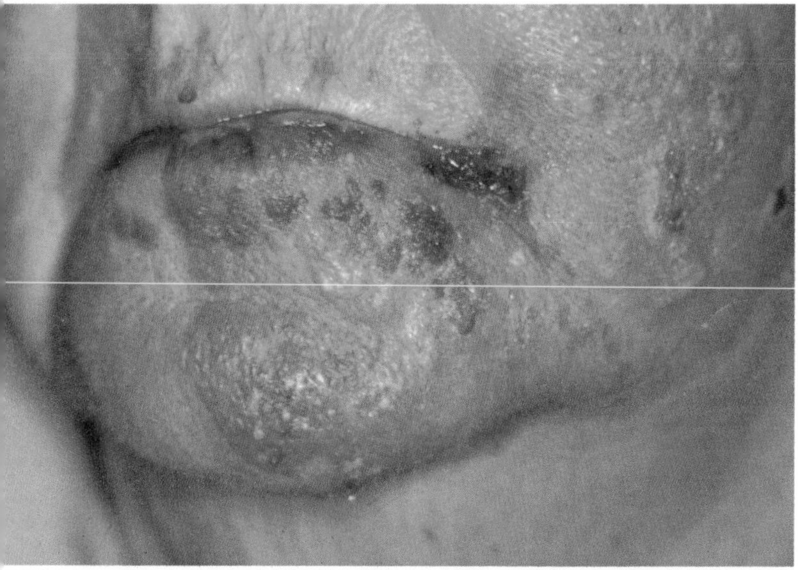

242

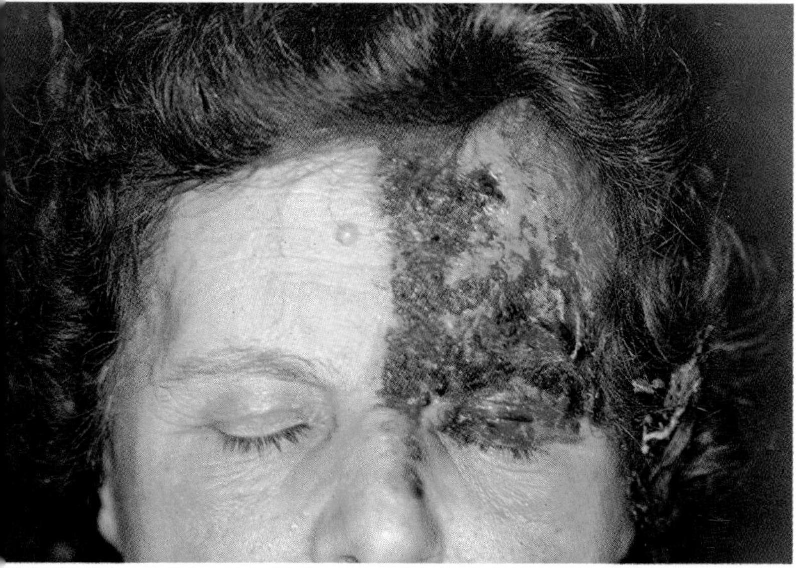

243 Evolution of rash — ulcers. In most attacks skin will heal without scars. Should the crusts separate and produce deep ulceration then scarring is inevitable. Heavy pigmentation may persist in the damaged area for many months.

244 Close-up of vesicles. The vesicles develop in clusters on an erythematous base.

245 Close-up of pustules. At a later stage the fluid in the blisters becomes turbid, and pustules are formed. This is not due to secondary bacterial invasion but to the activity of the virus itself. Adjacent lesions tend to run into each other, and already a central crust is appearing. Haemorrhage is common in severe attacks and produces bluish discoloration.

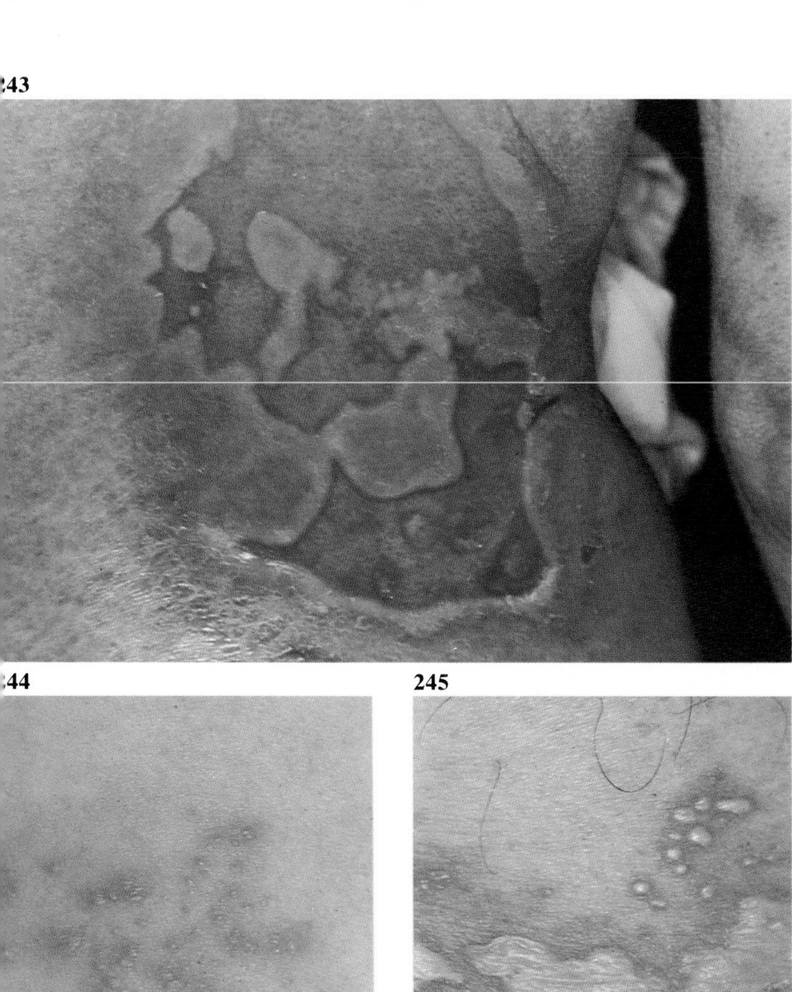

243

244

245

246 Distribution — cervical. The rash has sharply defined borders confined to the areas of skin supplied by cervical roots 4 and 5. This peculiar segmental distribution is a very helpful feature making it possible to distinguish herpes zoster from other similar rashes, particularly erysipelas (see **30**). Herpes simplex may simulate zoster, but pain is less troublesome, and the rash seldom conforms to a complete segmental distribution (see **284**).

247 Distribution — thoracic. Thoracic segments are affected in over 50% of patients with zoster. The rash is distributed in a band around the trunk. The term zoster is derived from the Greek meaning belt, and shingles from the Low Latin equivalent.

246

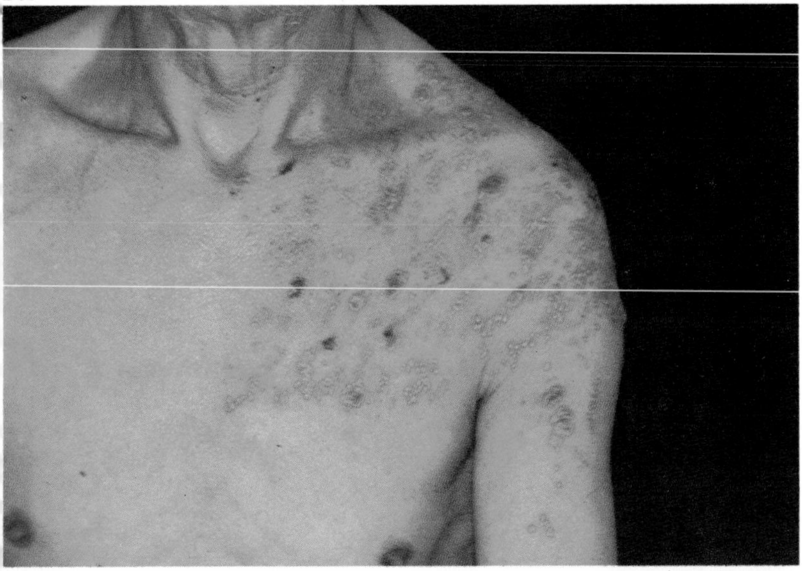

247

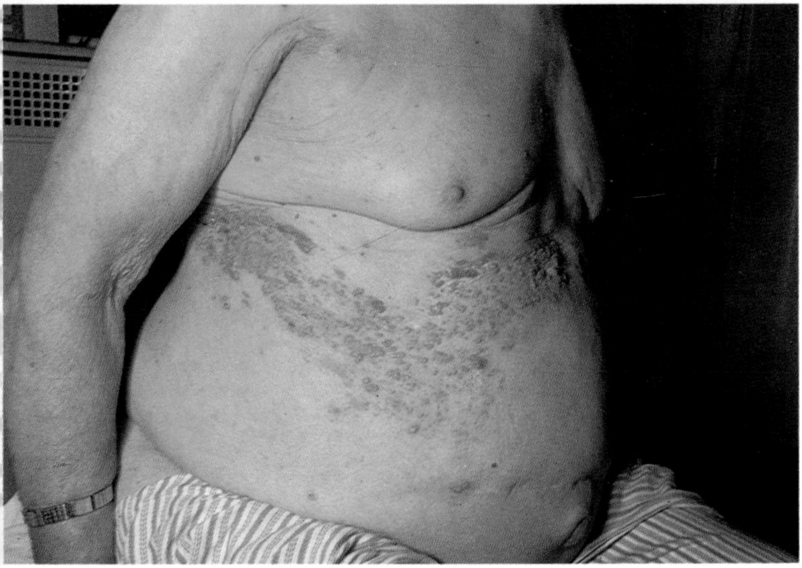

248 Distribution — thoracic. The rash seldom covers the entire area of skin in a dermatome. Lesions are grouped in clusters and generally form an unmistakeable pattern. The diagnosis may be difficult when the eruption consists of a single cluster, but a history of pain preceding the spots provides a helpful clue. In doubtful cases diagnosis can be established by demonstrating a rising antibody concentration in paired sera.

249 Herpes zoster with generalised rash. If patients with zoster are examined carefully, at least half will be found to have a sparse chickenpox rash. This emerges after the zoster, and the spots often abort at an early stage of development.

Moderate or heavy generalised varicella eruptions occur in 2 to 4% of cases, and are common when there is an underlying disturbance of immunity.

The standard sequence of events is reactivation of virus in the dorsal root ganglion with spread of virus along the sensory nerves to the skin segment, followed by dissemination into the blood stream resulting in a generalised rash.

250 Herpes zoster in a child. Herpes zoster is predominantly a disease of the middle-aged and elderly. Less than 5% of attacks occur in children below the age of 10 years. When zoster develops in very young children there is frequently a history of an attack of chickenpox in the mother during pregnancy. Post-herpetic neuralgia is seldom a problem in children.

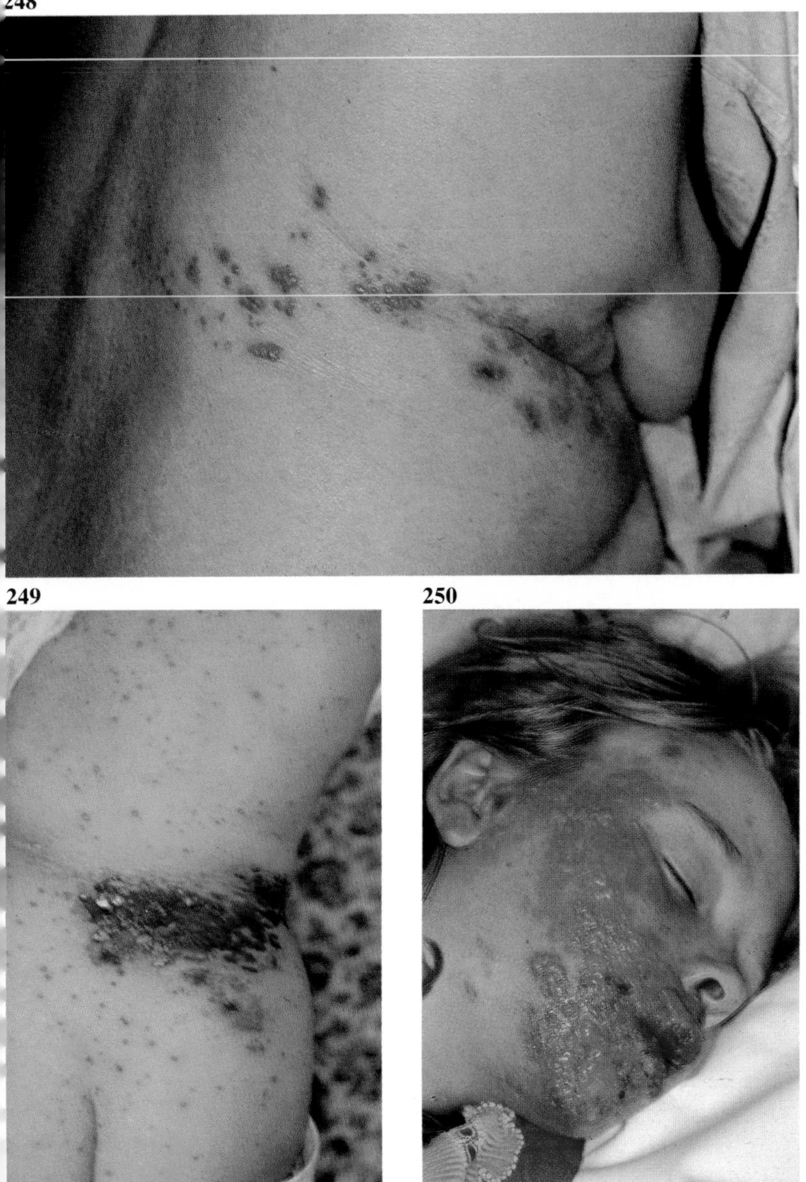
248
249
250

251 Herpes zoster of the palate. When an appropriate ganglion is affected lesions may be found on mucous membranes. Herpes zoster of the second division of the fifth cranial nerve affects the palate as well as the skin over the maxilla.

Complications

252 Conjunctivitis. Conjunctivitis may persist for several weeks after an attack of ophthalmic herpes, especially in the elderly, and may be associated with keratitis or iridocyclitis.

253 Corneal ulceration. During convalescence, after an attack of ophthalmic herpes, minor trauma to the anaesthetic cornea may abrade the surface and result in troublesome ulceration. Continual dabbing at the painful watering eye by an elderly confused patient may produce a penetrating ulcer that could perforate the anterior chamber. In these circumstances tarsorrhaphy may be required to protect the eye until the ulcer heals.

254 Chemosis. Unilateral ophthalmic herpes may be accompanied by oedema of the eyelids on both sides of the face and by striking oedema of the conjunctiva on the affected side (chemosis). When the eyelids are opened, the oedematous conjunctiva protrudes as a yellow gelatinous bag. The condition is not serious and resolves quickly.

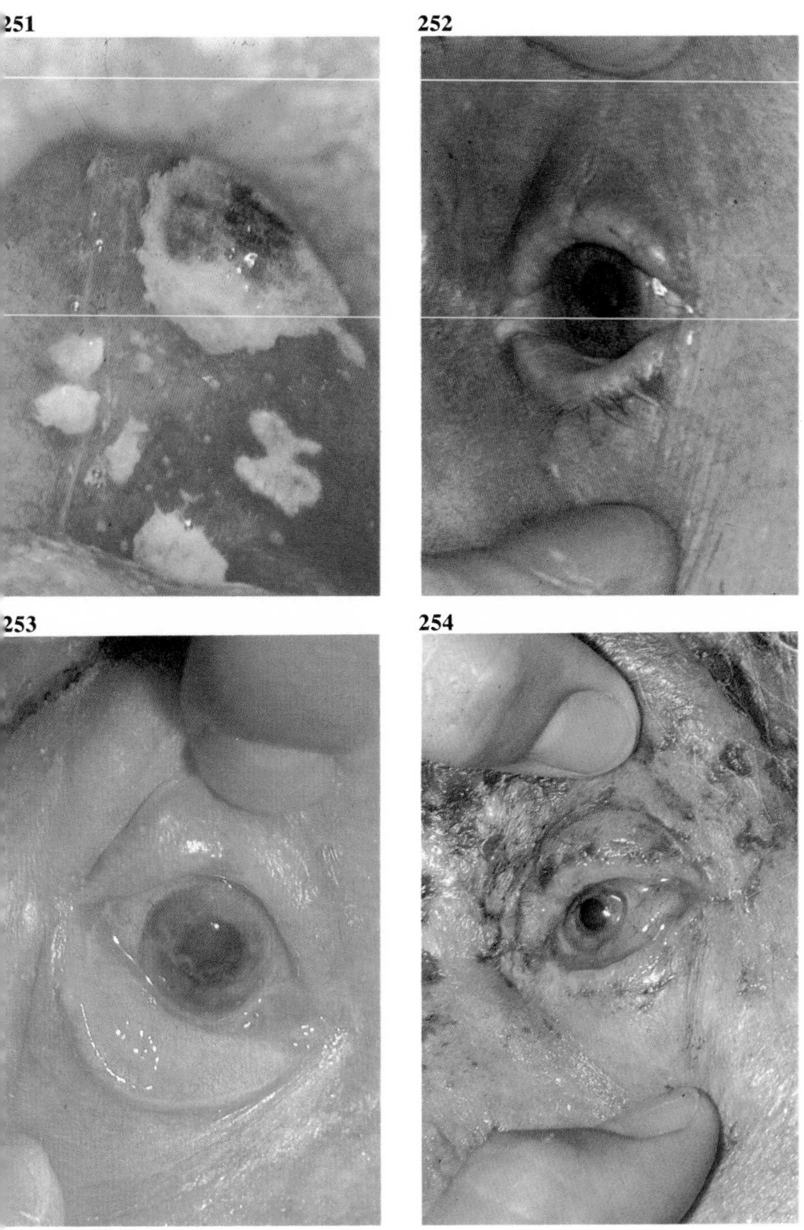
251
252
253
254

255 Iridocyclitis. The first division of the trigeminal nerve supplies the skin of the forehead and also the iris and ciliary body. A heavy rash on the side of the nose indicates that the nasociliary branch is severely affected, and iridocyclitis a strong probability.

The patient usually has difficulty in opening the oedematous eyelids so may not complain of defective vision. On examination the cornea is hazy and the pupil small. The reaction of the pupil is impaired, and the colour of the iris altered. When the pupil is dilated by a mydriatic the outline may be irregular as a result of adhesions between the iris and cornea.

256 Streptococcal impetigo. If herpetic lesions are kept dry, secondary bacterial infection is seldom a problem. Superimposed streptococcal infection may cause impetigo or erysipelas.

257 Secondary staphylococcal infection. A combination of zoster with a virulent staphylococcal infection may result in extensive damage to the corium and ugly scarring.

255

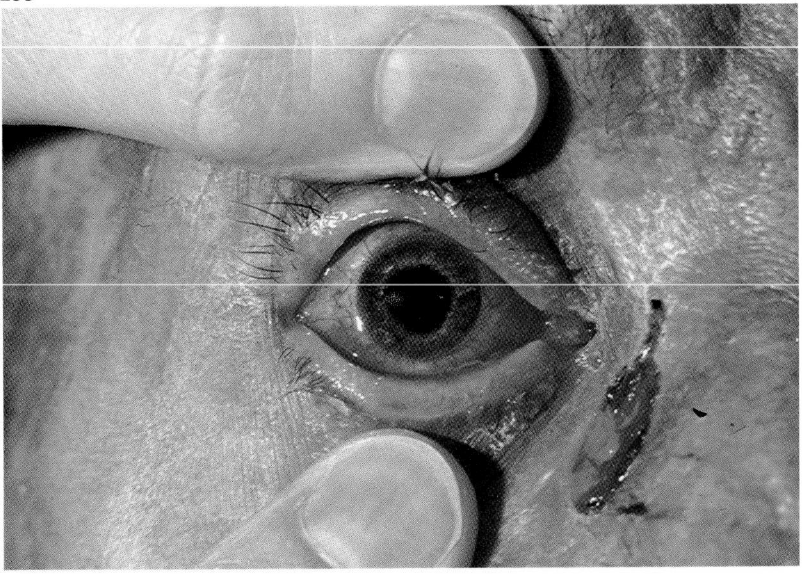

256

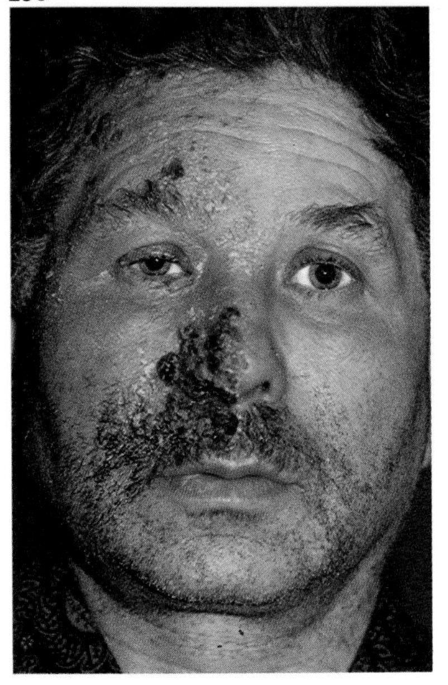

257

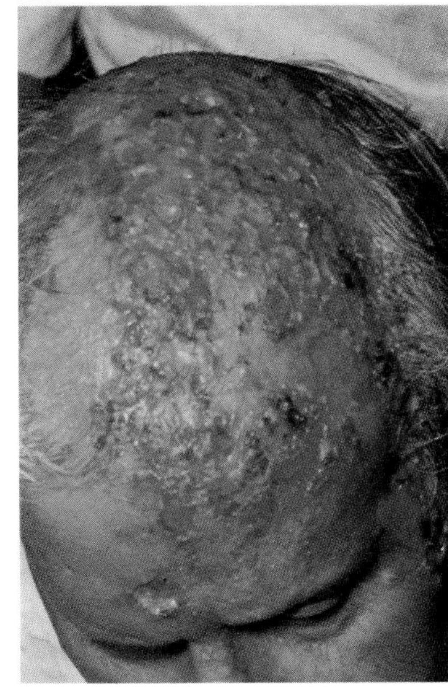

258 Herpes zoster with ophthalmoplegia. Spread of virus to lower motor neurone cells is not uncommon, and minor degrees of weakness are easily overlooked.

This patient had an attack of zoster involving the ophthalmic division of the fifth nerve complicated by ophthalmoplegia. He has ptosis and is unable to move his right eye. The conjunctiva is severely congested.

259 Facial paralysis complicating herpes zoster. Facial paralysis may follow herpes zoster of the trigeminal nerve, the geniculate ganglion of the seventh, or the second and third cervical roots. The exact pathways traversed by the virus are unknown.

This patient had zoster of the fifth cranial nerve, which resulted in facial weakness of lower motor neurone type and severe post-herpetic neuralgia.

258

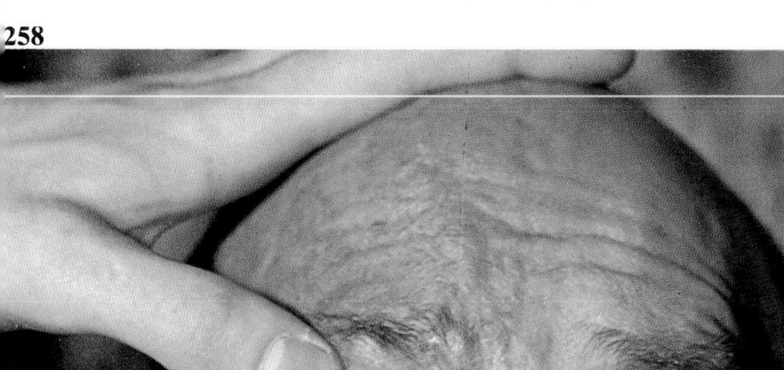

259

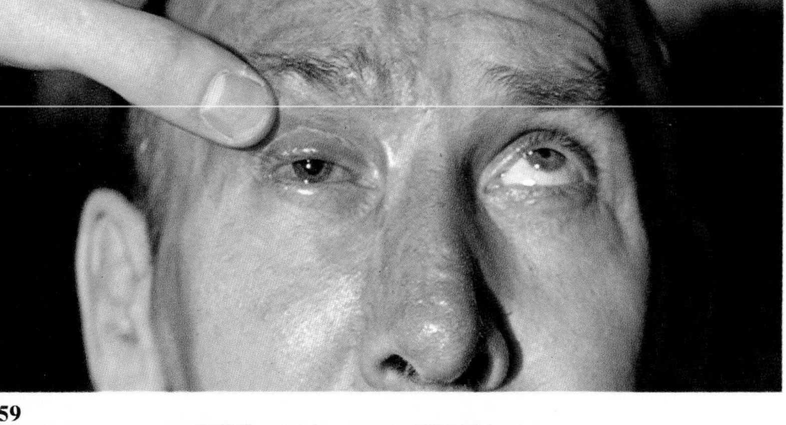

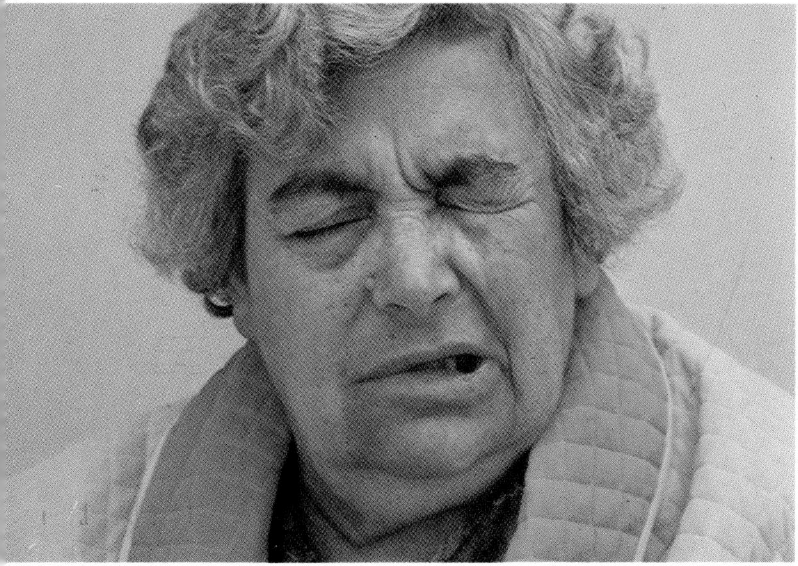

260 Geniculate herpes. Zoster of the geniculate ganglion of the seventh cranial nerve produces a crop of vesicles on the pinna and gives rise to facial paralysis accompanied by loss of taste over the anterior two-thirds of the tongue. Deafness may occur. The prognosis depends on the initial severity of the weakness.

261 Herpes zoster of C2 and C3 with facial paralysis. The patient has widespread zoster of the right side of her neck complicated by facial paralysis and deafness. She is unable to close her right eye, and her mouth is drawn over to the left. A year later the paralysis showed no improvement.

262 Herpes zoster of C4 and C5 with paralysis. During an attack of zoster affecting the fourth and fifth cervical roots, this elderly patient complained of 'rheumatism' in her right shoulder. Examination revealed that the stiffness was caused by weakness of the shoulder muscles. In attempting to abduct her arm the patient compensated for the deltoid paralysis by raising her shoulder and rotating her scapula.

260

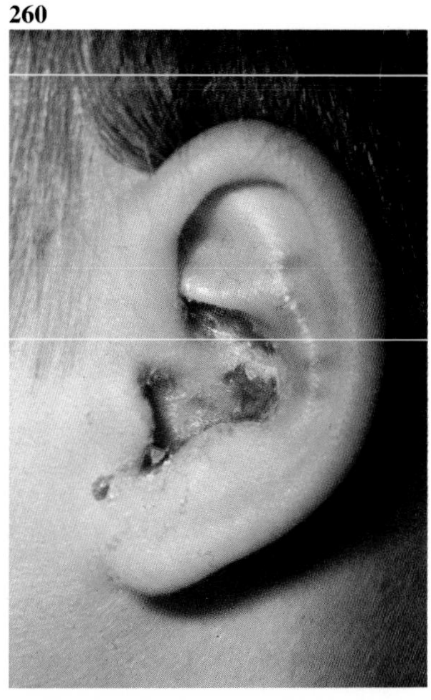

261

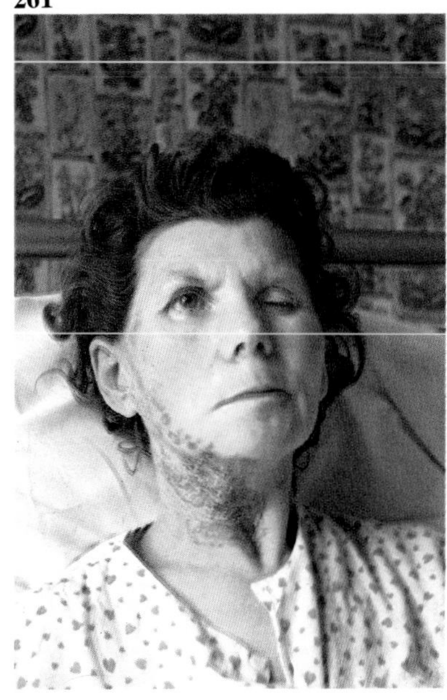

262

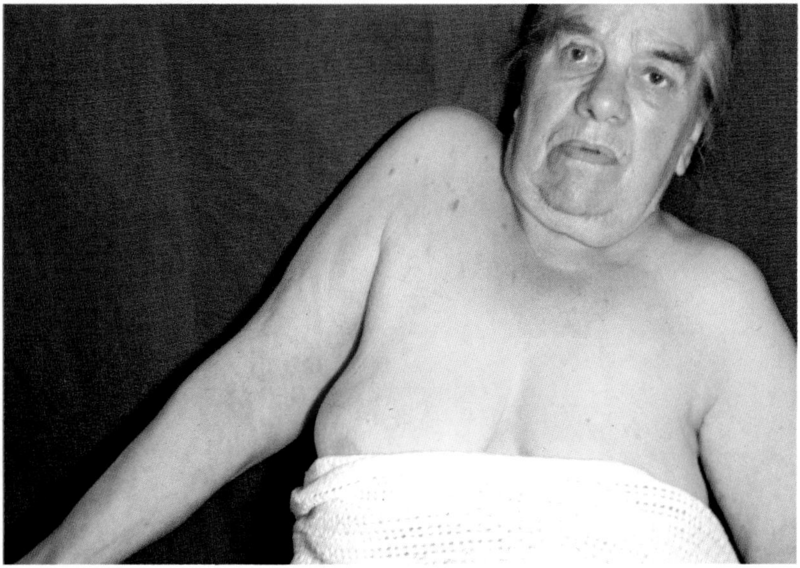

263 and 264 Horner's syndrome. The autonomic nervous system may also be affected by herpes zoster. This patient, with zoster of T2, developed Horner's syndrome on the affected side. Enophthalmos and a small pupil persisted for a few weeks then cleared.

263

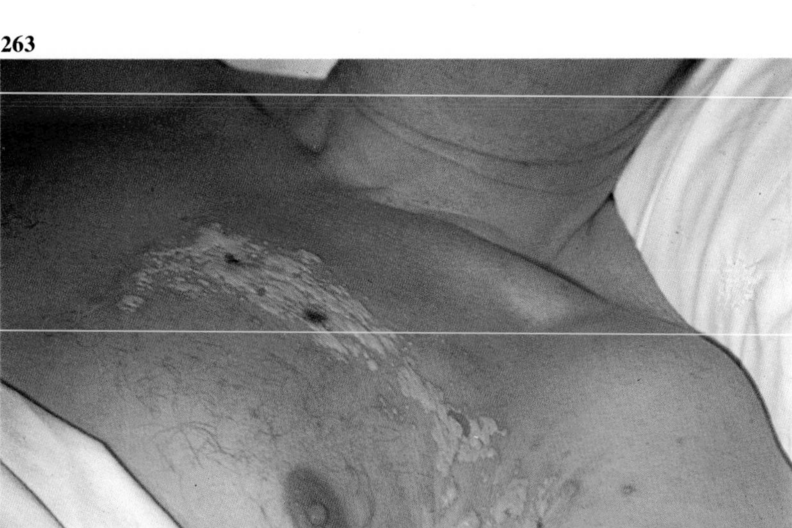

264

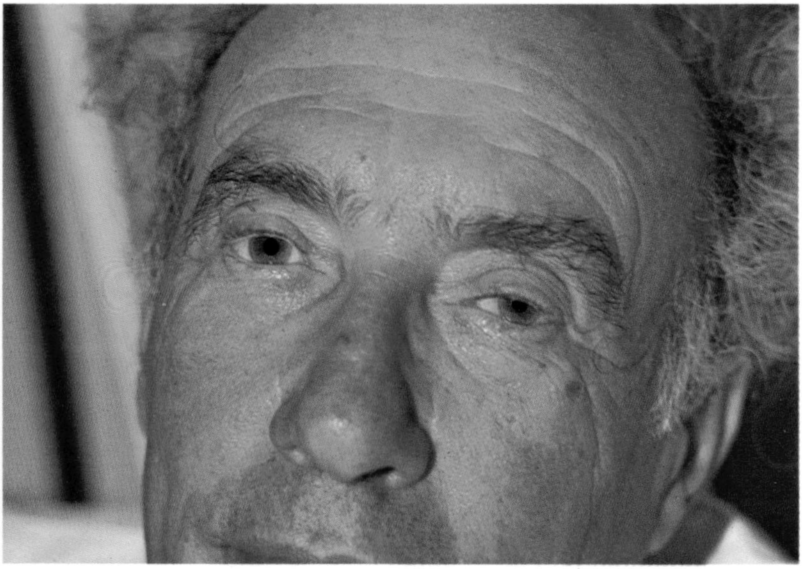

Associated diseases

265 Herpes zoster and leukaemia. An attack of herpes zoster may be precipitated by any condition that depresses immunity and allows the latent virus to emerge. All patients with zoster should be examined carefully for enlarged lymph nodes, splenomegaly, or hepatomegaly. The presence of undiagnosed lymphatic leukaemia may be signposted by an attack of shingles.

266 Herpes zoster and Hodgkin's disease. About 8% of patients admitted to hospital with zoster are found to have an underlying disease such as leukaemia, Hodgkin's disease, or carcinomatosis. Attacks may also be precipitated by immunosuppressive treatment. In such patients the skin lesions are often haemorrhagic and necrotic. The general disturbance is severe, and many patients die.

267 Herpes zoster and carcinomatosis. Metastases from surgically treated breast cancer were discovered when the patient developed a severe attack of herpes zoster and a heavy chickenpox rash. Many of the skin lesions are necrotic and the patient is jaundiced. The liver is enlarged and the abdomen distended by ascites. X-ray examination of the chest showed secondary deposits in the lungs.

265

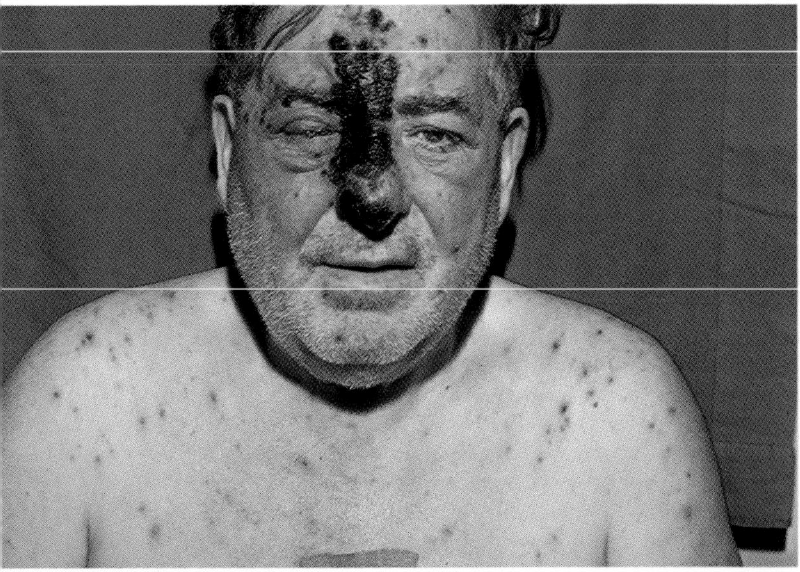

266

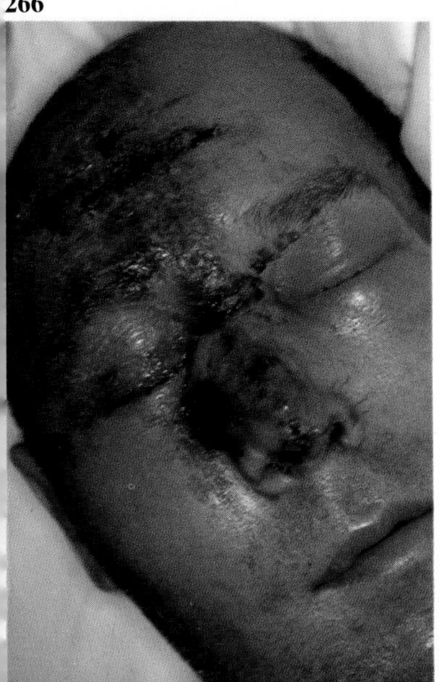

267

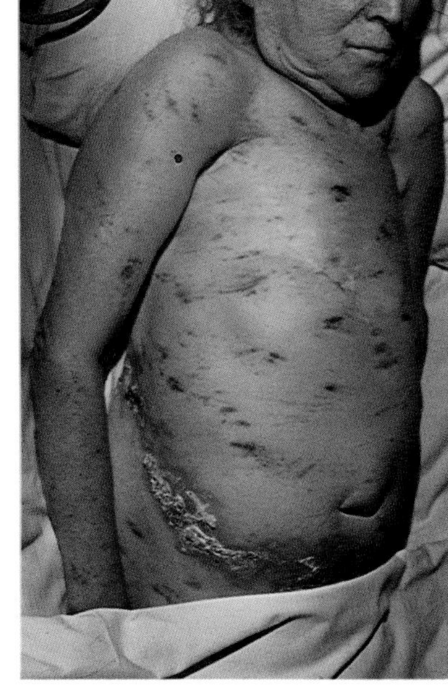

Herpes simplex infection

Primary infection with herpes simplex virus usually occurs in early childhood but may be deferred until adult life. In most children the reaction to the initial invasion is trivial with a few sores round the mouth, but a few develop acute gingivostomatitis and may be extremely ill. Subclinical infections are not uncommon. Once acquired, the virus may remain dormant for many years in cells of sensory nerve ganglia and has been detected in a high proportion of ganglia removed immediately after death.

Recurrent attacks are common and generally infect the skin around the mouth, although other sites may be affected. Herpes simplex virus is also responsible for infections of the central nervous system, eye and genital tract; it is suspected to be an etiological factor in squamous carcinoma of the lip and in carcinoma of the cervix of the uterus. Patients with eczema are especially susceptible to the virus and may succumb to generalised infection.

Herpes simplex virus of man is one of a large group of similar viruses naturally infecting many mammals and birds. Of these only B virus of monkeys is known to cause human disease. Herpes simplex virus can be separated into two types according to antigenic differences and biological characteristics. A small number of strains do not fall readily into either group.

Virology

268 Herpes simplex virus type 1 on chorioallantoic membrane. Type 1 viruses are usually isolated from the mouth or throat, from skin lesions, or from the brain of adults with encephalitis.

All human strains of the virus grow readily on chick embryo. Lesions appear on the chorioallantois within 24 to 28 hours after inoculation, and reach their maximum size in three to four days. The pocks produced by type 1 virus are smaller (less than 0.5 mm diameter) but more numerous than those produced by type 2. They are also more superficial.

269 Herpes simplex virus type 2 on chorioallantoic membrane. Type 2 viruses are usually isolated from the genital tract but may be recovered from brain and other organs in neonatal infection.

Fewer lesions are produced on chorioallantoic membrane by type 2 viruses but the lesions are large (more than 1 mm diameter) and more deeply seated.

268

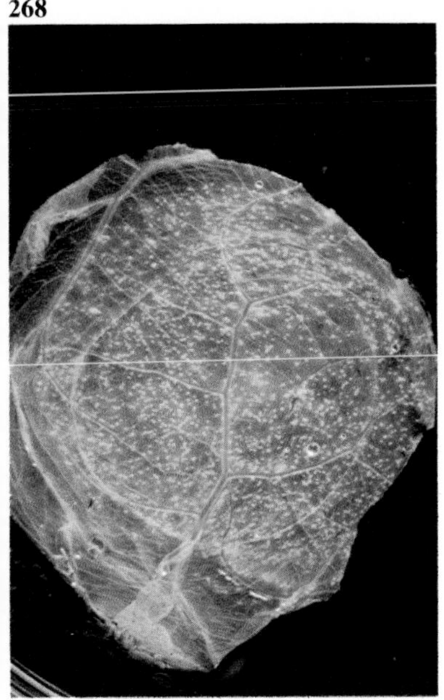

269

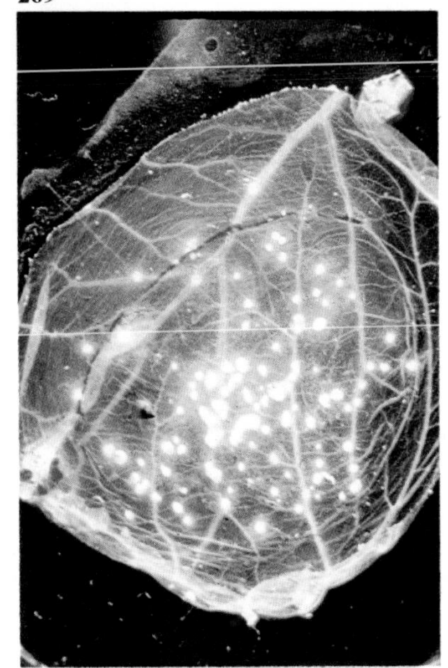

270 Normal monkey kidney cell culture.

271 Herpes simplex virus in monkey kidney cells. Chick embryo is no longer used for primary isolation of herpes simplex virus but is still used for confirming the type. Isolation of the virus is accomplished more easily in tissue cultures of primary rabbit kidney or primary human amnion cells, although many other cells are suitable. The growth of the virus can be recognised by cytopathogenic changes, which appear within 24 to 48 hours. These vary with the type of virus and the nature of the host cells. A lytic effect is produced in amnion cells and multinucleated giant cells may be found in HeLa cell cultures. In monkey kidney cell culture the infected cells degenerate and become rounded.

Clinical syndromes

272 Disseminated herpes infection in neonate. Focal necrosis of liver. Spread of infection from the mother's genital tract at birth or from an attendant may result in severe generalised infection culminating in death. Evidence of infection usually appears four to five days after birth. Local lesions may be found on the surface of the body but these are quickly overshadowed by the catastrophic general disturbance.

Foci of miliary necrosis are found in many organs and are particularly prominent in the liver. The condition may be mistaken for miliary tuberculosis. (Arrows = necrotic foci.)

273 Acute disseminated herpes — histology of liver. Intranuclear inclusion bodies are found in cells adjacent to areas of necrosis. When fully developed the inclusion is eosinophilic and Feulgen-negative. An unstained halo separates the inclusion from the nuclear membrane.

Around the edge of the lesion some of the cells show evidence of impending necrosis. These cells may be identified by their pyknotic nuclei.

Herpes simplex virus type 2 is found in 80% of neonates with disseminated infection. (A = intranuclear inclusion, B = pyknotic nucleus.)

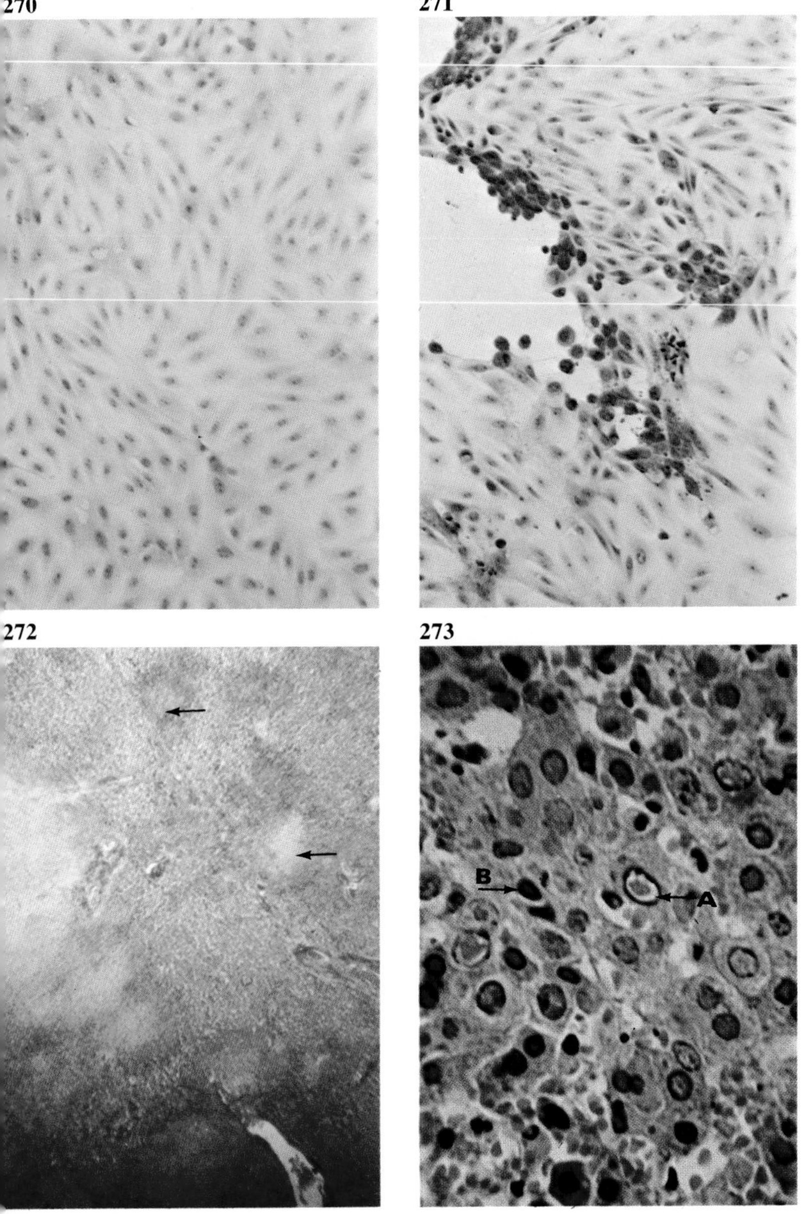
270
271
272
273
B
A

274 Herpetic encephalitis — section of brain. Infection of the central nervous system is more common than was previously thought. It may manifest as a meningo-encephalitis or encephalitis, generally associated with type 1 virus, or as aseptic meningitis, myelitis or radiculitis, generally associated with type 2 virus.

At autopsy there is intense engorgement of the brain and meninges with perivascular cuffing around the vessels in the cortex and subcortical white matter. The brain tissue is infiltrated with lymphocytes, plasma cells, and large mononuclear cells. Intranuclear inclusion bodies are found mainly in glial cells, but are also present in nerve cells.

Older children and adults may develop a localised form of encephalitis, mainly affecting the temporal lobe, which presents clinically as a space-occupying lesion. Necrosis is a striking feature of this localised form.

The section of brain shows perivascular cuffing with lymphocytes, plasma cells, and mononuclear cells. There are no polymorphonuclear cells or inclusions.

275 Neurones infected with herpes simplex virus. Fluorescent antibody staining shows viral antigens in nerve cells from a fatal case of herpetic encephalitis.

276 Acute disseminated herpes in older child — histology of liver. Fatal dissemination of the virus may occur in older children suffering from malnutrition. The changes in the tissues are similar to those found in neonatal infection. Type 1 virus is usually responsible.

This section of liver from an African child has been stained by fluorescent-antibody technique which indicates the presence of viral antigen along the portal tract.

74

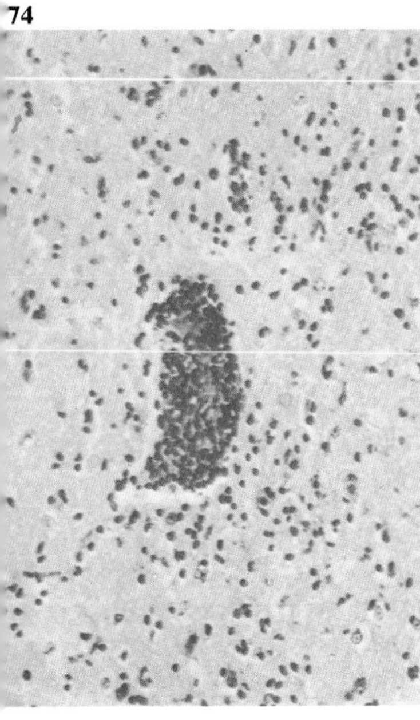

275

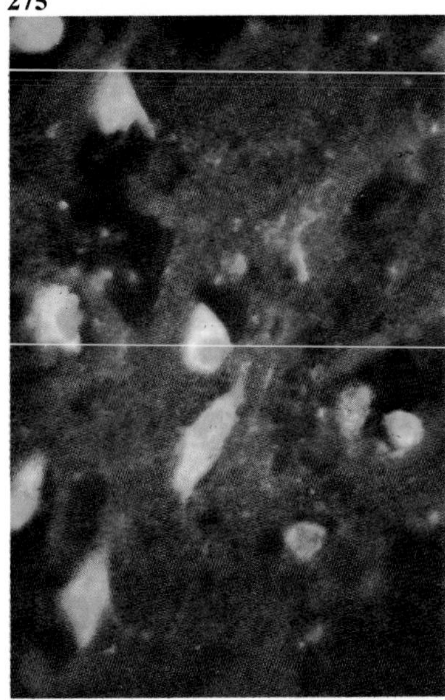

276

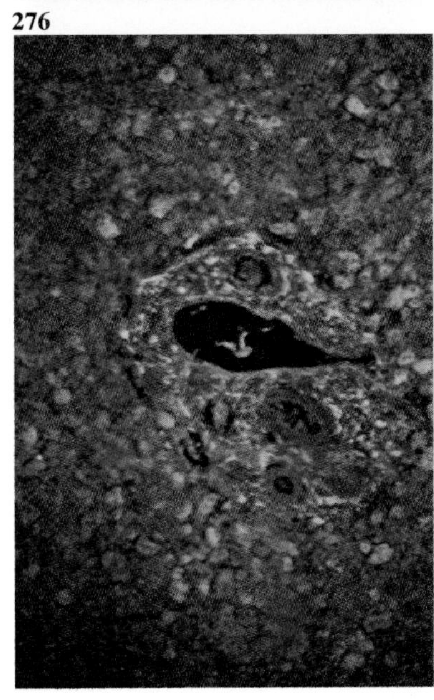

277 Histology of vesicle. At onset of infection cells in the deeper layer of the epidermis proliferate but degenerative changes soon follow. Th affected cells swell, become separated from each other and som eventually rupture. Multinucleated giant cells may form. The under lying dermis is infiltrated by moderate numbers of neutrophil poly morphonuclear cells and lymphocytes.

The section is from hairy skin and shows a superficial vesicle that ha destroyed the epidermis. The roof of the vesicle has collapsed and par of it may be seen at each side of the lesion. (A = edges of roof o vesicle, B = dermis, C = hair follicle, D = subcutaneous tissue.)

278 Primary gingivostomatitis in child. Herpes simplex virus is a ver successful parasite and infection is widespread. In most communitie about 60% of the population over five to six years old possess antibod against type 1 virus. Subclinical or mild infection is very common i early childhood, but primary infection in young children may occasion ally provoke severe gingivostomatitis.

After a short prodromal illness lesions appear in the mouth. Thes consist of thin-walled vesicles on an erythematous base that soo rupture to form typical shallow ulcers with a serpiginous edge. The gum are particularly inflamed and swollen.

277

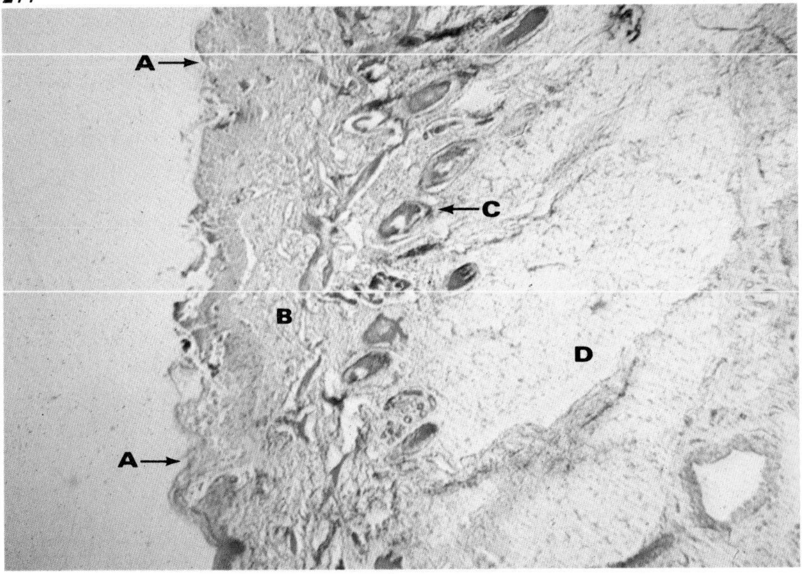

A
A
B
C
D

278

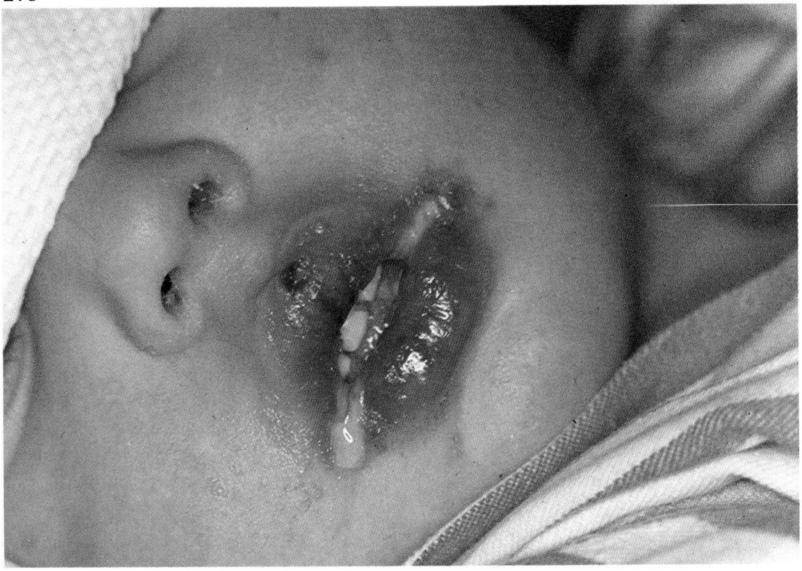

279 Stomatitis with secondary lesions on skin. In severe herpetic gingivostomatitis the young child becomes acutely ill with a high fever and is reluctant to eat or drink because of pain. Continuous drooling from the infected mouth transfers virus to the skin of the face, neck and chest. After a week the temperature usually returns to normal but another week or two may elapse before the mouth heals.

280 Herpetic gingivitis in adult. Adult patients with primary infection of the gums may be seen by the dentist rather than the physician. The gums are inflamed and swollen. Initially the vesicles are discrete, but soon run together and burst to form typical serpiginous ulcers. Primary infection in adults is found more commonly in higher socioeconomic groups.

79

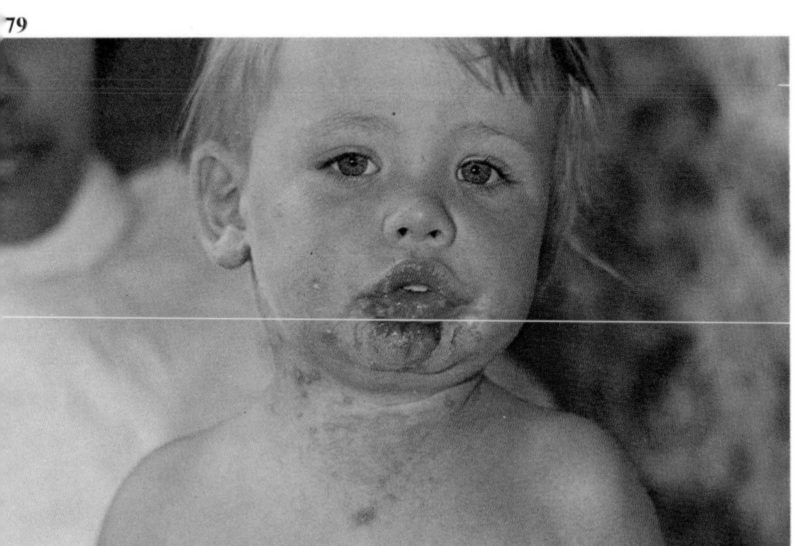

80

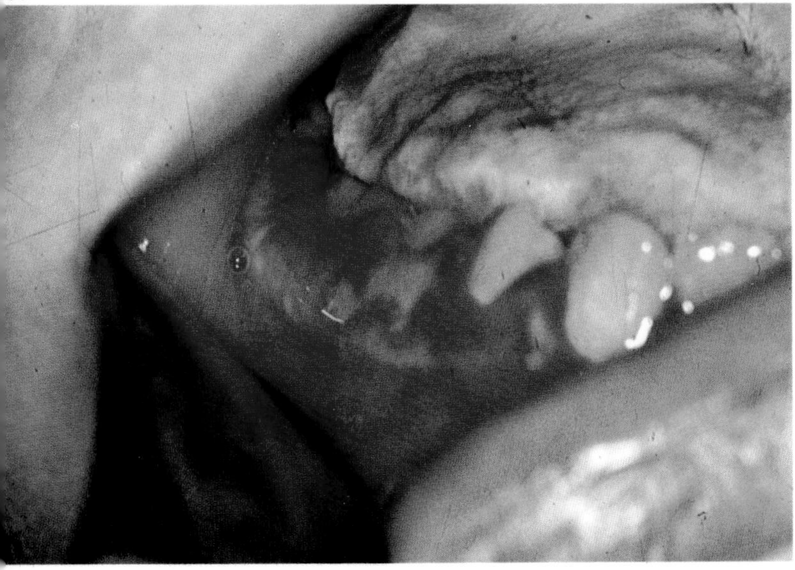

281 Acute gingivostomatitis in adult. Primary infection with herpe simplex virus may affect the mouth in adults as well as children. Th appearance is similar in both age groups, but the constitutional disturb ance is less in adults.

282 Herpetic lesions on tongue of adult. The tongue is heavily coate and small round vesicles are scattered sparsely over the surfac Herpetic stomatitis or glossitis should not be confused with aphtho stomatitis, which is an entirely unrelated condition. Palatal lesions ma be mistaken for herpangina (see **385** and **386**).

81

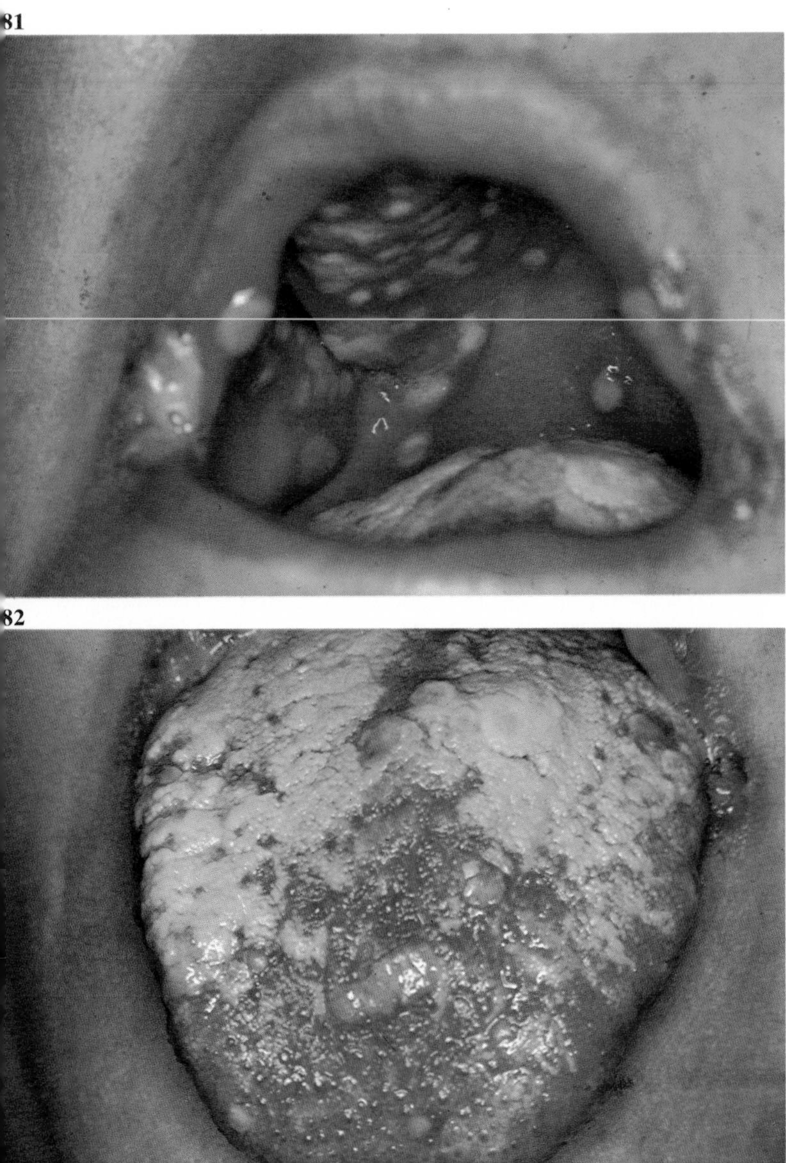

82

283 Primary infection of the skin. Primary infection of the skin is se more commonly in older children and adults. Spread is by direct conta to any part of the body. Outbreaks amongst wrestlers have bee dignified by the title 'herpes gladiatorum'.

284 Herpes simplex mimicking herpes zoster. In some patients herp simplex infection may closely simulate zoster, and there may even b mild sensory disturbance, but there is less pain and the distribution do not conform to a dermatome. Diagnosis is difficult when herpes zost affects only part of a root. In these circumstances the shorter prodrom period and the relative absence of pain in simplex infections are poin to be considered but, when doubt persists, the diagnosis will be decid by laboratory tests.

This rugby footballer developed a rash on his face after a game a was initially thought to have herpes zoster, but the rapid onset a unusual distribution aroused suspicion, and a diagnosis of prima herpes simplex infection was confirmed by growing the virus a demonstrating a rise in antibody titre.

285 Recurrent infection. Recurrent attacks of herpes simplex infectio differ from the primary attack. They occur in older children and adul with high antibody concentrations, and there is no subsequent rise titre. The attack is often precipitated by a trivial stimulus, but particularly common in pneumonia, meningitis and malaria. It is high probable that the virus lies dormant in cells of sensory nerve ganglia a spreads to the skin along cutaneous nerve fibres.

A sensation of tingling or tightness may be felt in the skin for a fe hours before the rash appears. Clusters of little vesicles develop rapid on an erythematous base, usually on the skin round the mouth. T vesicles quickly evolve through pustules to scabs, which separate a heal without leaving scars. Very rarely a squamous cell carcinom develops at the site of recurring herpes.

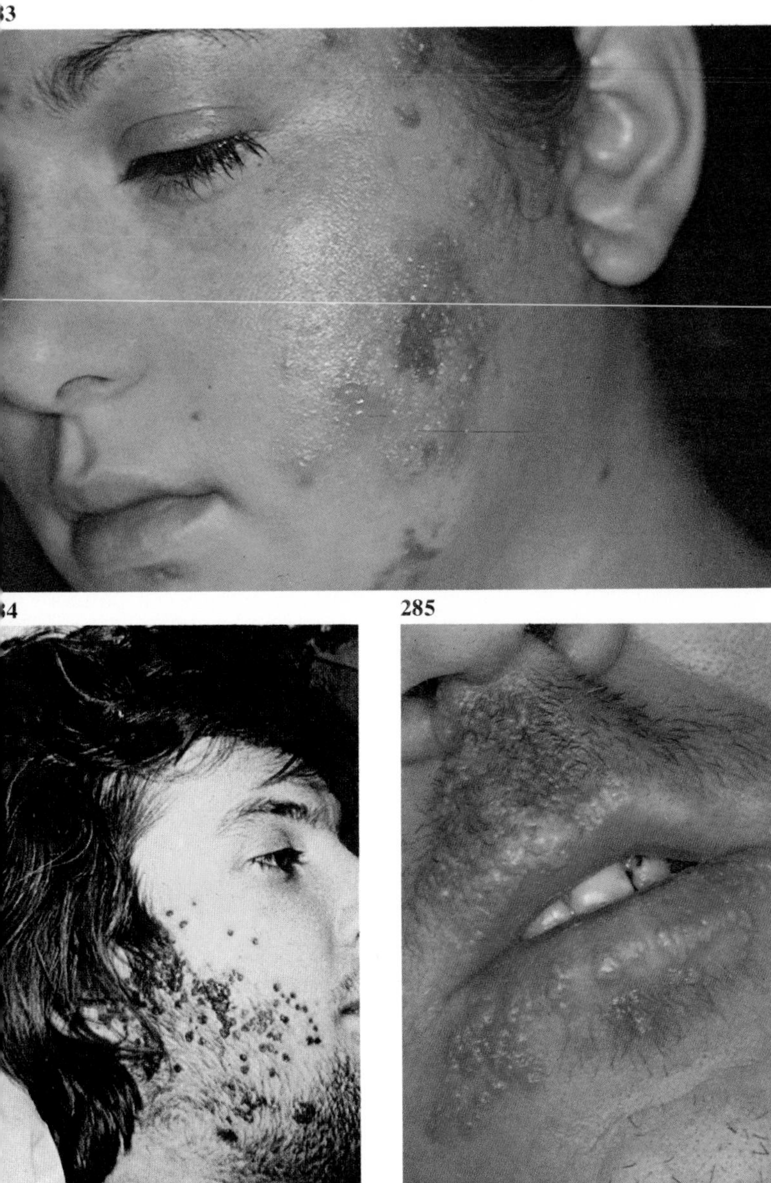
3
4
285

286 Herpetic infection of the eye. Herpetic infections of the eye ca occur at any age and may be primary or recurrent.

Neonatal eye infections are generally acquired from the mother genital tract at birth and may be the sole manifestation or else a min component of disseminated infection.

Primary infection of the eye is commonest in children and usual takes the form of unilateral follicular conjunctivitis with pronounce oedema of the conjunctiva and eyelids. Vesicles may be present on th eyelids. Associated infection of the cornea often results in coars punctate epithelial opacities.

Recurrent herpes is usually seen in adults and may prove exceeding troublesome. The cornea is predominantly affected, and follicul conjunctivitis is exceptional. Herpetic keratitis varies greatly in severit from superficial dendritic ulceration to inflammation of the deep layers of the corneal stroma. Topical applications of corticostero preparations are dangerous and may convert simple dendritic ulceratio into deep amoeboid ulceration with risk of perforation and hypopyon.

The dendritic ulcer in the illustration has been stained with fluorescein.

287 Herpetic whitlow. Nurses and doctors lacking specific antibody ar especially susceptible to primary herpetic infection of the fingers. Th virus is acquired from patients and readily penetrates the skin throug minor cuts and abrasions. Infection is often derived from catheters use for clearing tracheostomy tubes. Herpetic infections of the finger als occur in children and may be secondary to gingivostomatitis.

Herpetic whitlows may take the form of pulpitis or of clusters c blisters on the skin. The lesions are painful and there may be a gener reaction with fever and headache.

86

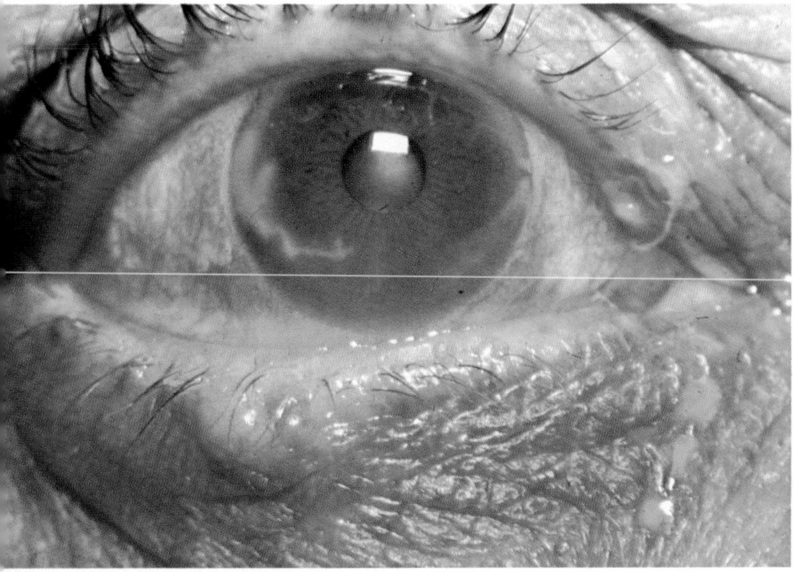

87

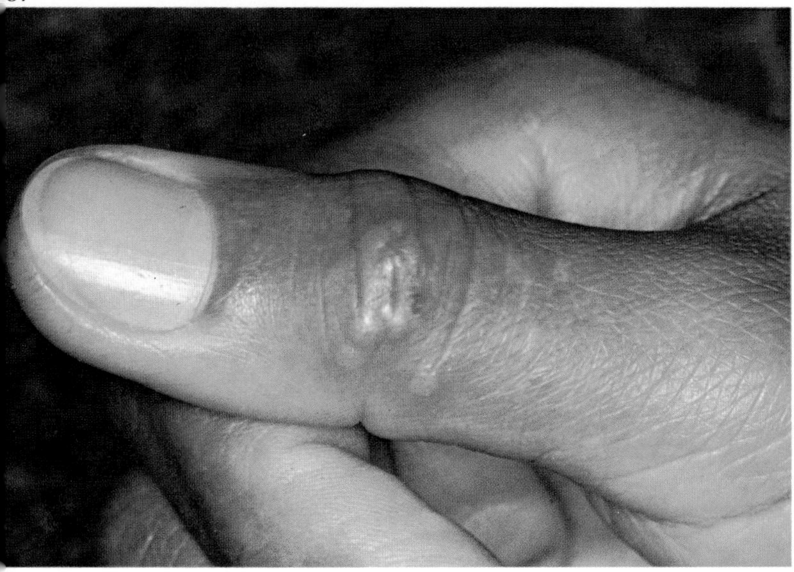

288 Eczema herpeticum — trunk of adult. Patients with eczema are particularly vulnerable to infection with herpes simplex virus. Infection spreads readily in the eczematous skin, producing crops of small superficial vesicles. These evolve through a pustular stage to form crusts that separate, leaving shallow necrotic ulcers. These eventually heal with a variable degree of scarring.

Systemic invasion may lead to generalised infection and death. Eczema herpeticum is seen most frequently in young children, but occurs occasionally in older children and adults.

289 Eczema herpeticum — close-up.

290 Genital herpes — adult male. Genital herpes is usually caused by type 2 virus. Infection is commonly transmitted by sexual intercourse but not invariably. The prevalence is much greater in women.

Lesions are detected most often on the prepuce or in the coronal sulcus. They also occur on the shaft of the penis or in the urethra. Latent infection with type 2 virus seems to be common in men but not women. Heaviest infection is found in the vas deferens.

288

289

290

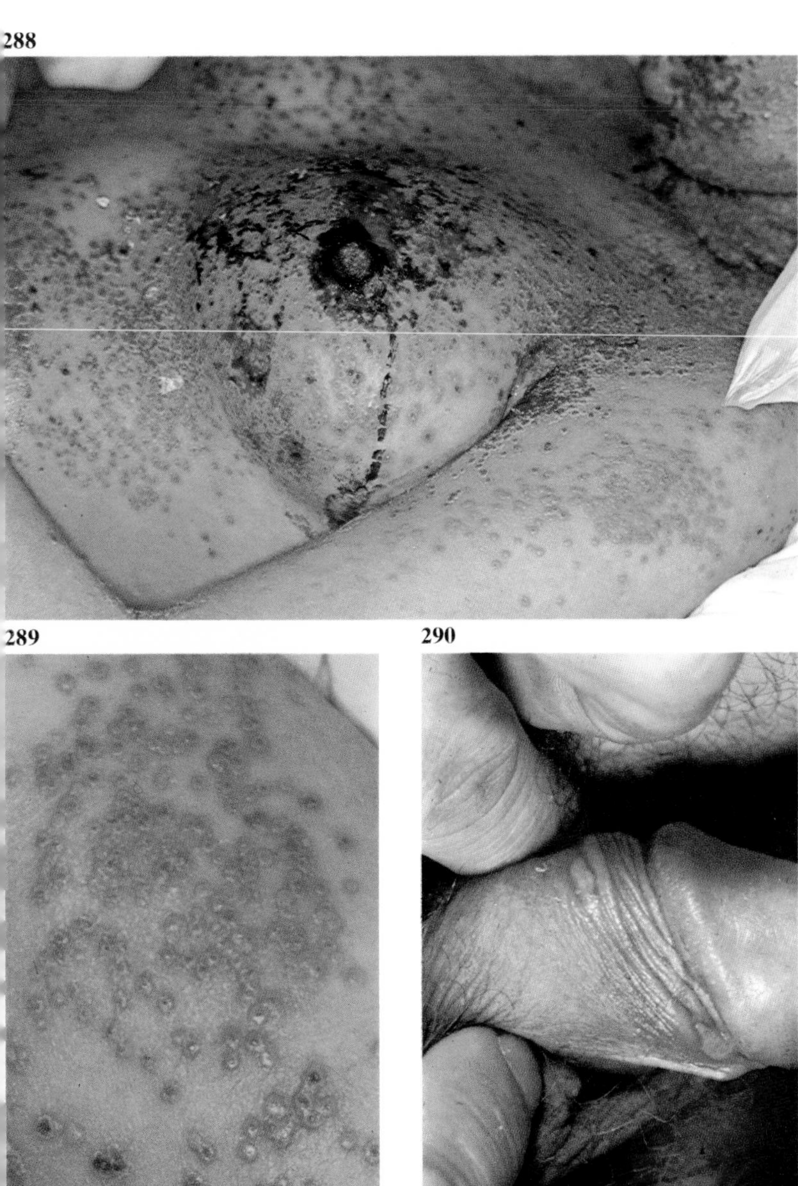

291 Genital herpes — adult woman. Herpetic lesions may be found on the vulva, vagina or cervix, and may appear on the perineum or buttocks. Genital herpes in pregnancy may cause overwhelming infection in newborn babies, particularly when they are premature. This extremely high mortality necessitates the investigation of all vesicles or ulcers on the genital tract of pregnant women.

292 Genital herpes — adult woman. Herpetic cervicitis may result from a primary infection or follow reactivation of latent infection. The genital lesions in women tend to ulcerate rapidly and become covered with exudate. It has been suggested that there may be an association between type 2 virus infections and invasive carcinoma of the cervix.

293 Vulvovaginitis in child. Primary infection of the skin may be found at any site. When the vulva is infected in infants, a diagnosis of 'nappy rash' may be made and the possibility of herpetic infection overlooked.

In herpetic vulvovaginitis the skin is macerated and the labia stuck together by gummy exudate. Vesicles may be inconspicuous.

291

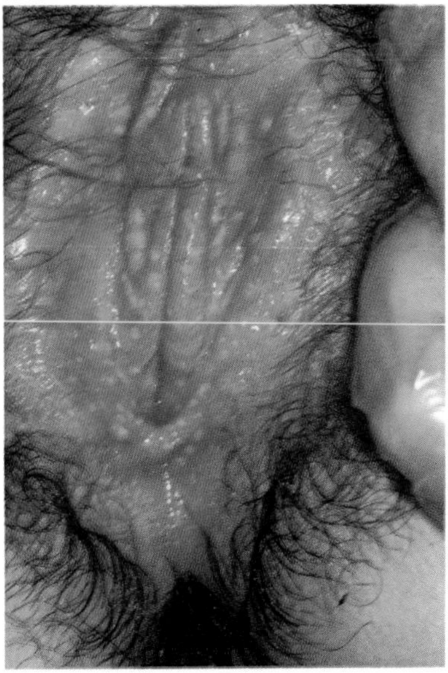

292

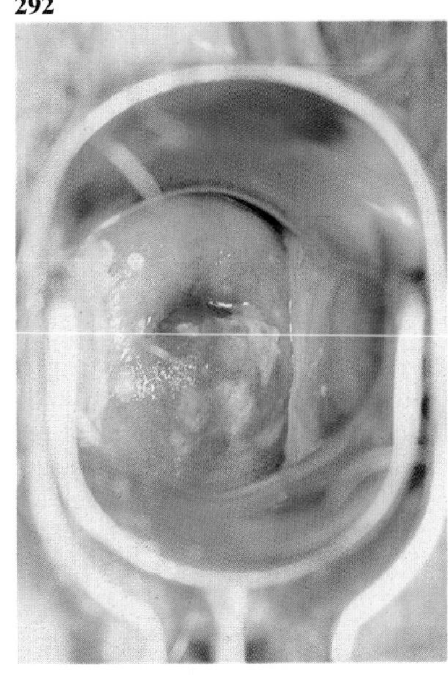

293

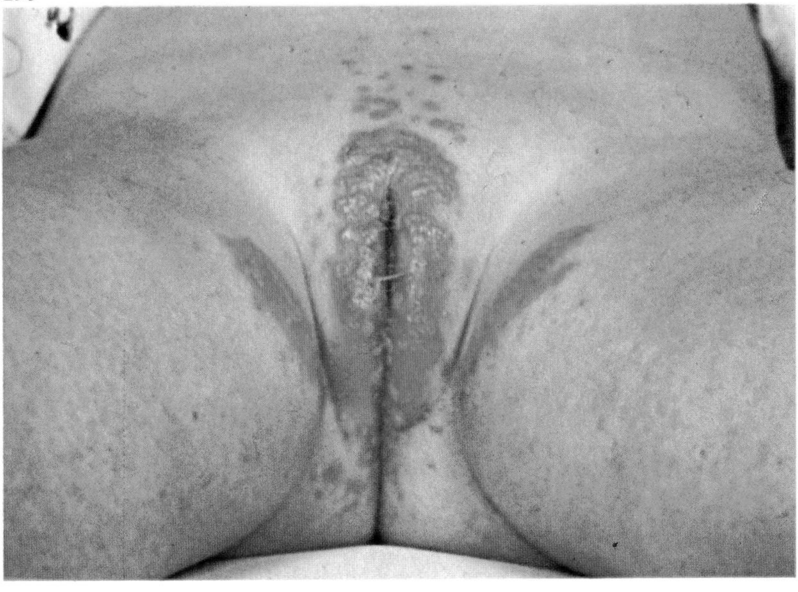

Cytomegalovirus infection

Primary infection of the mother during pregnancy may occasionally result in death of the fetus or serious generalised disease in the newborn child that closely simulates toxoplasmosis. Erythroblastosis, thrombocytopenia with purpura, jaundice and hepatomegaly, are striking features of the illness. More commonly, however, congenital cytomegalovirus infections appear to follow a benign course, though roughly 10% of affected children may subsequently be mentally retarded.

In children, infection acquired after birth may cause chronic liver disease but is more often asymptomatic and latent throughout childhood and adolescence. Primary infection in adults may be subclinical or may present with a variety of syndromes, including cytomegalovirus fever, hepatitis, or Paul–Bunnell-negative infectious mononucleosis. Patients with disorders of immunity or those receiving immunosuppressive drugs may develop generalised disease with severe infection of the lungs.

294 Electron micrograph of cytomegalovirus. Cytomegaloviruses are found in man and various animals. On electron microscopy the virus has the characteristics of a herpesvirus, with a capsid approximately 96nm in diameter. The virus is icosahedral in shape and has 162 elongated hollow capsomeres. Enveloped particles have a diameter of about 180nm.

295 Cytomegalovirus. Section of parotid gland showing inclusion bodies. Cytomegaloviruses have a particular affinity for salivary glands. Large acidophilic intranuclear inclusion bodies ('owl eye') are found in a small proportion of cells lining the ducts of the salivary glands in 5 to 25% of babies dying in early infancy. The affected cells are large, with a diameter of up to 40μm. Small basophilic granules may be found in the cytoplasm. (Arrow = large cell with 'owl eye' inclusion.)

294

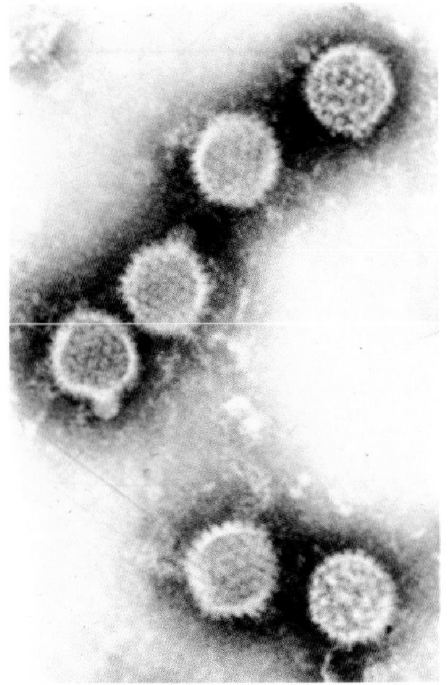

295

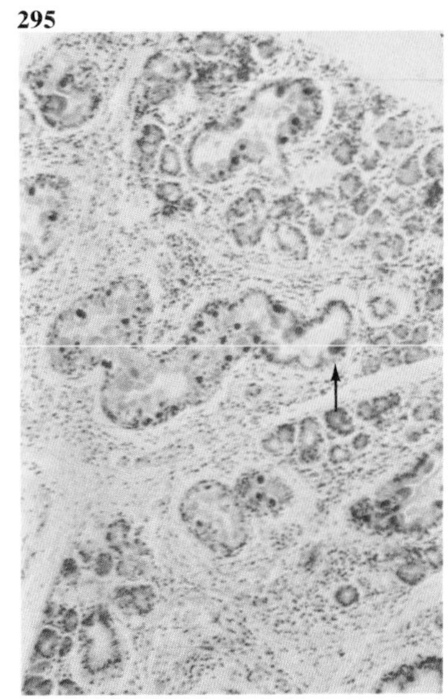

296 Cytomegalovirus. Section of kidney showing inclusions. In generalised disease large cells containing inclusions may be found in the lungs, kidneys, pancreas and other organs. A dilated tubule can be seen in the centre of the renal section. The lining epithelial cells contain large intranuclear inclusions. Enlarged cells with inclusions may be detected in the urine, and virus can be recovered on tissue culture. Infection in children results in prolonged excretion of the virus and, therefore, it is essential to assess such findings carefully in relation to the clinical picture. Virus excretion in adults is associated with active disease. (Arrow = tubule with characteristic large cell containing intranuclear inclusion body.)

296

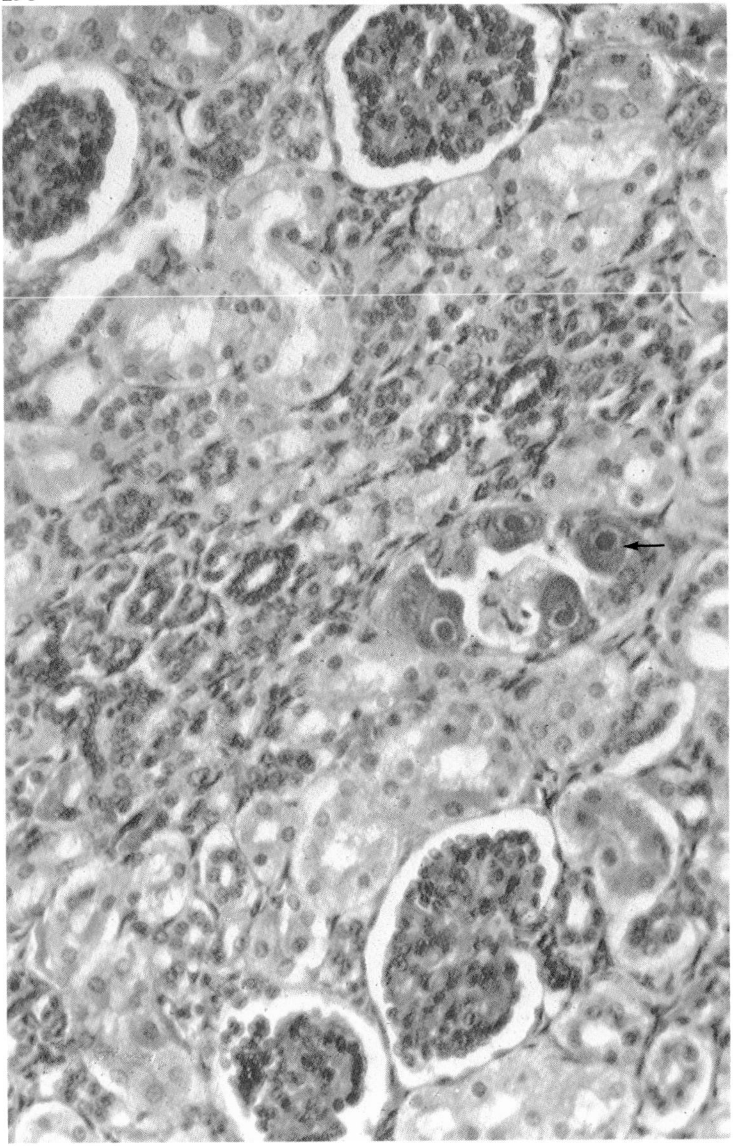

297 Radiograph of chest — cytomegalovirus infection in immune-deficient patient. A high proportion of patients with renal or bone marrow transplants, or with malignancies such as leukaemia or Hodgkin's disease, develop active cytomegalovirus infection either because of primary infection or reactivation of latent infection. In many the infection remains subclinical; in others it may result in fever, infectious mononucleosis or pneumonitis. Cytomegalovirus infection of the lung is difficult to diagnose and may be associated with other opportunistic infections, such as candida and pneumocystis. Fever, dyspnoea and a non-productive cough are common among patients with serious pulmonary infection.

The radiological appearance of cytomegalovirus pneumonitis is not characteristic. In many patients there is an interstitial pattern of shadowing; in others there is a nodular pattern. The chest x-ray film of this leukaemic child shows a large pneumatocele in the right lung caused by staphylococcal pneumonia, and diffuse interstitial shadowing caused by cytomegalovirus pneumonitis. The diagnosis was confirmed virologically.

297

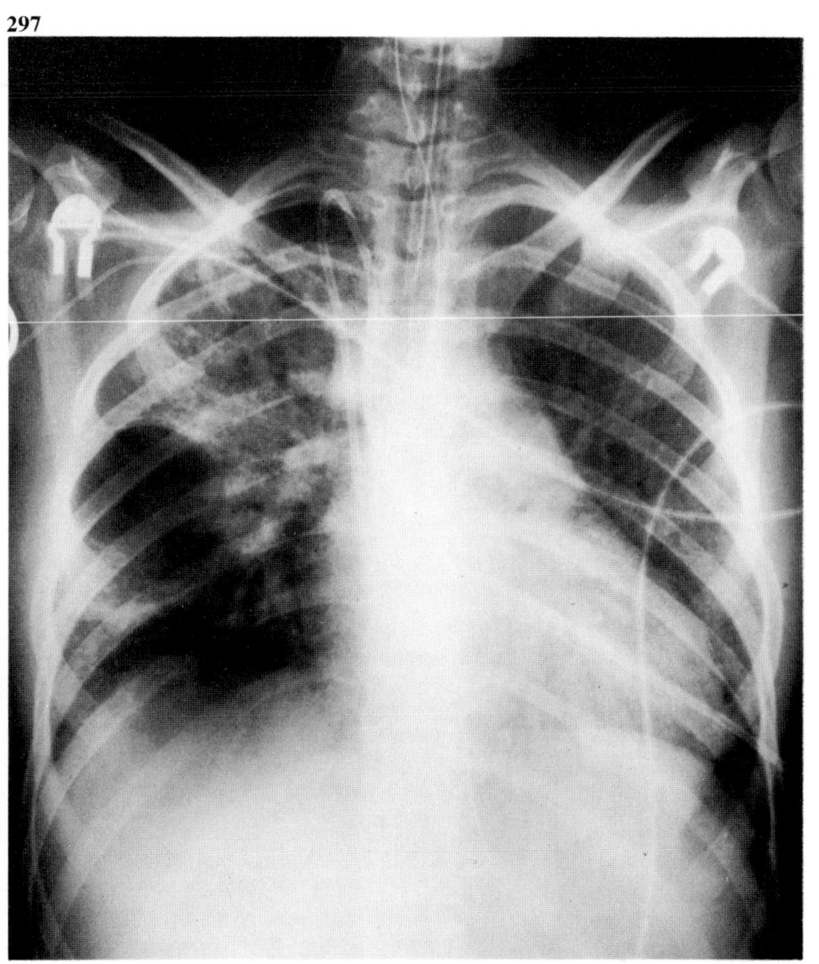

Infectious mononucleosis

Acute infectious mononucleosis is a generalised disease which adopts many guises. The anginose variety is most commonly seen in young adults, but any organ may be affected, and clinical syndromes are not sharply demarcated. Characteristic changes are found in blood: a high proportion of abnormal mononuclear cells and many 'inappropriate antibodies' are seen. The diagnostic Paul–Bunnell–Davidsohn test detects a heterophil antibody, which agglutinates sheep red blood cells but is not adsorbed on guineapig kidney. There are several simplified variants of this test.

The disease is endemic in most countries and has a striking predilection for young people between the ages of 15 and 20 years. The agent is transmitted in saliva from cases or carriers and there appear to be many subclinical infections. The incubation period is not certain but is thought to lie between 33 to 49 days. For many years the causative agent escaped detection, but Epstein–Barr virus (EBV) is now known to be responsible.

Virology and pathology

298 Electron micrograph of Epstein–Barr virus. EBV was originally detected in cells derived from Burkitt's lymphoma. It has the morphology of a herpesvirus with an electron-dense core of DNA. Subsequent surveys have shown infection with EBV to be worldwide. Most infections are acquired in early childhood and are not associated with recognisable clinical syndromes.

Patients with infectious mononucleosis have been found to develop antibodies to EBV, and EBV has been recovered from throat swabs of patients with infectious mononucleosis. The virus has also been linked with nasopharyngeal carcinoma, Hodgkin's disease, leukaemia and lymphoma. Studies of family or social contacts of patients with infectious mononucleosis have shown that spread occurs, but infectivity is low.

298

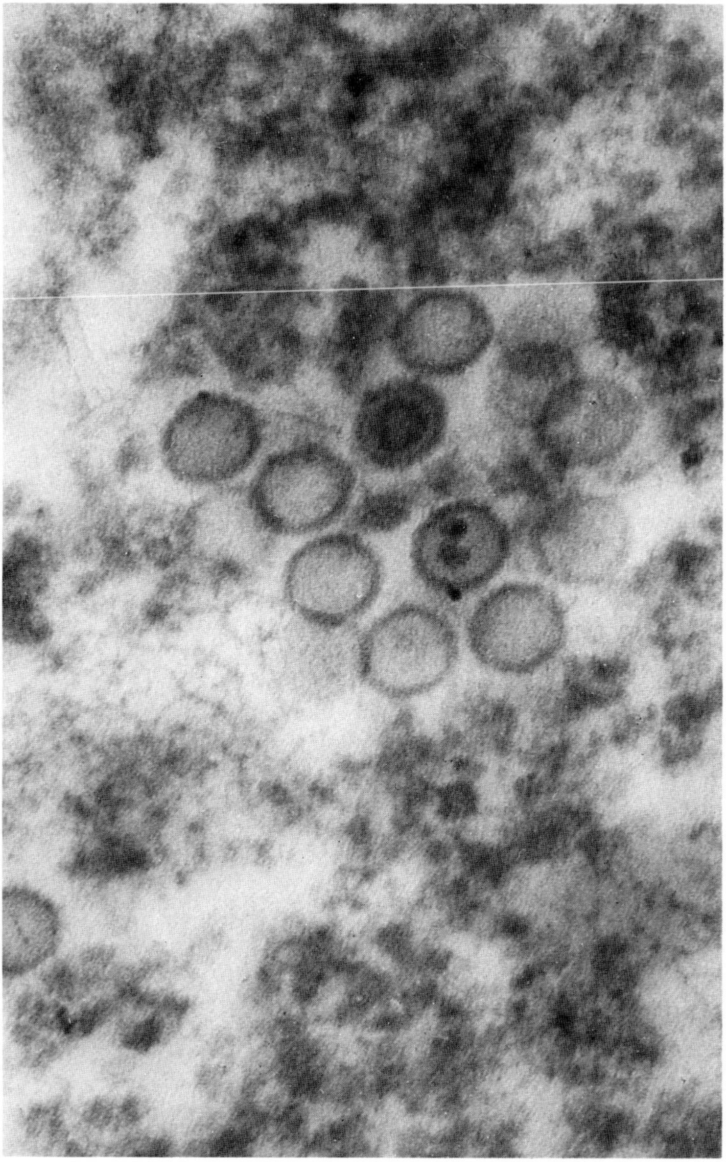

299 Blood film — abnormal mononuclear cells. The total white blood cell count is usually normal or slightly increased during the first week, but a few patients may have a neutropenia. A moderate leucocytosis develops towards the end of the first or the beginning of the second week, reaching a peak during the third. This leucocytosis is a result of an absolute increase in the circulating lymphocytes, many of which are abnormal. The virus is present in B lymphocytes.

The large number of atypical mononuclear cells found in the peripheral blood of patients with infectious mononucleosis is one of the characteristics of the disease. The cells vary greatly in size and shape. The nucleus may be round, bean-shaped or lobulated; the cytoplasm is vacuolated and more basophilic than usual. Dividing cells are found in the peripheral blood, and mitotic activity is greatly enhanced, but cellular structure is not fundamentally deranged. The nuclear chromatin in most abnormal mononuclear cells is too coarse and the cytoplasm too abundant for confusion to arise with lymphoblasts.

Clinical features

300 Appearance of face. Many patients with infectious mononucleosis have slight puffiness of the eyelids and a pinkish flush to their cheeks.

301 Enanthem — petechiae. Various rashes have been found on the palate. A cluster of small haemorrhages at the junction of the hard and soft palate is almost invariably present in the anginose variety of infectious mononucleosis but is not pathognomonic, as similar lesions are found in other infections of the respiratory tract.

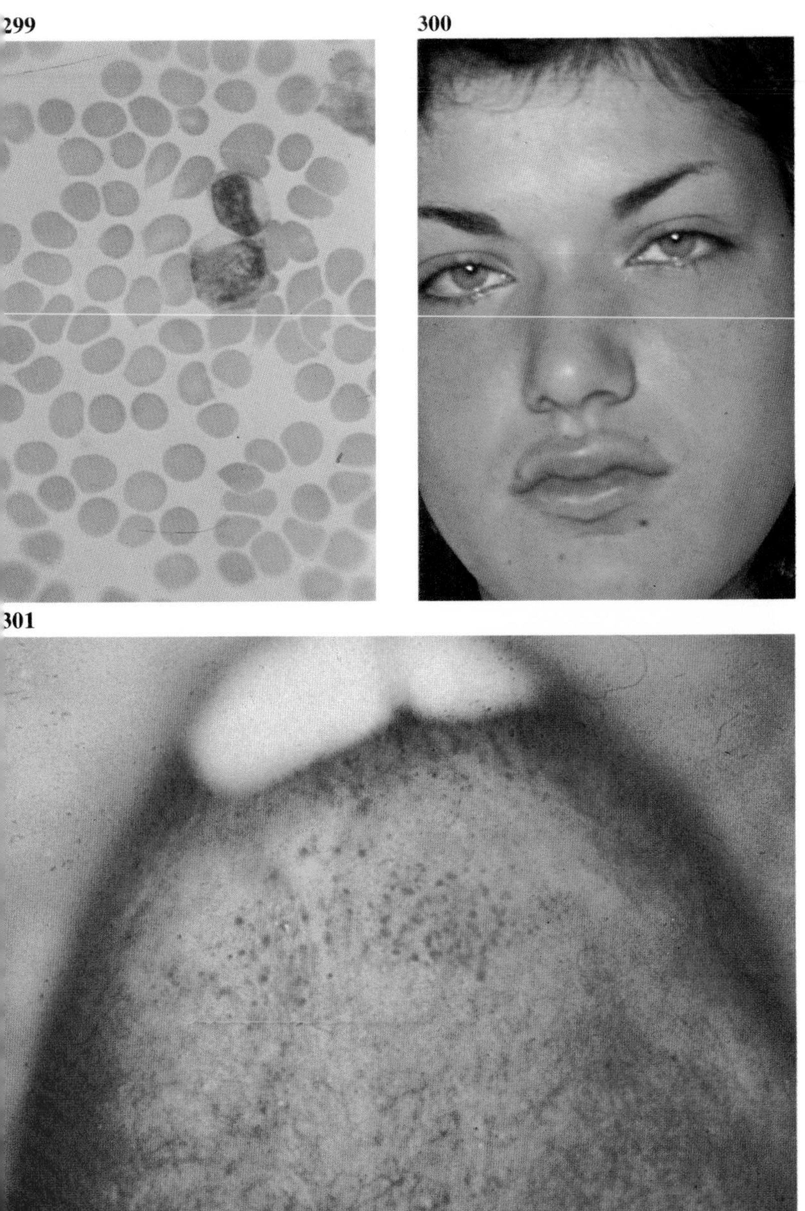
299
300
301

302 Anginose variety — inflamed throat without exudate. Shortly after onset of illness the patient may complain of a sore throat. The fauces are inflamed, but there is no exudate on the tonsils, and it is not possible from the appearance of the throat alone to make a diagnosis of infectious mononucleosis.

303 Anginose variety — follicular exudate. As the illness progresses patches of white exudate appear on the tonsils, which may be very swollen. The uvula is red and oedematous.

304 Anginose variety — typical exudate. The patches of exudate run together, forming thick plaques of opaque white membrane. The degree of inflammation varies considerably.

302

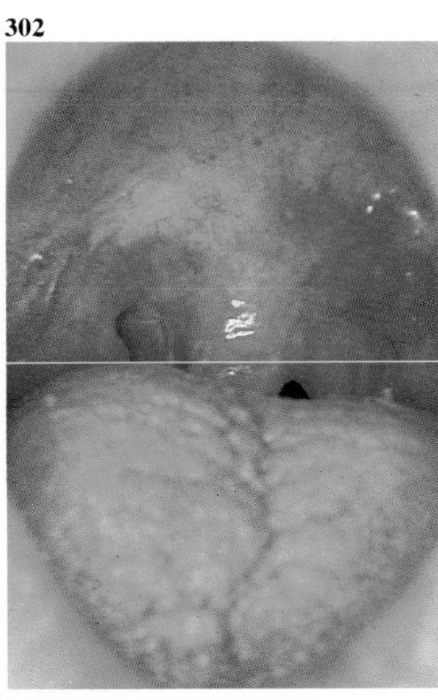

303

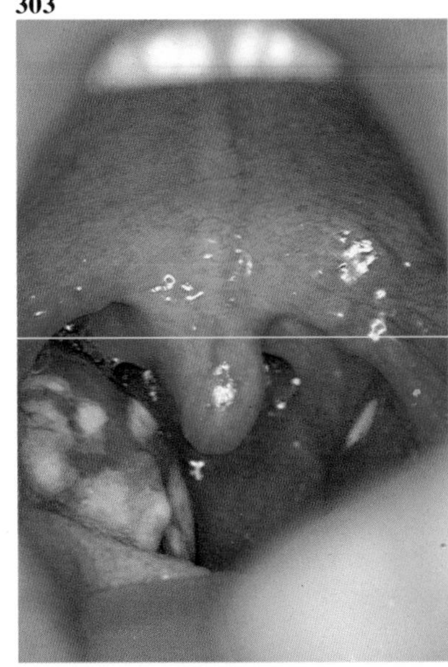

304

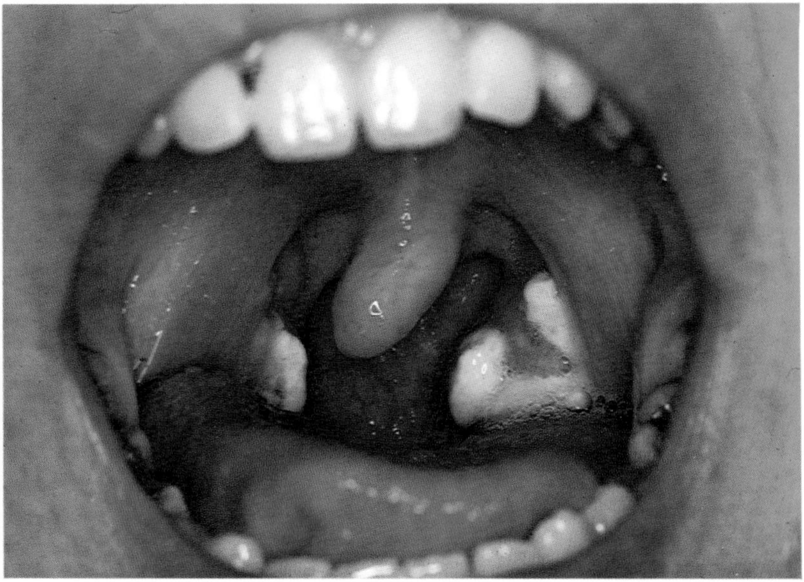

305 Anginose variety — late stage. The exudate persists for seven to 14 days or even longer, and may completely cover both tonsils; however, the patient's general condition remains good. The membrane often retains its pristine whiteness as it matures, but the colour may alter. Note the enanthem on the palate.

306 Anginose variety — obstruction. In the severest cases there may be so much congestion from inflammatory oedema that swallowing and breathing become difficult and life is endangered from respiratory obstruction.

It is difficult to recognise the normal anatomical landmarks. The tonsils are grossly swollen and covered with thick membrane, which obscures the uvula. The appearance of the throat might easily be mistaken for diphtheria, but the presence of splenomegaly and generalised enlargement of lymph nodes indicates the correct diagnosis. If doubt persists the matter can be settled by finding characteristic cells in the blood and a positive Paul–Bunnell test. If facilities for these tests are not available it would be advisable to give diphtheria antitoxin.

305

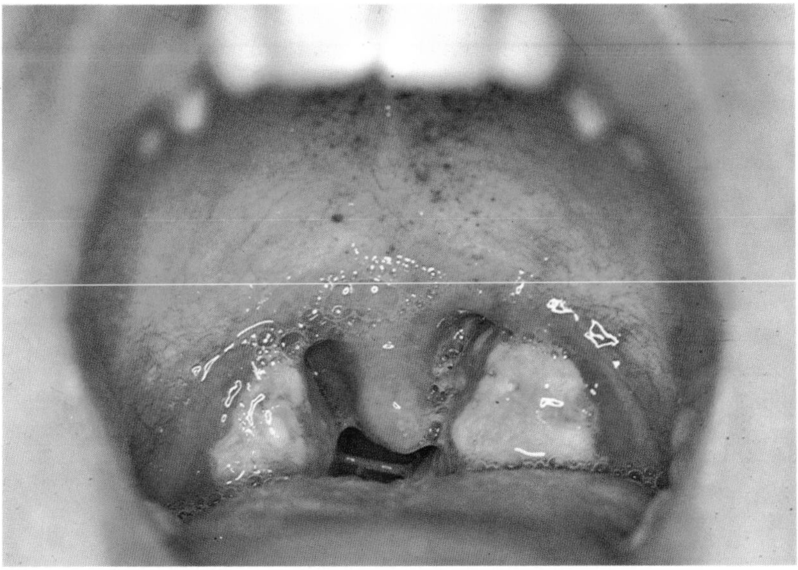

306

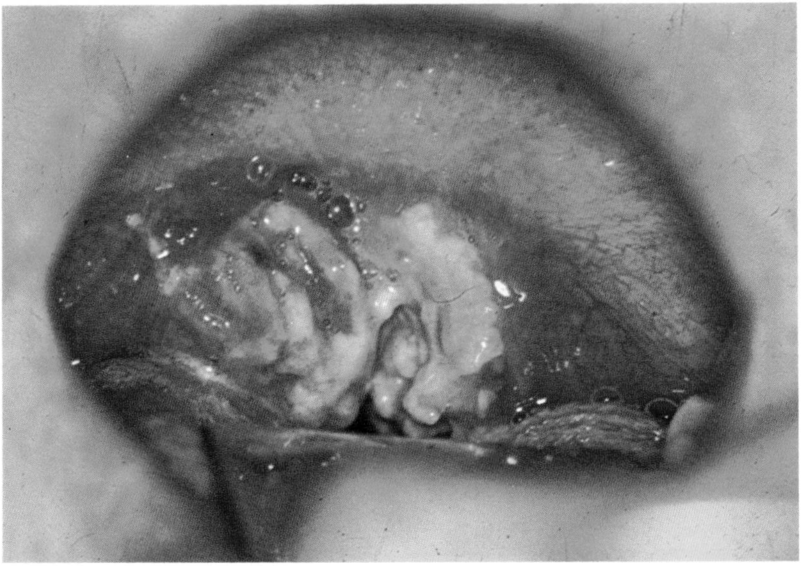

307 Rash on trunk. There is a high incidence of drug-related rashes among patients with infectious mononucleosis, but rashes also appear in those who have not been treated with drugs. The rash of infectious mononucleosis usually emerges during the second week and with its pinkish maculopapular character may be mistaken for rubella. The duration of the prodromal period is a helpful guide.

308 Rash on upper limb. The distribution of the rash tends to be patchy and is heavier on the limbs. Contrast with the rash of rubella (**364** to **367**).

309 Ampicillin rash. The incidence of rashes is exceptionally high (about 60%) in patients given ampicillin for the treatment of infectious mononucleosis. The rash resembles measles but has a bluish tinge. The individual lesions vary from one patient to another; some lesions have a pale and others a dark centre.

307

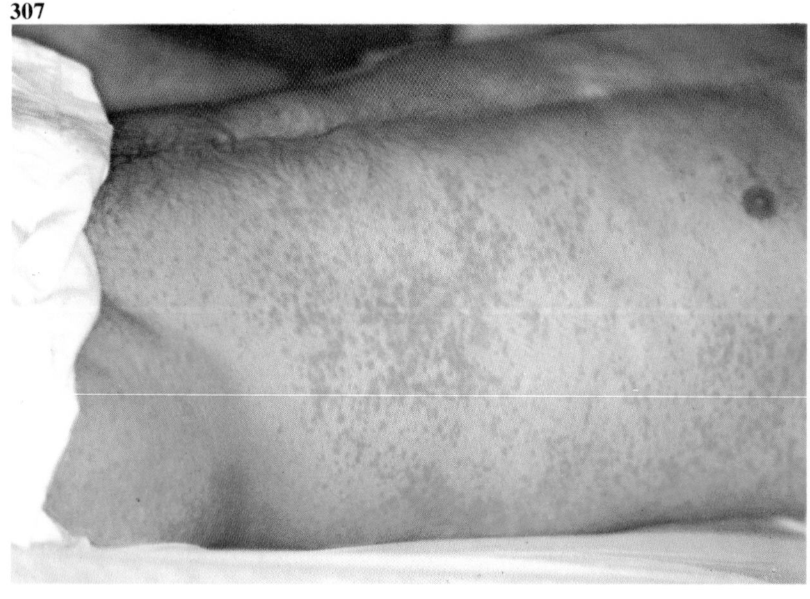

308

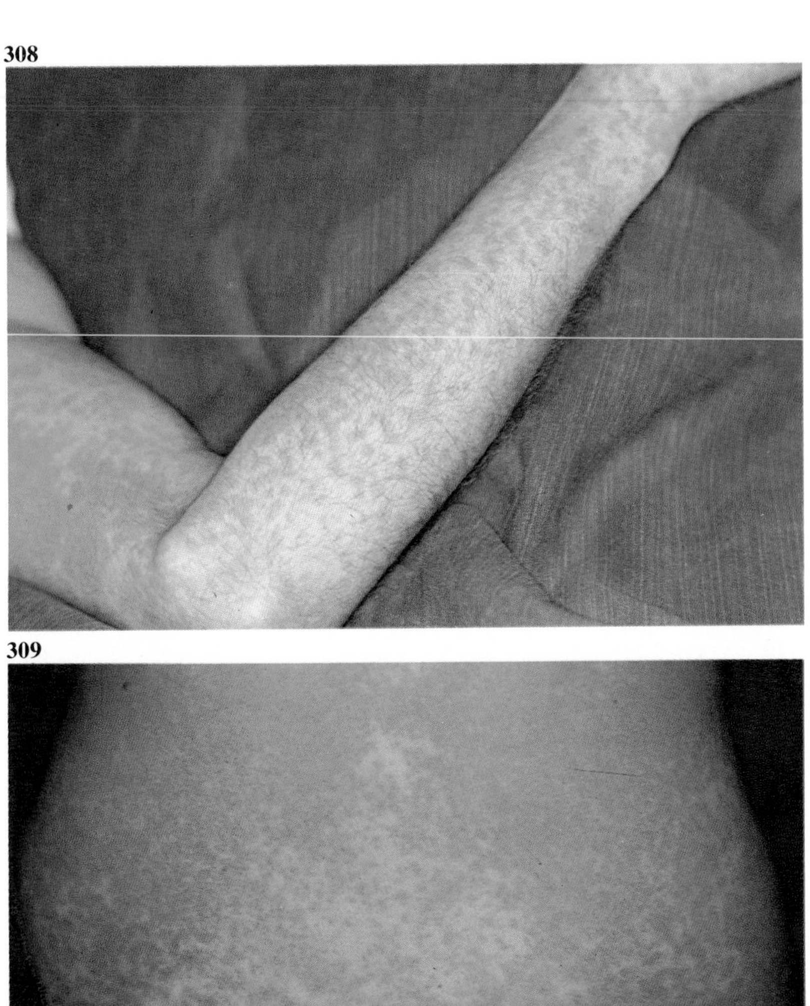

309

310

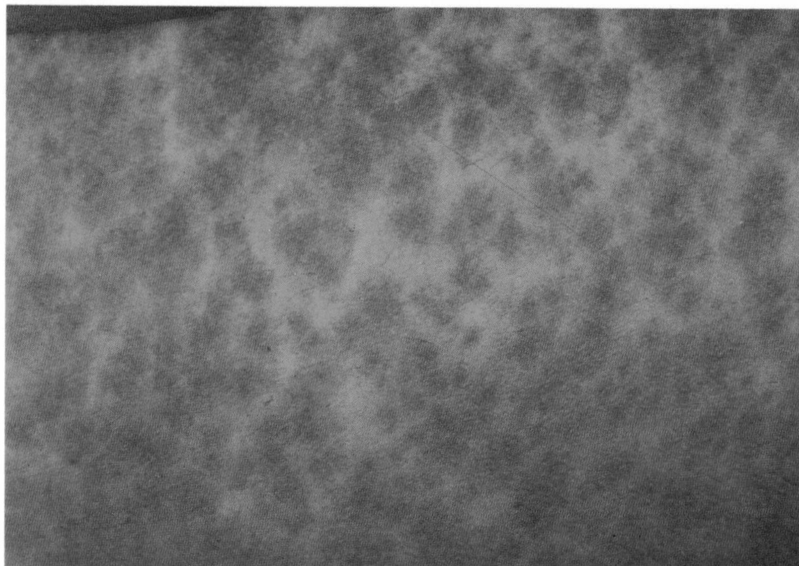

310 Ampicillin rash — close-up. Contrast with measles rash in **347**. Diagnosis is simple when exudate is present on the tonsils, but when exudate is absent there may be some confusion. The character of the individual components of the rash and the lack of respiratory catarrh exclude a diagnosis of measles.

Viral hepatitis

Many parasites, ranging in complexity from viruses to metazoa, are capable of causing hepatitis in man. Viral infections of the liver are particularly common throughout the world. Several viruses are known to produce hepatitis in man. The two most important so far identified are virus A of short incubation period (infectious hepatitis) and virus B of long incubation period (serum hepatitis). The use of sensitive immunoassays for the diagnosis of these two forms of hepatitis has revealed the existence of at least two other agents responsible for non-A, non-B hepatitis. Less commonly, hepatitis is caused by other viruses, including yellow fever virus, cytomegalovirus, herpes simplex virus, and some strains of enteroviruses. A mild degree of hepatitis is also a very frequent finding in acute infectious mononucleosis.

Virus A hepatitis predominantly affects children and young adults. The virus is usually transmitted by the faecal–oral route, but in some instances infection may be derived from blood or its products. Several large outbreaks have been traced to water contaminated by sewage. Outbreaks caused by food-borne infections may result from direct contamination by a carrier, or indirectly from foodstuff contaminated by infected water. Shellfish are particularly dangerous. Many infections are subclinical: young children tend to have anicteric attacks, presenting with a mild gastrointestinal disturbance, whereas older children and adults become jaundiced.

Virus B is usually transmitted parenterally by infected blood or serum, but may occasionally be spread by inhalation or ingestion. The incubation period of virus B hepatitis overlaps that of virus A but is generally considerably longer. There is a high incidence of long-incubation hepatitis among drug addicts and homosexuals, and this variety of hepatitis may be a major problem in transplant and dialysis units. There is no cross-immunity between the two infections. Passive immunisation with human normal immunoglobulin affords protection against virus A but not against virus B, for which hyperimmune globulin is necessary.

Non-A non-B hepatitis is now the most common form of post-transfusion hepatitis in many parts of the world, and a significant problem in renal dialysis and other specialised units. The viruses responsible may be transmitted by whole blood or blood products such as factor VIII. Infection is endemic in some communities, and sporadic outbreaks have been reported unrelated to inoculation. In these circumstances the mode of transmission is not known but may be by ingestion.

Pathology

311 Electron micrograph of negatively stained preparation of virus B hepatitis serum. Serum from patients with virus B hepatitis has been found to contain three distinct particles — Dane particles, spheres and tubules. All three are agglutinated by antiserum to hepatitis B surface antigen (HBsAg). The larger double-shelled Dane particle has a relatively constant diameter of 42nm and a distinct 27nm core, which is believed to be the virus. Virus-like particles, similar to the internal component, have been found in the liver of patients who have died during the acute stage of virus B hepatitis. The amorphous spheres and tubules appear to be incomplete particles of viral coat. During the early stage of hepatitis the particles are evenly dispersed, but as the illness progresses they clump together with antibodies to form large immune complexes. In chronic carriers the particles remain discrete.

HBsAg has been found in most body fluids, but only serum, saliva and semen are infectious. HBsAg appears in the circulation between one and three months after infection and persists for a few weeks in self-limiting infections. The production of antibody to HBsAg (anti-HBs) is very variable in relation to clearance of HBsAg. Anti-HBs may persist for years and is associated with protection against reinfection.

HBsAg varies in antigenic structure and at least eight subtypes have been recognised. These variations have proved useful in epidemiological studies. Hepatitis B core antigen (HBcAg) is present in the nucleus of infected hepatocytes and is only present in the circulation as an internal component of the Dane particle. Anti-HBc can usually be detected three to five weeks after HBsAg appears in serum, persists throughout the clinical illness and for several years afterwards. HBeAg in serum is associated with high concentration of Dane particles and is a marker of infectivity.

In most patients with virus B hepatitis, HBsAg clears within four to six weeks but can persist indefinitely. Most healthy carriers of HBsAg have never been jaundiced. Many patients receiving dialysis treatment for chronic renal failure become carriers, and there is a high carrier rate in patients with Down's syndrome, and in patients with immunity disorders. HBsAg is comparatively rare among the general population in Western Europe and North America, but is much more common in Japan and many tropical countries.

In parts of Africa and south-east Asia, where there is a high incidence of HBV infection, primary liver cancer is often found in adults of all ages. Those at particular risk appear to be chronic carriers of the virus,

311

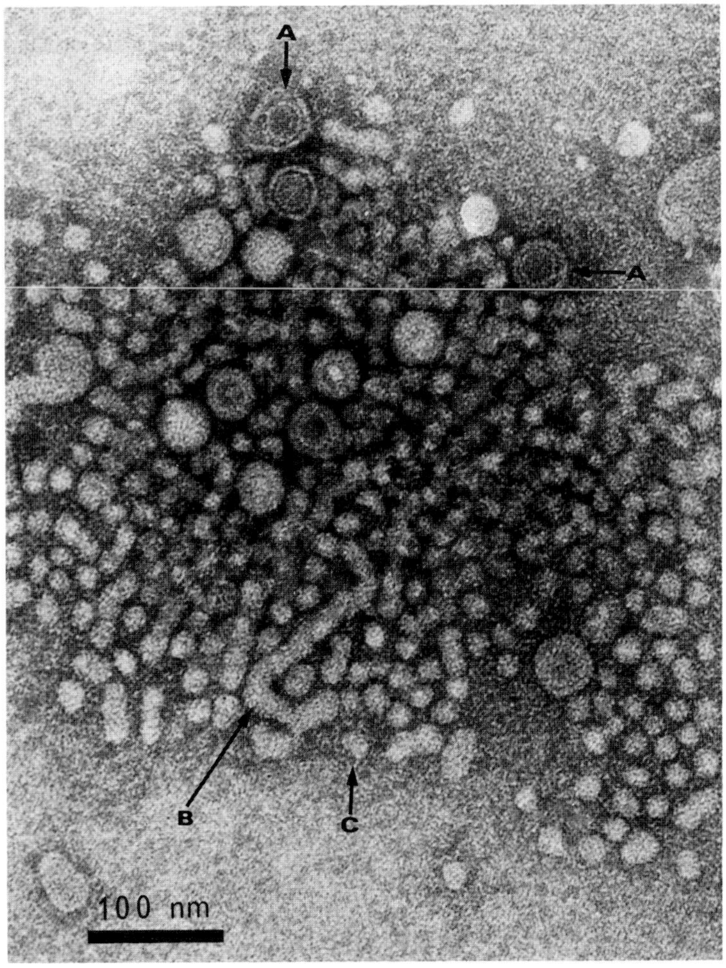

who were infected in early childhood. The cancer is commonly associated with hepatic cirrhosis. Although there is strong epidemiological evidence that this form of cancer is linked to HBV infection, environmental and other factors probably play a part in determining the high incidence of neoplasia. Primary liver cancer is thought to be the commonest fatal neoplasm of man. (A = Dane particle, B = tubule, C = sphere.)

312 Histology of acute hepatitis (H and E). There are no differences in the appearance of the liver in the two main types of viral hepatitis. The entire liver is affected, and the degree of impairment corresponds roughly to the severity of the histological changes.

During the acute stage parenchymal cells in any part of the liver may undergo necrosis. The affected cells are shrunken and rounded, with an intensely eosinophilic cytoplasm. The nucleus degenerates and disappears, leaving a globular eosinophilic structure. In the regions most distant from the portal tracts the liver cells become swollen, the nuclei disintegrate, and the affected cells disappear.

The Küpffer cells enlarge and increase in number. There is heavy infiltration with lymphocytes, plasma cells and histiocytes round the portal tracts. In uncomplicated cases the Küpffer cell reaction begins to subside after a month, and the inflammatory reaction in the portal tracts has disappeared by the end of two months. The normal structure of the liver is fully restored.

In the section shown here the architecture of the liver is intact. A dying liver cell is easily recognised in the centre of the picture by its eosinophilic appearance and pyknotic nucleus. The Küpffer cells are prominent, but at this early stage there is little infiltration by inflammatory cells. (A = degenerate hepatocyte with pyknotic nucleus, B = Küpffer cells.)

313 Chronic persistent hepatitis. Section of liver (H and E). Occasionally, mild symptoms may persist for more than a year after an acute attack of hepatitis, and the liver remains enlarged with a normal or firm consistency. Minor abnormalities are usually found on liver function tests.

On biopsy the liver characteristically has a normal reticulin framework, but there is conspicuous round cell infiltration of the portal tracts and patchy necrosis of the liver cells. Although the histological appearance may remain unaltered for years, the outcome is generally favourable, with minimal scarring in the portal zones. Very rarely, the process terminates in cirrhosis.

In the section shown here a dense pattern of round cells and fibrous cells is seen in the portal tract. Some of the parenchymal cells show evidence of incipient necrosis with darkly stained cytoplasm and pyknotic nuclei. (A = portal tract, B = parenchyma.)

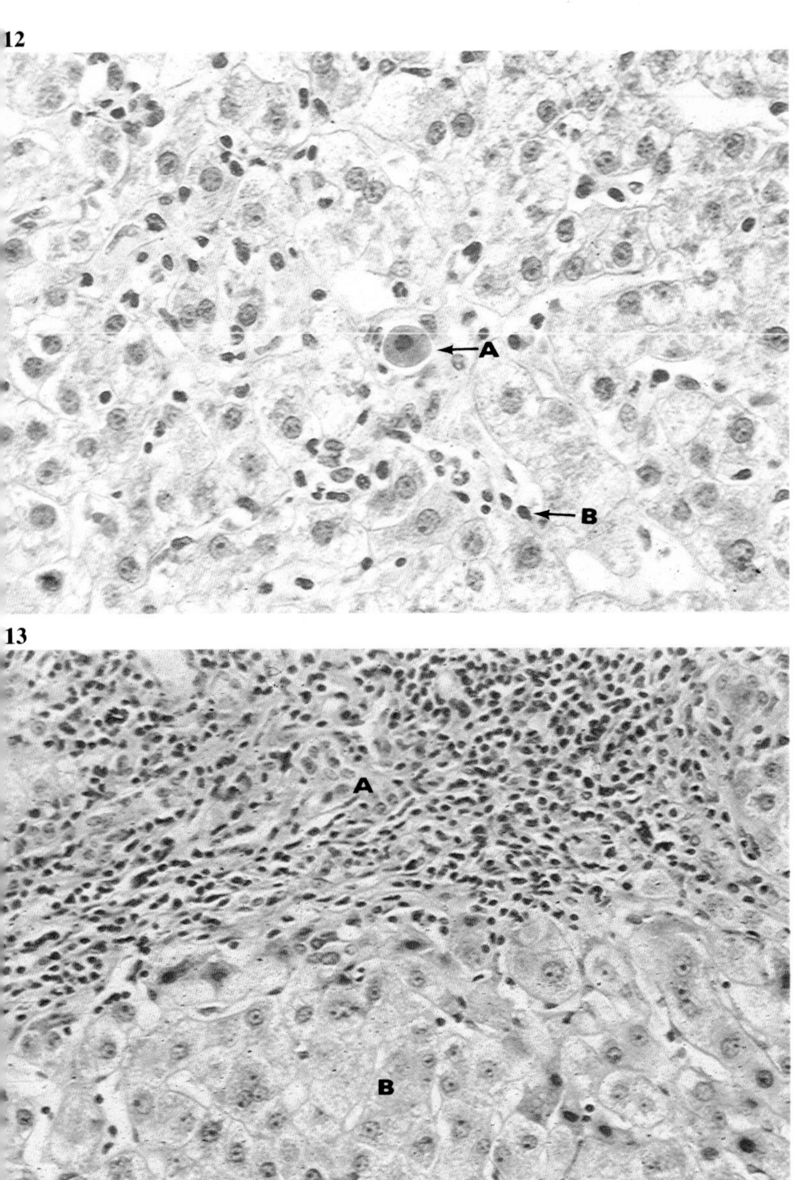
12
A
B
13
A
B

314 Hepatic necrosis. Histology of liver (H and E). In a few patien with severe hepatitis, recovery may be accompanied by extensiv scarring. During the acute stage of the illness widespread destruction c parenchymal cells leads to collapse of the reticulin framework an approximation of adjacent portal tracts. As recovery takes place th destroyed liver cells are replaced by fibrous tissue, which separate nodules of regenerated liver cells. With time, the fibrous tissue contrac and becomes less cellular. The final stage is a coarsely scarred nodul liver.

The section shows an early stage of the process with a band of fibro tissue and lymphocytes separating nodules of parenchymal cells. (A fibrous tissue and lymphocytes, B = parenchymal cells.)

Clinical features

315 Appearance of urine in hepatitis. In acute viral hepatitis bilirubi appears in the urine before the patient becomes jaundiced. Urobilin found in the urine during the early stages but disappears at the height c the illness and returns as liver function improves.

Urine containing bile is greenish or brownish-yellow in colour. Th surface tension is altered and the froth, which forms on top afte shaking, is usually permanent. Conjugated bilirubin is excreted in th urine but unconjugated bilirubin is not. Urine containing an excess c urobilin develops a warm orange colour on standing.

The colour of the faeces in virus hepatitis varies with the degree c intrahepatic obstruction.

316 Jaundiced sclera. Elastic tissue has a special affinity for bilirubi so structures with a high content of elastic tissue, such as skin, ocul sclera and blood vessels, readily become jaundiced and retain th pigment even after the serum bilirubin has returned to normal.

Compare the jaundiced eye of viral hepatitis with the suffused eye c leptospiral jaundice in **170**.

4

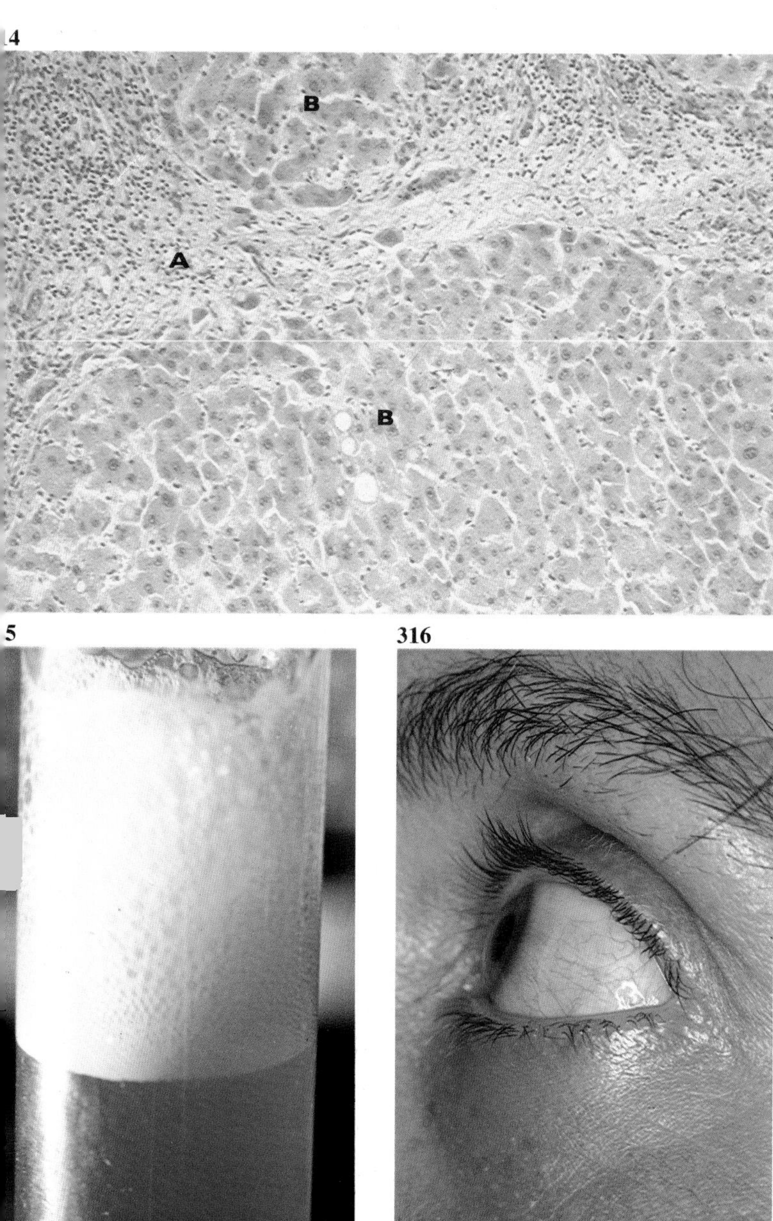

5

316

317 Jaundiced skin. The water-soluble conjugated bilirubin, found
patients with hepatocellular and cholestatic jaundice, produces a mo
intense colour in the skin than the unconjugated pigment of haemolyt
jaundice. The skin of patients with long-standing obstructive jaundi
may have a greenish tinge, possibly as a result of biliverdin and oth
pigments.

In this illustration the colour of normal skin is contrasted with t
yellow skin of a patient with acute hepatitis.

318 Rash in viral hepatitis. Rashes are found in 5% of patients wi
viral hepatitis. They are seen more commonly in HBsAg-positi
hepatitis, particularly in the pre-icteric phase, when they may
associated with arthralgia. The rash may be erythematous, macul
papular, or urticarial. Purpuric rashes are common in patients with liv
failure.

The illustration shows an erythematous rash on the leg of a patie
with virus B hepatitis.

319 Virus B hepatitis. Long-incubation (virus B) hepatitis is general
transmitted by blood or blood products. As little as 0·004 ml of seru
has been known to cause infection. Patients and staff in renal dialys
units are particularly vulnerable to this disease, and there is also a hi
incidence in drug addicts and homosexuals.

The patient shown here was one of a group of young men infect
from a tattooing needle. The intensity of the jaundice is shown by t
contrast with the normal colour of the physician's hand.

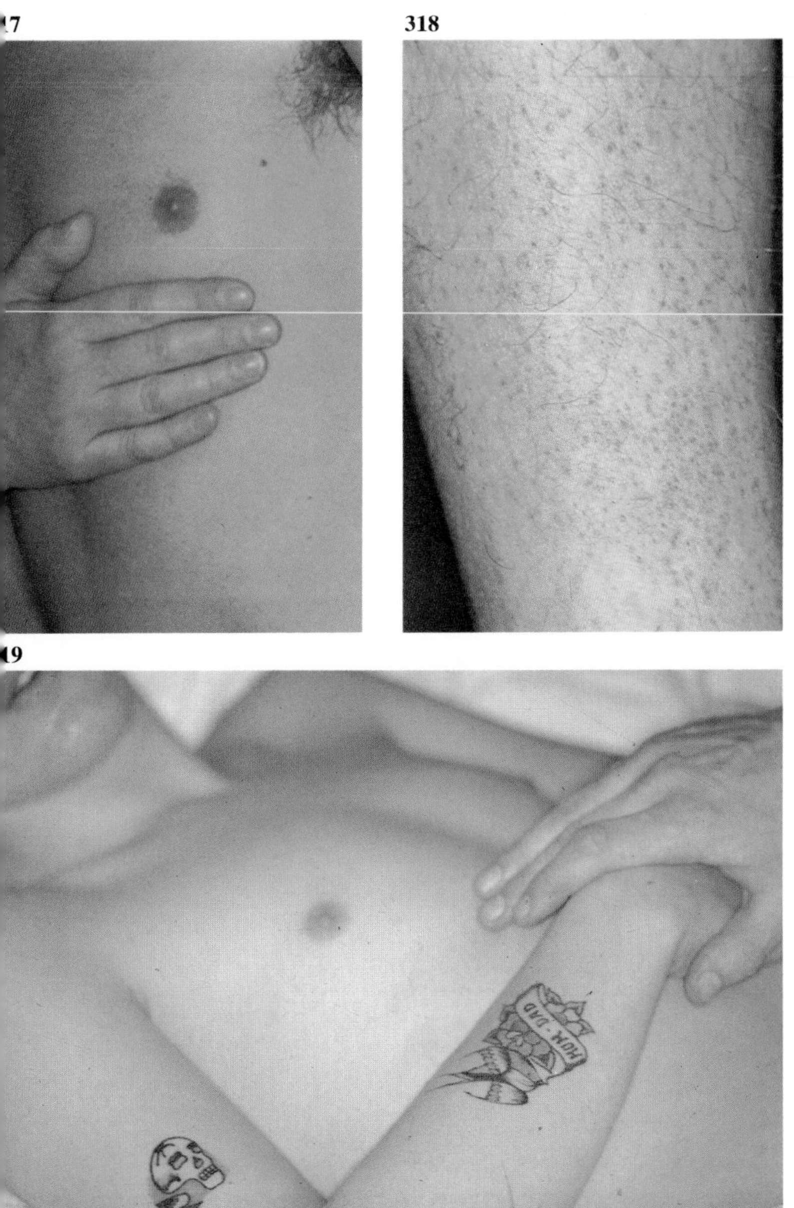
17
318
19
MOM · DAD

Myxovirus infection

Myxoviruses are responsible for many respiratory diseases of mar other mammals, and birds. They are so-named because they possess special affinity for mucin. The viruses contain a core of RNA, wit protein capsomeres arranged along its coils. The outer membrane has lipid component, so the viruses are sensitive to ether. Most myxoviruse possess haemagglutinins, and some also possess haemolysins. Th viruses are easily deformed and therefore difficult to measure, bu commonly range in size from 80 to 150nm. They may be spherical c filamentous in shape. Myxoviruses can be divided into two subgroup but only those members affecting man will be considered.

a) Orthomyxoviruses — influenza viruses A, B and C. These are sma and have filamentous forms. The internal structure of RNA is slende They lack haemolysins.

b) Paramyxoviruses — measles virus, mumps virus, parainfluenz viruses 1, 2, 3 and 4. These are large and vary in size. The RN structure is thicker. Filamentous forms are not found. They posses haemolysins as well as haemagglutinins.

Influenza

Influenza is a highly infectious disease caused by *Myxovirus influenzae*; there are three distinct serotypes (A, B and C), each containing antigenic strains. Although the illness caused by the two main viruses, A and B, cannot be distinguished clinically, the epidemiological pattern is different. Virus A causes both pandemics and localised outbreaks, whereas virus B is found in limited epidemics and sporadic cases. Influenza shows the phenomenon of antigenic drift, and the emergence of a new antigenic strain may herald a pandemic. Infection is airborne and the virus gains access through the respiratory passages.

A short incubation period of one to four days is followed by abrupt onset of fever with headache and myalgia. The virus damages the respiratory mucosa causing nasal obstruction, sore throat and a dry hacking cough. Sweating is a marked feature. In uncomplicated influenza there are few physical signs. The duration of the illness is very variable, but the temperature generally returns to normal on the third or fourth day. In severe attacks bronchiolitis and pneumonia may be caused directly by the virus or by secondary bacterial invasion of the lungs. Although mortality is low, the attack rate is high and pandemics with new antigenic strains may result in millions of deaths.

Virology

320 Electron micrograph of influenza virus. Particles from infected allantoic fluid are spherical in shape and measure 80 to 120nm in diameter. Recently isolated virus A may be filamentous and have the same diameter, but measures several microns in length. The virion consists of a hollow, helically arranged nucleoprotein thread, 800nm in length and 9nm in diameter, coiled in a central mass. The viral nucleoprotein is formed within the nucleus of the host cell. The outer membrane has rod-like projections containing haemagglutinin, and neuraminidase is also present on the surface.

Influenza viruses can be grown on embryonated hen eggs and cultures of mammalian cells. The virus causes agglutination of human and fowl red blood cells. Each type of influenza virus is characterised by its specific nucleoprotein (soluble) antigen. Antigens present in the envelope (V-antigens) give subtype or strain-specific reactions.

Pathology

321 Influenza — appearance of trachea and lungs. When death occurs during the early stages of influenza, before secondary bacterial invasion the lungs are brightly mottled with subpleural haemorrhages, and blood-stained fluid runs freely from any cut surface. The trachea and bronchi are congested and there is considerable destruction of the epithelial lining. On section, the lungs are haemorrhagic and solid, a finding that readily explains the extreme respiratory distress and cyanosis preceding death. Pneumonia developing at a later stage is caused by secondary bacterial infection, often staphylococcal. (A = larynx, B = trachea.)

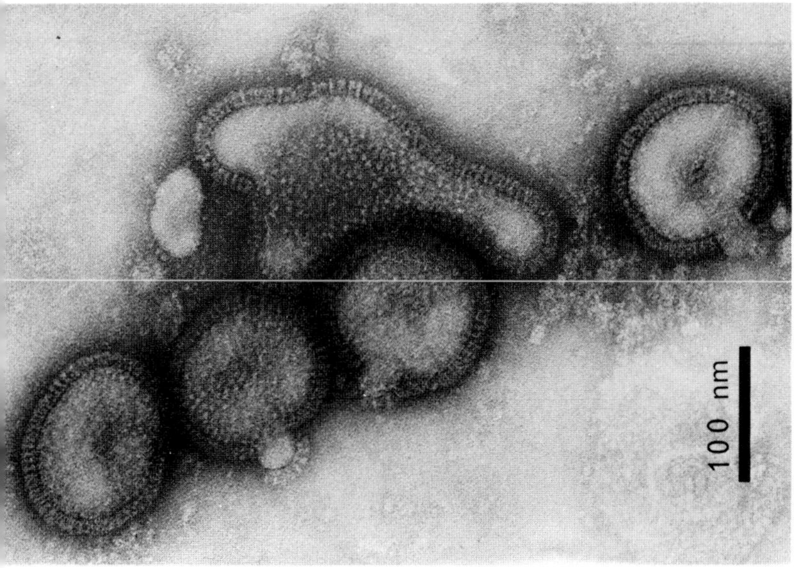

321

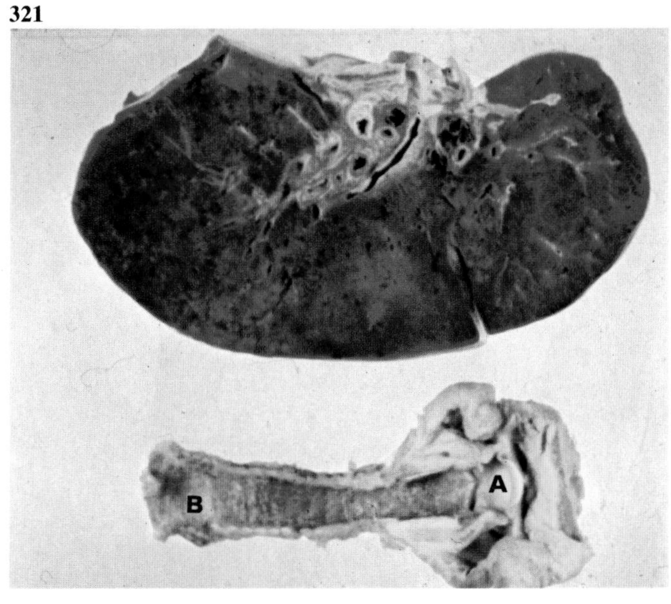

322 Section of trachea (H and E). The trachea and bronchi bear the brunt of the initial damage to the respiratory tract by influenza virus. The submucosa is swollen and infiltrated by mononuclear cells, while the ciliated columnar epithelium has been shed from the basement membrane. This injury to the lining of the trachea and bronchi paves the way for secondary invasion by bacteria from the upper respiratory passages. (A = desquamating epithelium, B = basement membrane, C = submucosa with mononuclear cells, D = cartilage ring.)

323 Section of lung in influenza (H and E). The alveolar walls are thickened and infiltrated by mononuclear cells. The air sacs are free from exudate. There is congestion around the small bronchus in the centre of the section, and the lumen is plugged with mononuclear cells. (A = air sac, B = thickened alveolar wall, C = bronchus with plug.)

324 Section of lung in influenza (H and E). Under higher magnification it can be seen that the alveolar structure is retained but the walls are notably thickened and infiltrated by mononuclear cells. The air sacs are free from exudate, but there is a heavy deposit of hyaline material on the surface, which would greatly impede the absorption of oxygen. A similar appearance is found in hyaline membrane disease of neonates and in radiation pneumonitis. (A = air sac, B = alveolar wall, C = hyaline material.)

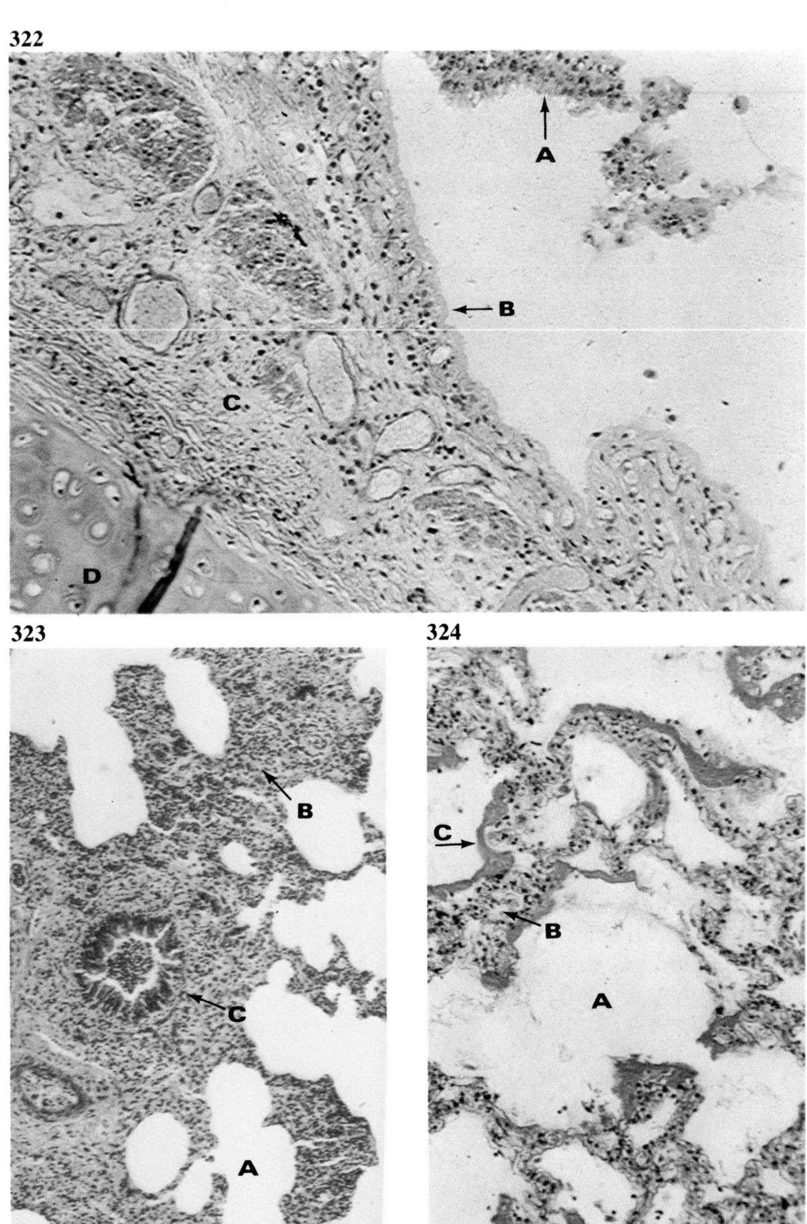

322
A
B
C
D
323
B
C
A
324
C
B
A

Mumps

Mumps is a generalised viral infection with a predilection for the salivary glands, but many other structures may be affected, and inflammation of the testes, pancreas or central nervous system may be the only manifestation. Subclinical attacks are very common and account for about 30% of all cases of mumps.

Mumps is only moderately infectious, and man is the sole reservoir of infection. The virus is disseminated by infected saliva and gains access through the respiratory passages. Virus may also be found in urine, but there is no evidence that this is important in the spread of mumps.

Myxovirus parotidis possesses haemagglutinin and haemolysin. Filamentous forms are not found. It is a single antigenic entity distinct from other myxoviruses. Mumps virus has two complement-fixing antigens, V (viral antigen) and S (soluble antigen). Following active infection, V antibody develops slowly but persists, whereas S antibody appears during the first week of illness, reaches a peak, and then declines.

Virology

325 Normal monkey kidney cell culture.

326 Mumps virus in monkey kidney cells. Mumps virus grows rather more slowly in chick embryo than does influenza virus. It does not have a cytopathogenic effect, but may be detected in the amniotic fluid by agglutination of fowl red blood cells.

Isolation of the virus may be best achieved in cultures of HeLa, human amnion, or monkey kidney cells, in which it produces a cytopathic effect with formation of giant cells and cytoplasmic inclusions. The presence of virus may be shown by haemadsorption with chick, human, guineapig, or sheep red blood cells. The supernatant fluid will agglutinate fowl or human red cells.

The diagnosis of mumps is most readily confirmed by complement-fixation tests on paired sera.

325

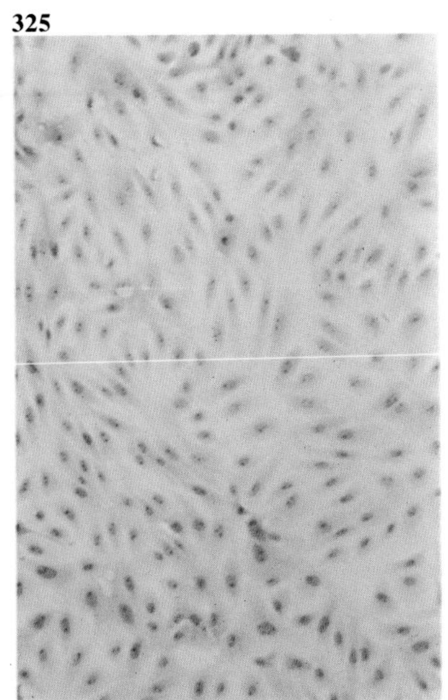

326

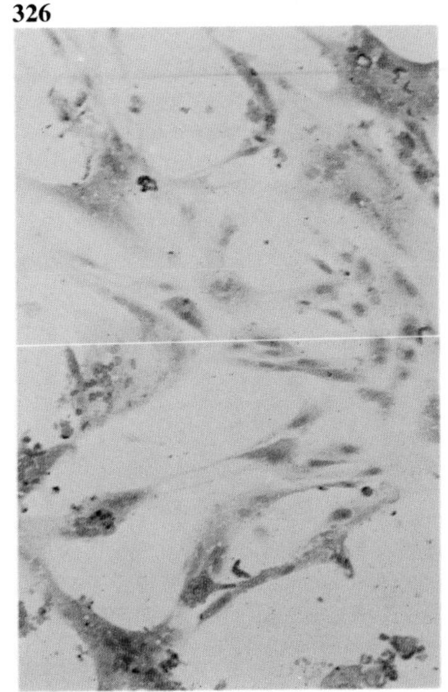

Clinical features

327 Parotitis in child. Mumps is a generalised infection with a wide range of clinical manifestations. Parotitis is common and may be accompanied by inflammation of other structures. Both parotid glands are involved in 70% of patients with parotitis.

The illness begins with fever and malaise, quickly followed by trismus and pain behind the angle of the jaw. Within 24 hours the parotid gland begins to swell, the hollow behind the angle of the mandible fills, and the swelling extends over the ramus. Confusion sometimes arises with enlarged lymph nodes, but these are usually sited below the parotid gland and the posterior border of the ramus can be sharply defined.

328 Parotid papilla in mumps. Redness of the parotid papilla is a helpful early sign. Any fluid discharged from the parotid duct is clear.

329 Parotid papilla in suppurative parotitis. In suppurative parotitis a bead of pus may drip or be expressed from the duct. This form of parotitis is common in debilitated patients but may be found occasionally in previously healthy individuals.

327

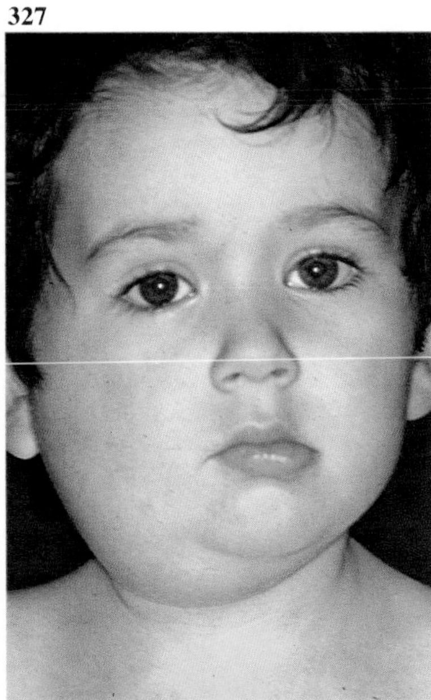

328

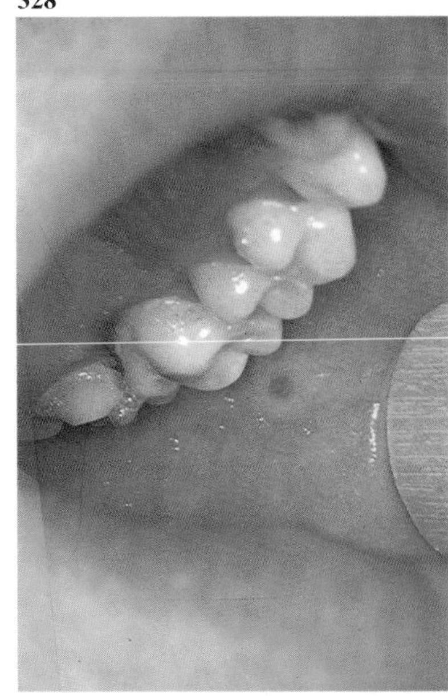

329

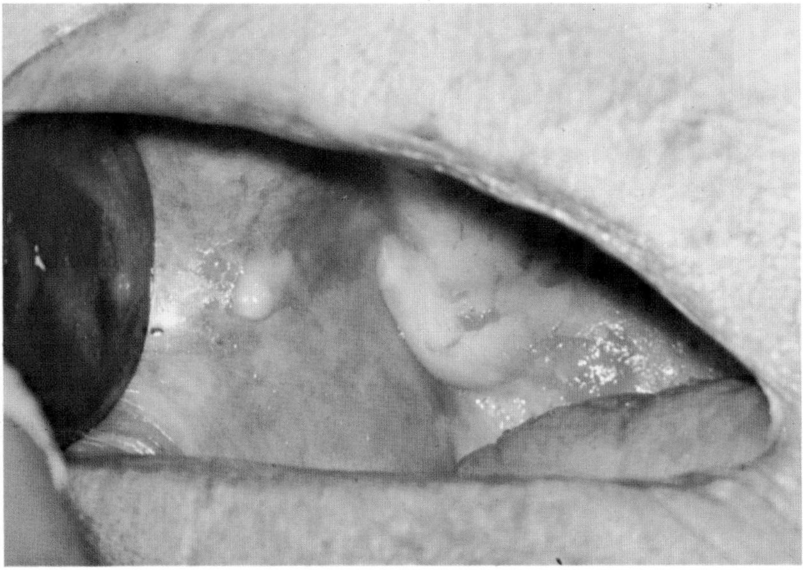

330 Parotitis in adult. Although only 60% of adults are aware of having had an attack of mumps, serological tests show a much higher incidence. The illness tends to be more severe in adults, and the swelling is more painful. Parotitis in the elderly is usually caused by bacterial invasion along the parotid duct.

331 Acute parotitis — oedema of tissues. Swelling of the parotid gland may be accompanied by oedema of the surrounding tissues, which extend into the floor of the mouth and downwards in the neck to the insertion of the deep cervical fascia in the manubrium sterni. This gelatinous oedema is particularly common in black people and a sharp tap will produce a jelly-like quivering in the affected tissues.

332 Appearance on recovery. The oedema has subsided and normal appearance has been restored.

330

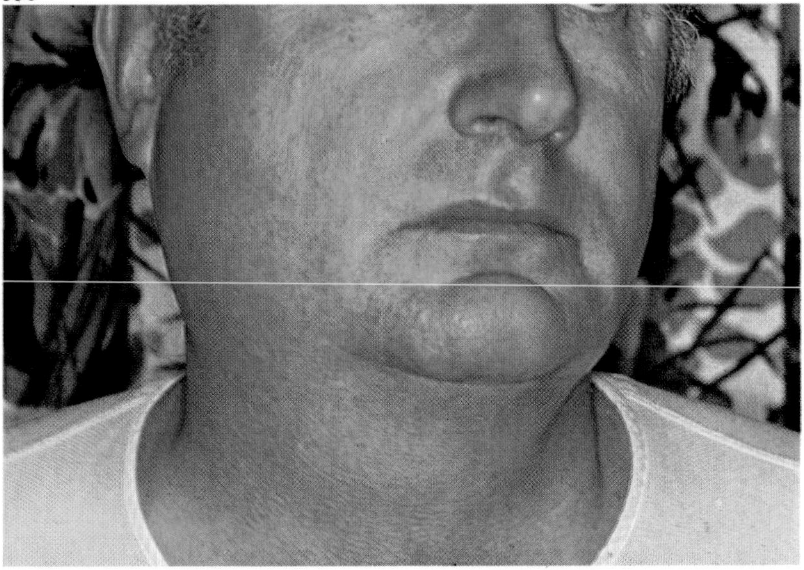

331

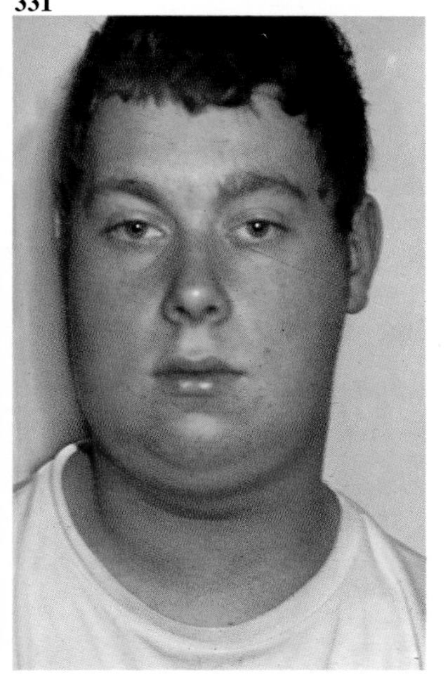

332

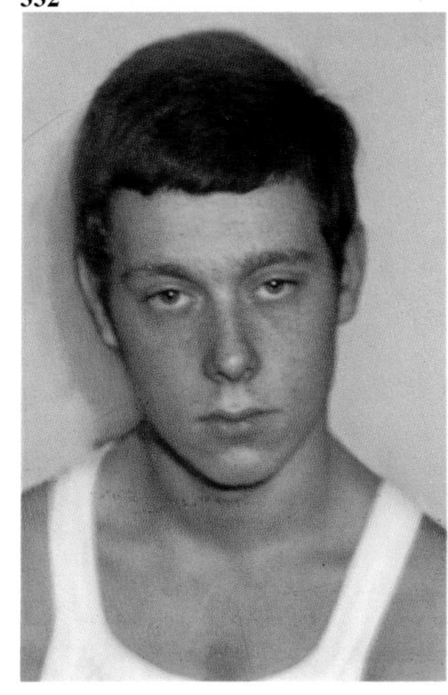

333 Submaxillary mumps. The submaxillary glands are affected in 10% of patients with mumps. The diagnosis is easy when the parotid glands are also swollen, but otherwise may be exceedingly difficult. A white blood cell count, serum amylase estimation, or complement-fixation tests are helpful in distinguishing submaxillary salivary adenitis from submaxillary lymphadenitis.

334 Orchitis. Mumps orchitis seldom occurs before puberty. It is usually associated with parotitis, but may be the sole manifestation. The incidence varies considerably in different epidemics but averages 20 to 25% in adolescent and adult males with mumps. It is unilateral in 80% of cases. The testicular swelling may be aggravated by a hydrocele or by oedema of the scrotum.

335 Electrocardiographic changes in mumps. During the acute stage of the illness electrocardiograms are found to be abnormal in 5 to 15% of cases. The common abnormalities are flattening or inversion of T waves, and depression of the ST segment. The cardiograms return to normal during convalescence. Clinical evidence of myocarditis is rare, but pericarditis may occasionally be detected. Similar electrocardiographic changes are found in many other infections.

The tracings opposite (V_4) were taken from a 10-year-old boy with mumps but no clinical evidence of heart involvement. The first ECG was taken during the acute stage, the second two weeks later, and the third after 10 weeks. The myocardial damage has steadily improved.

333

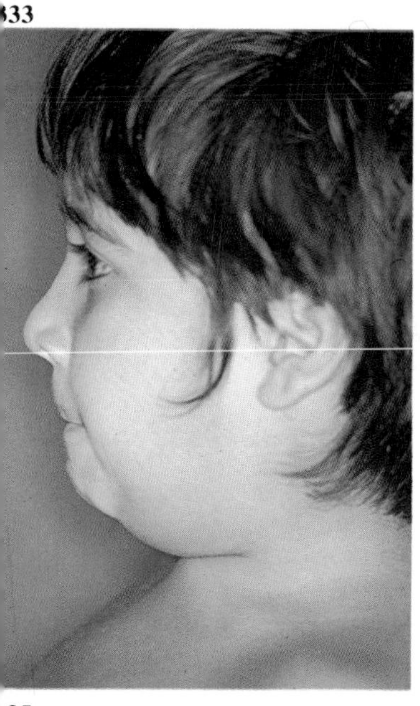

334

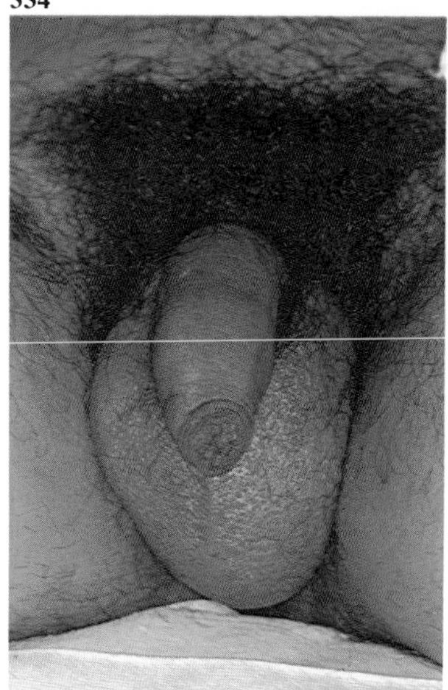

335

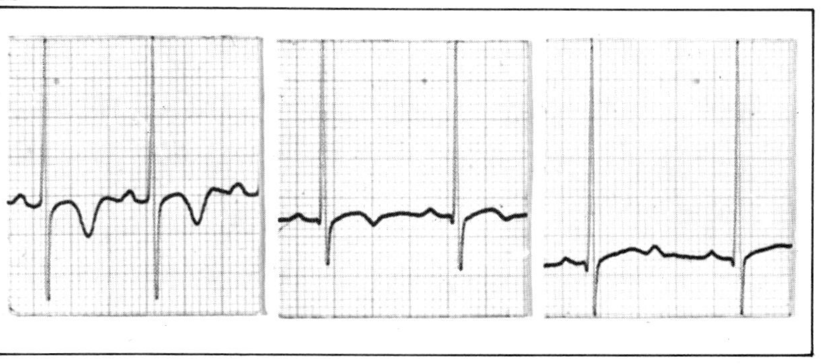

Measles

Measles is a highly infectious disease caused by a virus closely related to the larger myxoviruses. Patients are infectious during the acute stage of the illness, and virus is transmitted by the airborne route. There are no carriers, so spread is by direct case-to-case contact. The illness is characterised clinically by a catarrhal prodromal stage, followed by a florid, generalised maculopapular eruption. Damage to the respiratory mucosa facilitates secondary bacterial invasion of the middle ear or lungs. Cerebral disturbance is common and may take several forms. Immunity is life-long.

Virology

336 Electron micrograph of measles virus. Measles virus belongs to the genus *Morbillivirus,* which includes the viruses causing distemper in dogs and rinderpest in cattle. On electron microscopy the virus is roughly circular in outline and measures 120 to 140 nm in diameter. The outer envelope contains lipid and protein. Haemagglutinin is present but neuraminidase is lacking. Spikes may be seen radiating from the surface. The nucleocapsid contains RNA and has a helical structure.

337 Normal monkey kidney cells.

338 Measles virus in monkey kidney cells. Primate kidney cells are most effective for primary isolation, but higher concentrations may subsequently be obtained in other tissues. Once isolated, the virus can easily be adapted to continuous cell lines of human origin. It has also been adapted to growth on chick amnion.

The nature of the cytopathic effect varies with the strain of the virus, the type of cell, and the composition of the medium. In primary culture the affected cells form syncytia, but on serial passage the principal change is alteration in the shape of cells from polygonal to spindle. Intranuclear inclusions are a constant finding. Compare with normal monkey kidney cells in **337**.

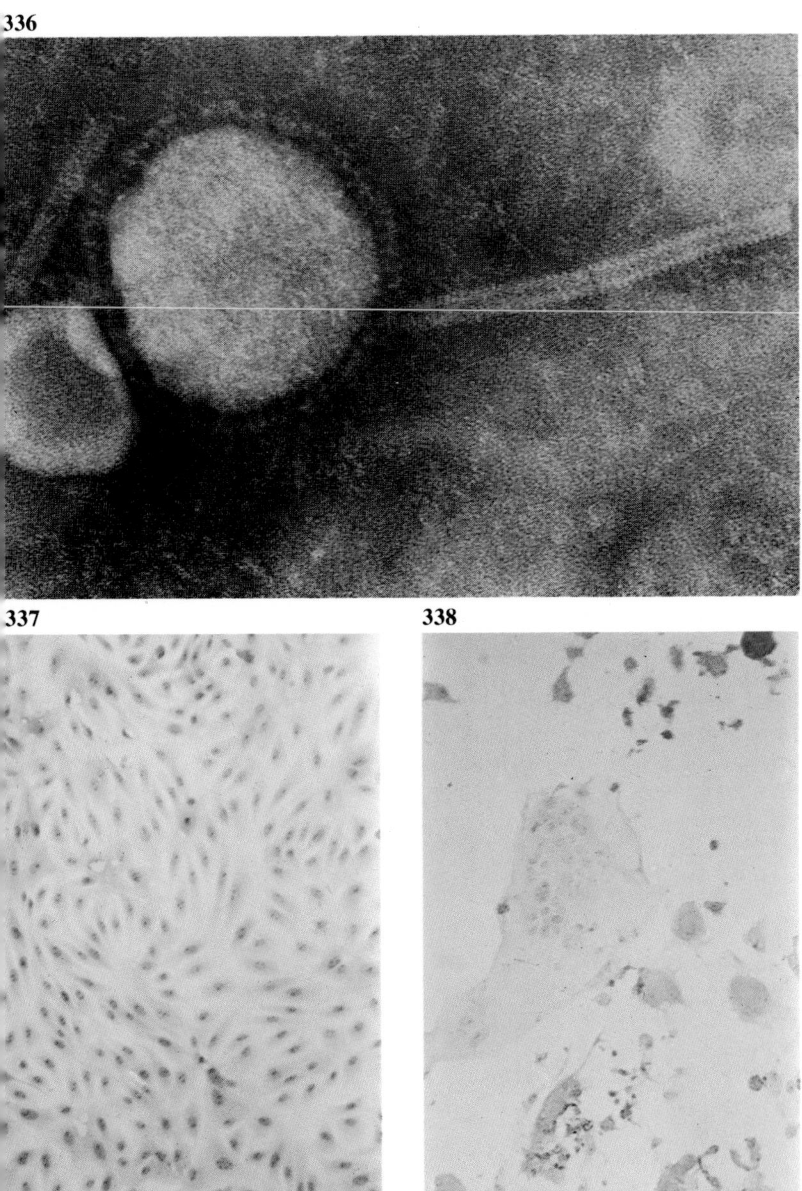

336

337

338

339 Histology of lung in measles (H and E). During the acute stage of measles the virus may give rise to an interstitial pneumonia resulting in severe respiratory distress. Secondary bacterial invasion of the lungs usually occurs at a later stage, when the rash is fading, and produces a patchy bronchopneumonia.

In the lung section shown here the alveolar pattern has not been disturbed, but the air sacs are packed with mononuclear cells. Very little fibrin is present. Some of the alveoli are lined with hyaline membrane, which can interfere seriously with gaseous exchange. Note the large multinucleated giant cells. (A = air sac with mononuclear cells, B = hyaline material, C = multinucleated giant cell.)

340 Measles pneumonia (histology of lung, red and yellow stain). A large multinucleated giant cell can be seen in the centre of the section. The viral nucleic acid has stained pale pink.

In patients with leukaemia, mucoviscoidosis, and Letterer–Siwe disease, where cell-mediated immunity is defective, infection with measles virus may not result in the classical disease but give rise to giant-cell pneumonia, a prolonged and usually fatal illness. (A = giant cell, B = viral nucleic acid.)

341 Histology of appendix (H and E). In the prodromal catarrhal stage of measles, vomiting and diarrhoea are common in young children. The appendix and colon at this stage are infiltrated with mononuclear cells, and giant cells are formed. The congestion of the appendix may be sufficient to cause symptoms of appendicitis. As the rash emerges the multinucleated cells disappear. (A = mucosa, B = lymphoid follicle, C = giant cell.)

339

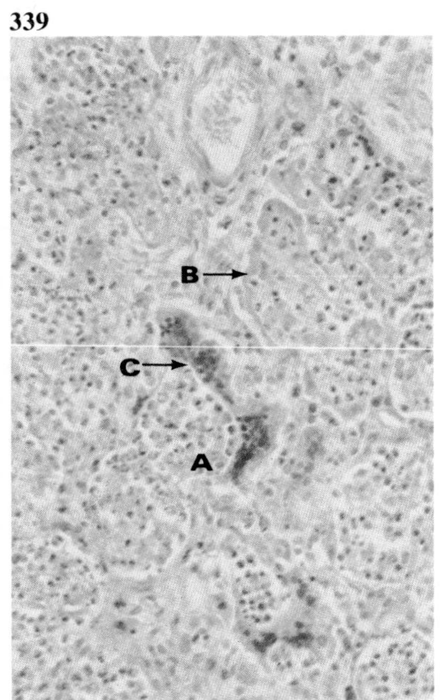

340

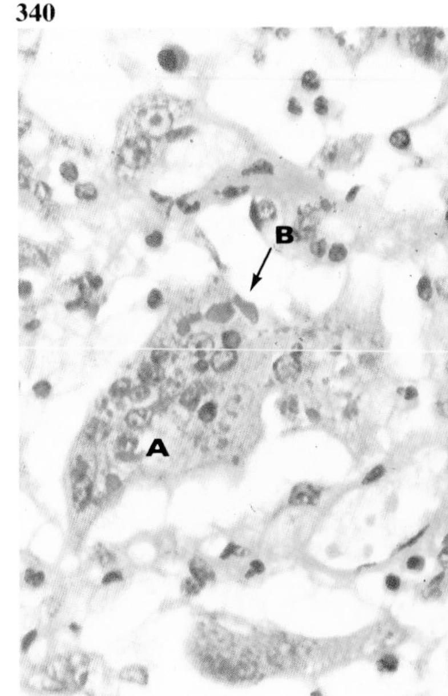

341

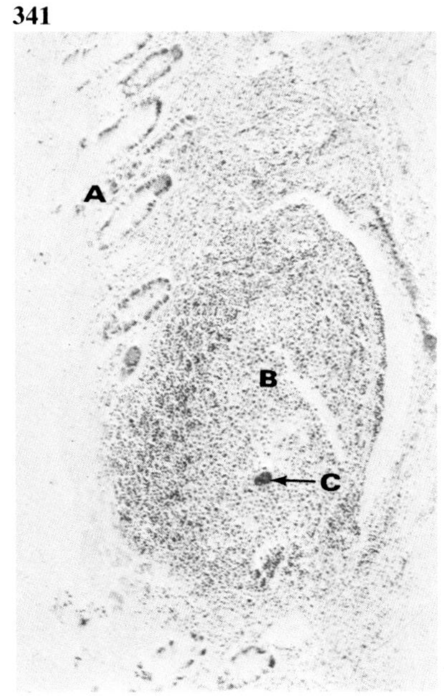

342 Appearance of brain in encephalitis. Post-infectious encephalitis usually develops three to four days after onset of the rash. The incidence is roughly one in 1,000 cases. The brain is congested and the essential lesion is demyelination accompanied by microglial proliferation.

Note the severe inflammation of the meninges, the intense congestion of the cortex, and the dilated blood vessels in the white matter.

Clinical features

343 Koplik's spots. Koplik's spots are pathognomonic of measles. They are found on mucous membranes during the prodromal stage and are easily detected on the mucosa of the cheeks opposite the molar teeth, where they resemble coarse grains of salt on the surface of the inflamed membrane. Histologically the spots consist of small necrotic patches in the basal layers of the mucosa with exudation of serum and infiltration by mononuclear cells.

342

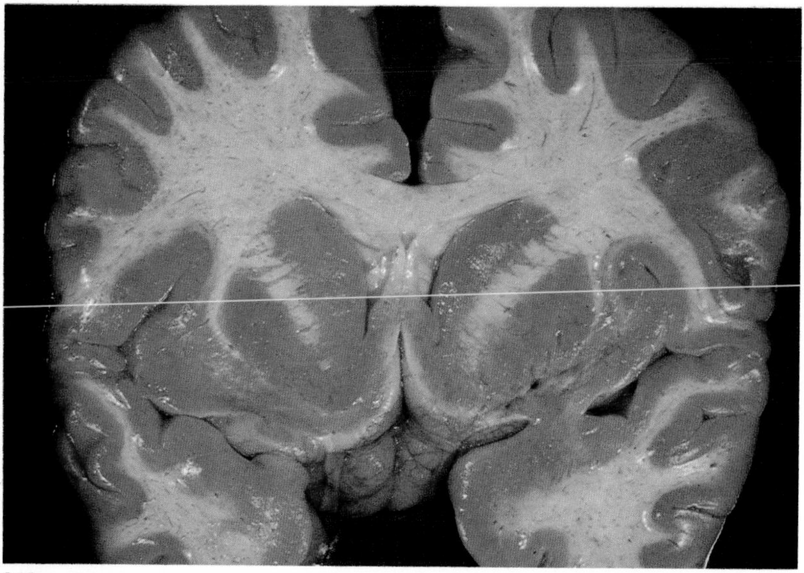

343

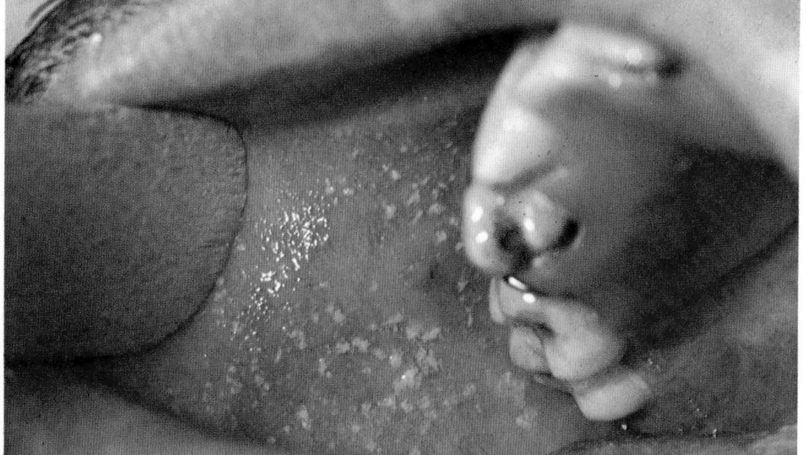

344 Koplik's spots and exanthem. Koplik's spots are nearly always present during the early catarrhal stage of measles but disappear as the rash emerges and cannot be seen after the first or second day of the exanthem.

The child in the illustration has a well-developed rash on her face, and Koplik's spots are still visible inside her mouth.

345 Appearance of face in measles. The face has an unmistakeable appearance, with suffusion of the conjunctivae, congestion of the buccal cavity, and a dusky-red blotchy rash on the skin.

346 Measles rash on first day. A transient erythematous rash during the prodromal period may be confused with scarlet fever, but careful inspection of the mouth will usually disclose Koplik's spots.

The true rash appears behind the ears and along the hairline, quickly affects the face, and spreads progressively from above downwards. On the first day of the rash the face is heavily covered, but elsewhere the spots are scanty.

344

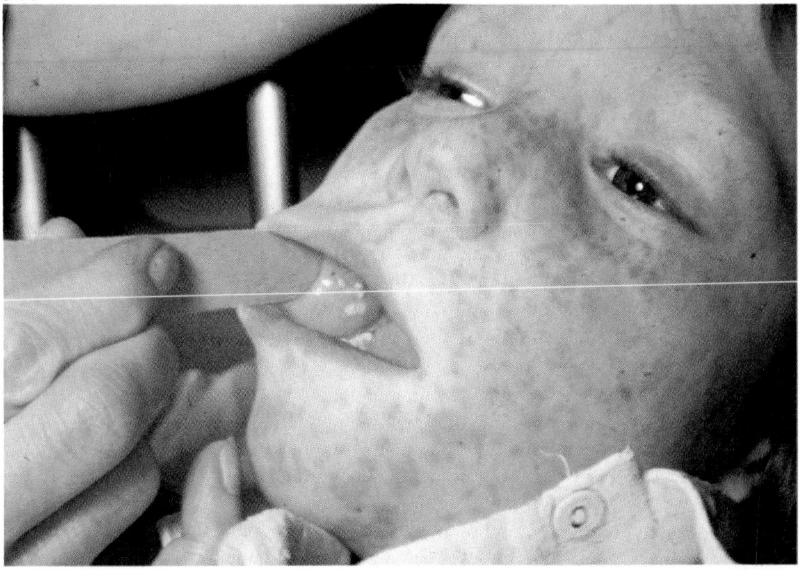

345

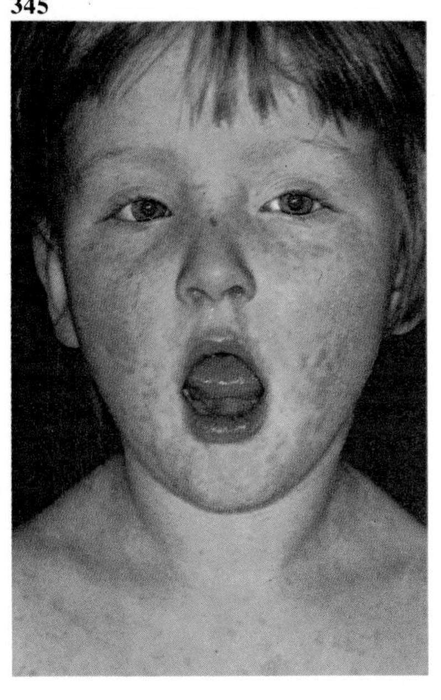

346

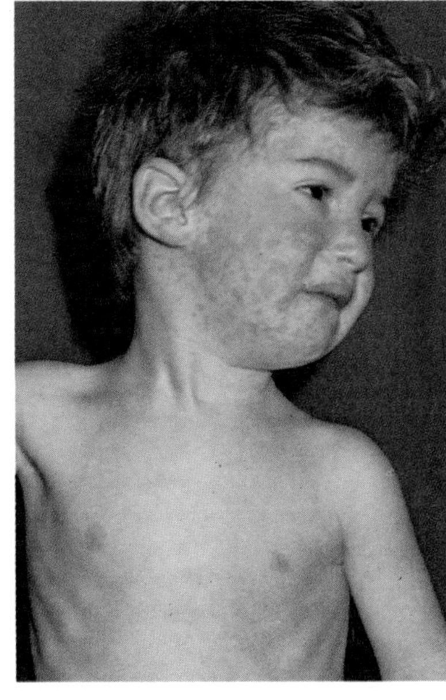

347 Close-up of rash. The rash consists of large macules or slightly raised lesions called maculopapules. These run into each other to form irregular blotches.

348 Rash on second day. Large blotches appear on the trunk during the second day of the rash. The evolution of the exanthem from above downwards is helpful in distinguishing it from drug eruptions of a similar nature that seldom follow this course.

349 Rash on third day. By the third day the rash may have become confluent over most of the body, but some discrete spots remain, especially on the limbs.

347

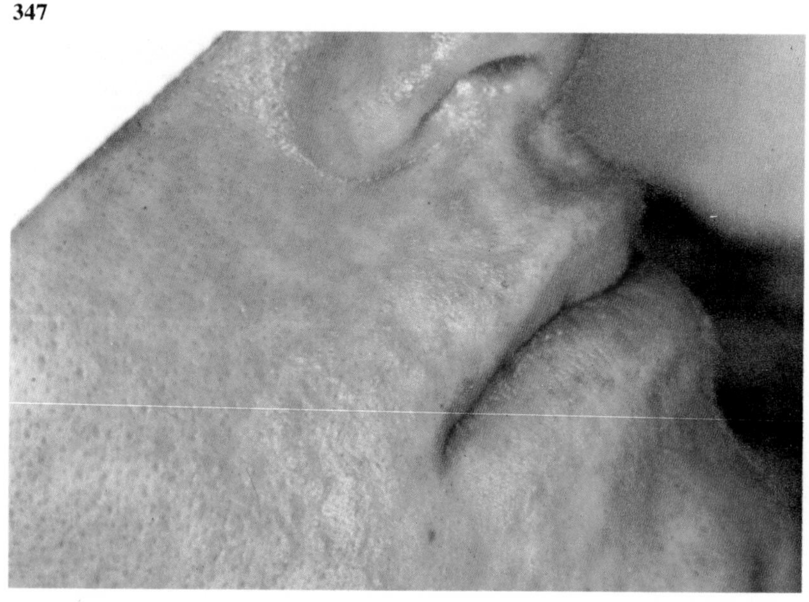

348

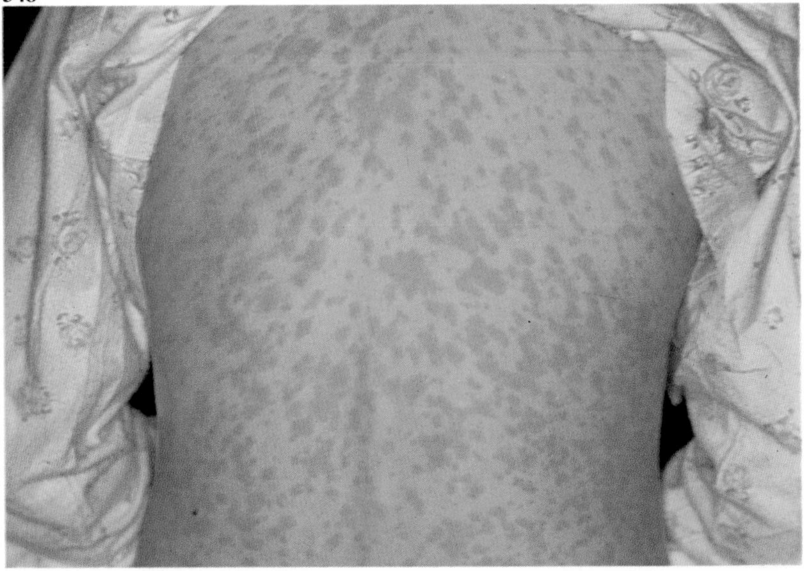

349

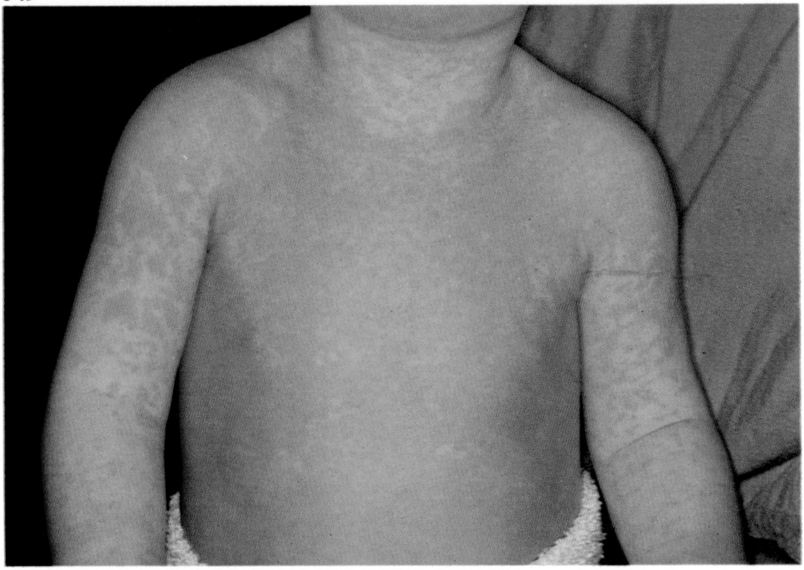

350 Measles in a black child. Measles may be difficult to diagnose in a dark-skinned patient. Catarrh remains a striking feature and Koplik's spots may be found during the prodromal period.

351 Rash in a black child. The erythematous element of the rash is much less conspicuous on a dark skin. The papular component can be thrown into relief by viewing the skin in oblique light.

352 Severe measles. In a severe attack the rash may be confluent over large areas, and fine desquamation may develop. Note the excoriation round the eyes.

350

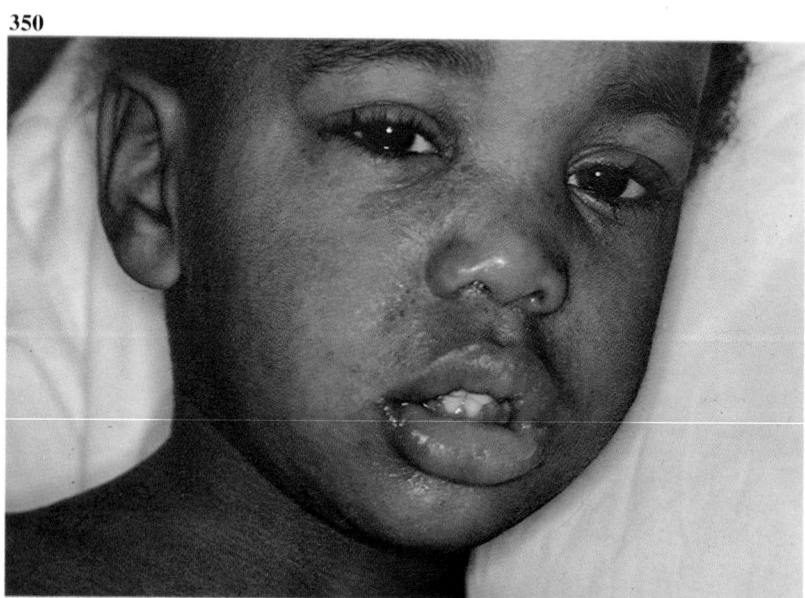

351

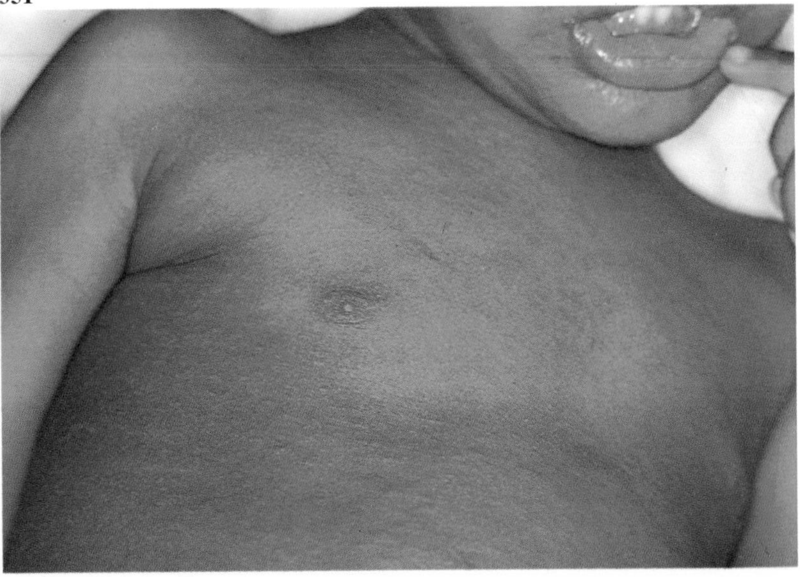

352

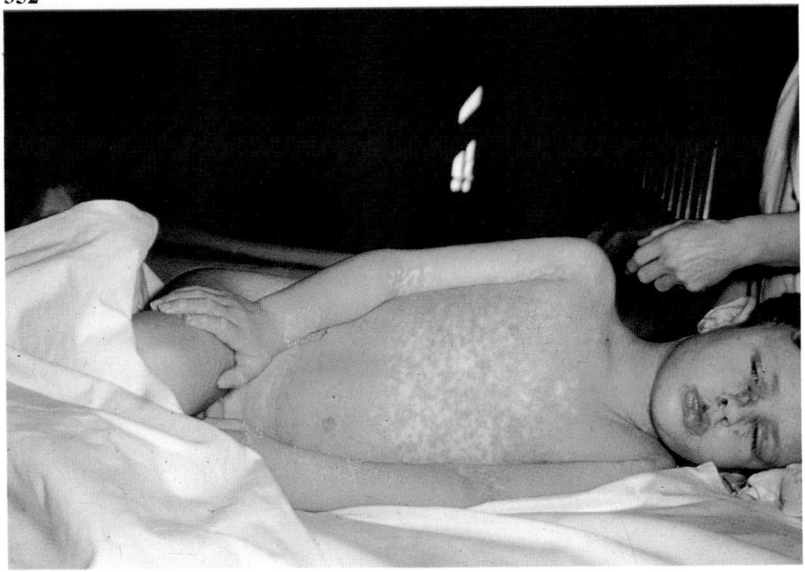

353 Staining. The rash fades in the same order as it appears, leaving a brownish pigmentation of the skin called staining. This may be generalised but sometimes has a patchy distribution. In contrast to the original maculopapular rash, the discoloration does not blanch on pressure. Staining may persist for a week or 10 days, then fades without trace.

354 Rash of secondary stage of syphilis. In secondary syphilis the combination of fever, enlarged lymph nodes, and a heavy maculopapular rash may trap the unwary into diagnosing measles. The history and careful clinical examination will usually point to the correct diagnosis, but in doubtful cases it is wise to check the possibility of syphilis by serological tests. The early macular rash of meningococcal septicaemia may also be confused with measles (**71**).

355 Erythema multiforme. Erythema multiforme may be mistaken for measles, especially when accompanied by conjunctivitis and stomatitis. The rash in erythema multiforme is pleomorphic, and the individual lesions have a pale centre and a bluish tinge. The rash persists for much longer than that of measles.

353

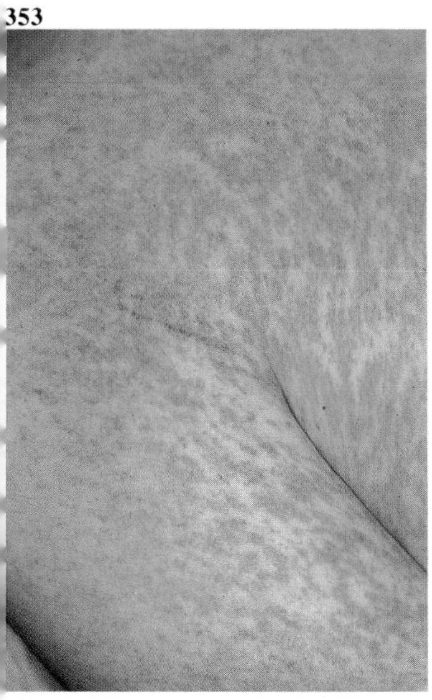

354

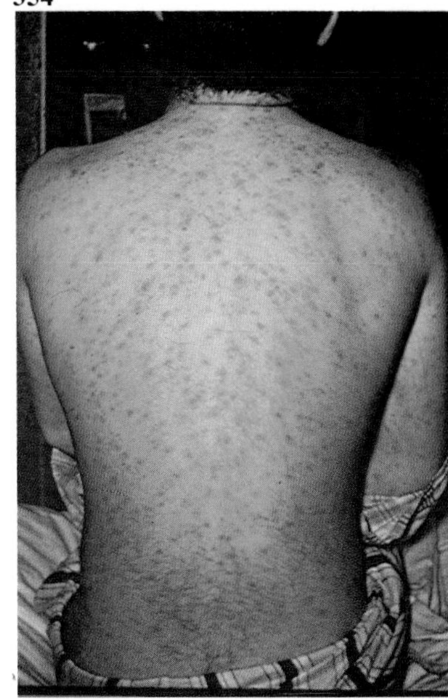

355

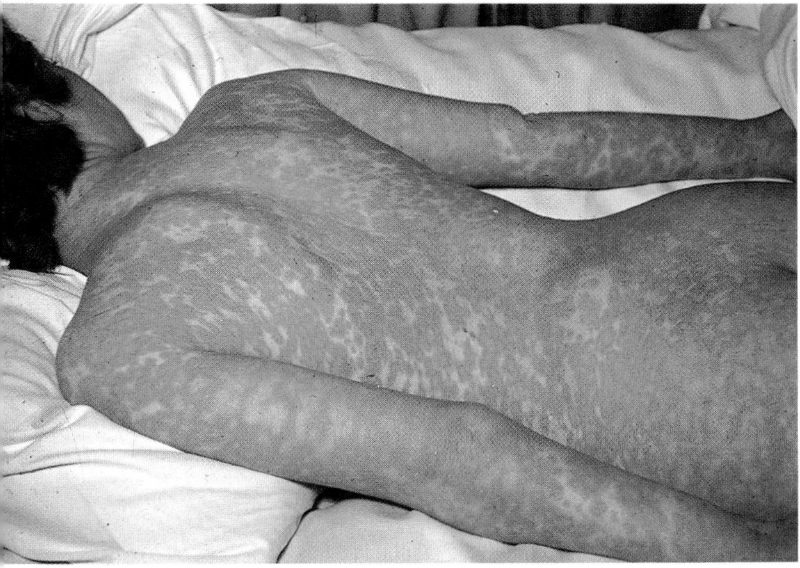

Complications

356 Cancrum oris. Children suffering from protein deficiency as a result of malnutrition are exceedingly vulnerable to measles and have a high death rate from gastroenteritis and pneumonia. Necrotic ulceration of the mouth may sometimes complicate measles in these children.

357 Secondary bacterial pneumonia. Chest radiograph. Respiratory symptoms during the prodromal and early eruptive stages of measles are caused directly by the virus, which is responsible for catarrhal inflammation of the whole respiratory tract. In young children laryngitis may give rise to alarming symptoms of obstruction, but surgery is seldom required. Acute bronchitis is an integral component of measles and x-ray examination during the eruptive phase may show evidence of viral pneumonitis.

As the rash fades the temperature falls and respiratory distress subsides. Damage to the respiratory mucosa, however, may pave the way for secondary bacterial invasion of the lungs, and the expected defervescence may not take place. Respiratory symptoms increase and x-ray examination may reveal patchy opacities of bronchopneumonia. The white blood cell count may switch from a leucopenia to a polymorphonuclear leucocytosis.

356

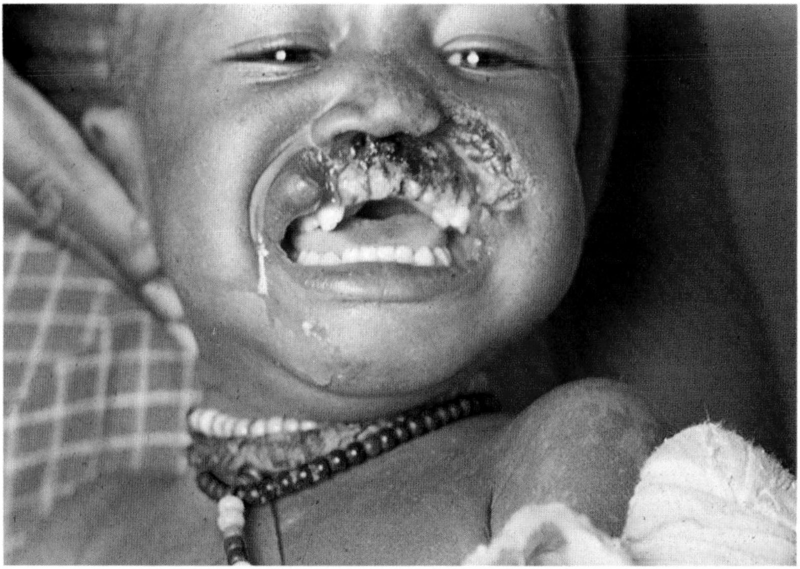

357

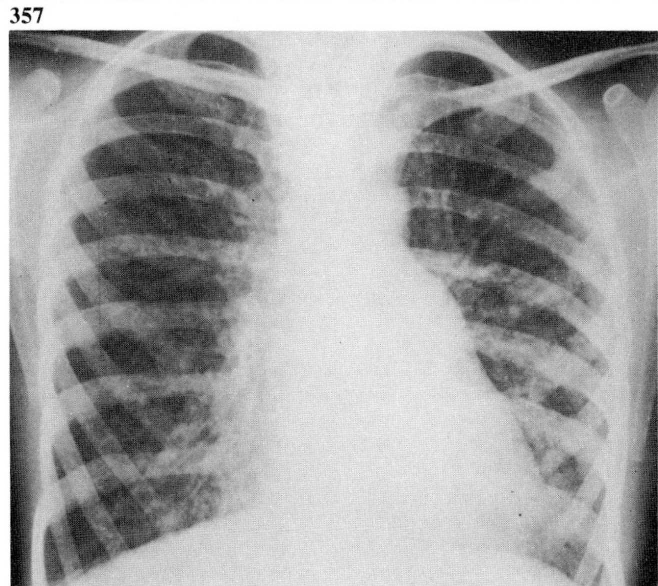

358 Encephalitis — electroencephalogram. Drowsiness and irritability are constant features with measles, and convulsions are common in young children. Transient abnormalities, with an excess of slow wave patterns, are commonly found in electroencephalograms taken during the acute state of the illness. The EEG quickly returns to normal during convalescence. The incidence of abnormalities is higher in children with febrile convulsions, but is unrelated to the height of the fever. EEG changes are appreciable in encephalitis after measles and may persist after clinical recovery.

The tracings shown here were obtained from a five-year-old boy who developed mild encephalitis with drowsiness and neck stiffness three days after the onset of the measles rash. Symptoms persisted for eight days, followed by an uneventful recovery. The EEG returned to normal after two weeks.

359 Post-measles encephalitis. Post-infectious encephalitis varies greatly from transient drowsiness to profound coma, resulting in death or severe disability. The child in the illustration has quadriplegia with paralysis in extension caused by this type of encephalitis. The essential lesion is demyelination accompanied by microglial proliferation, possibly the result of damage from an immunological reaction.

Subacute sclerosing panencephalitis is a rare disease that develops several years after an attack of measles. Virus persists in brain tissue after the original attack, causing severe brain damage with proliferation of microglia but minimal demyelination. The illness evolves slowly and inevitably proves fatal within two years.

358

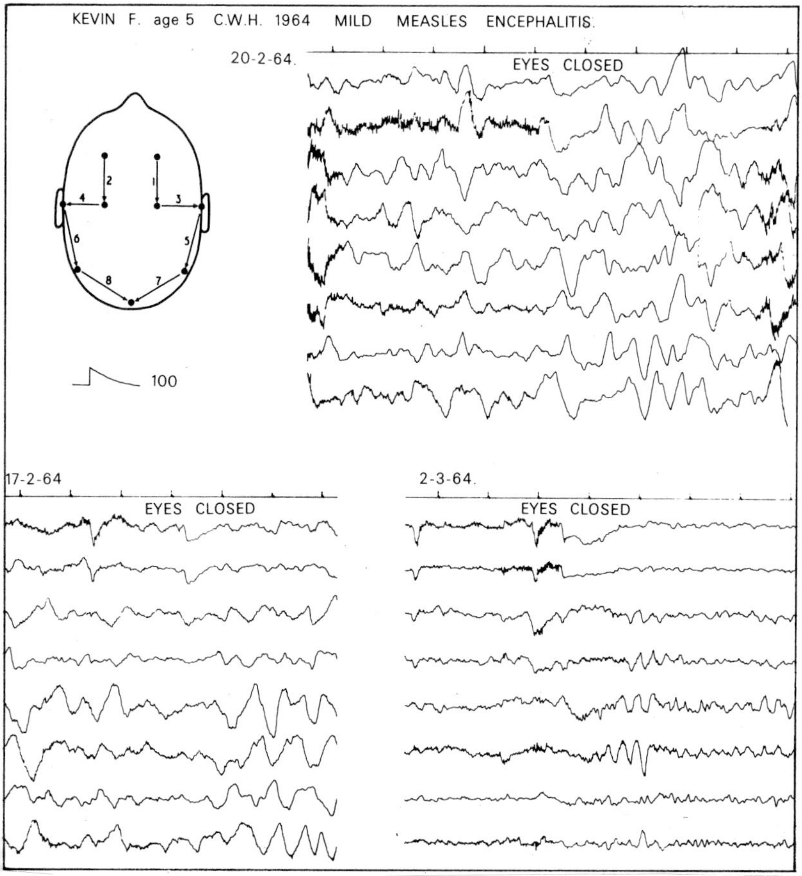

KEVIN F. age 5 C.W.H. 1964 MILD MEASLES ENCEPHALITIS.

20-2-64.

EYES CLOSED

100

17-2-64

EYES CLOSED

2-3-64.

EYES CLOSED

359

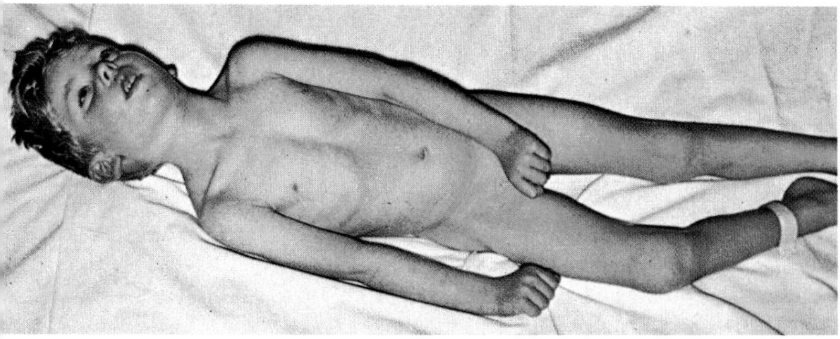

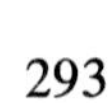

Rubella

Rubella is a virus disease with a worldwide distribution. Epidemics occur at irregular intervals of six to nine years, and the pattern of disease tends to vary from one epidemic to another, suggesting the existence of more than one strain of the virus. In most countries over 80% of the population have developed antibodies against rubella by early adult life.

Postnatal rubella is usually a trivial illness and may occur with or without a rash. Clinical diagnosis is very difficult and often impossible because many other viral infections produce a similiar pattern of disease. For accurate diagnosis, antibody tests should be performed on paired sera or specific antibody should be demonstrated in IgM. Virus is present in the throat for at least a week before and after the onset of the rash, and infection is usually transmitted by droplets.

Active infection with rubella during pregnancy results in congenital rubella. The consequences are varied and unpredictable, ranging from fetal death to birth of an infected, but otherwise normal child. The risk to the fetus is greatest in early pregnancy, and the timing of the attack is critical in determining the site of maximal damage. Virus may be shed from the respiratory passages and urine for many months after birth.

Virology

360 Normal rabbit kidney cells (RK13).

361 Rubella virus in RK13 cells. Rubella virus is rounded or ovoid in shape and measures 120 to 180nm in diameter. It contains RNA and its infectivity is readily destroyed by ether or chloroform and extremes of pH.

The virus grows on primary and continuous cultures of many mammalian cells and produces subclinical infection in several species of laboratory animal. Vervet monkey kidney cells are widely used for isolating the virus, but there is no cytopathic effect, and activity of rubella virus is recognised by interference with growth of a challenge dose of an enterovirus or by indirect immunofluorescent or immunoperoxidase techniques.

In a line of rabbit kidney cells (RK13) the virus regularly produces a cytopathic effect with focal changes and inclusions within the cytoplasm. Cells, destroyed by the virus, pile up as islets on the uniform culture sheet to form characteristic microfoci.

360

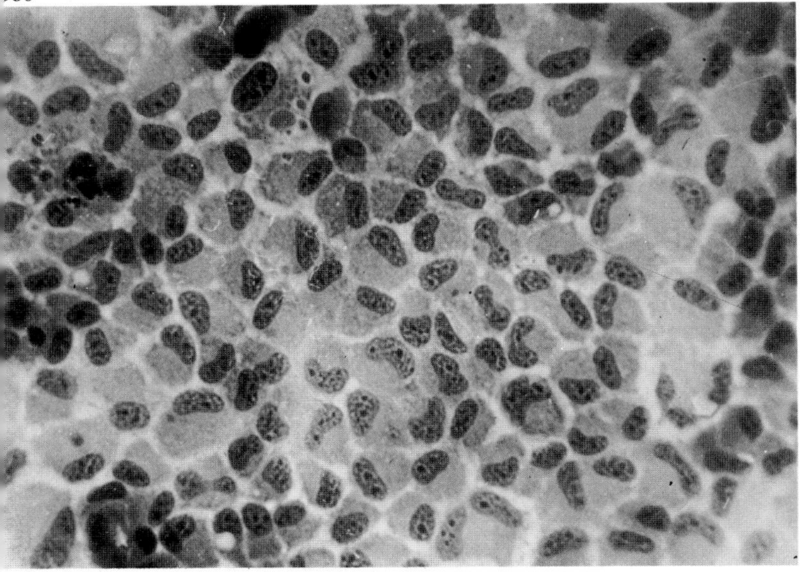

361

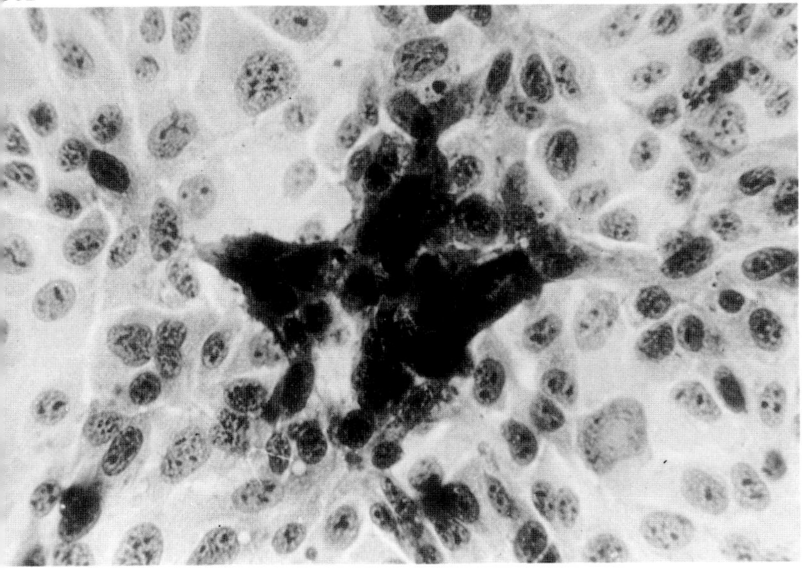

Postnatal rubella

362 Throat in postnatal rubella. Rubella acquired after birth is usually a trivial illness and may manifest with or without a rash. The throat may be painful and slightly inflamed, but exudate is seldom present. There is complete absence of coryza, and the buccal cavity is clean and pale. Koplik's spots are never found.

Rubella in young children often occurs without a rash and is indistinguishable from the numerous other viral infections to which they are prone. Such children form an important reservoir of infection for pregnant women.

363 Conjunctivitis in rubella. The conjunctival injection in rubella is not as marked as in measles and there is no discharge from the eyes. The degree of congestion of the conjunctivae and buccal cavity is of value in differentiating rubella from measles and scarlet fever. In rubella the eyes are suffused but there is no congestion of the buccal cavity; in measles both are inflamed; in scarlet fever the buccal cavity is congested but the eyes remain clear.

364 Rubella rash on first day. The rash consists initially of discrete, delicate pink macules, but sometimes maculopapular and haemorrhagic elements may be found. The severity of the rash varies considerably and is easily missed when lesions are sparse.

Similar rashes may be found in many other virus infections, notably ECHOvirus infections. The clinical diagnosis of rubella is most unreliable and less than half the suspected cases are confirmed when antibody tests are performed on paired sera.

362

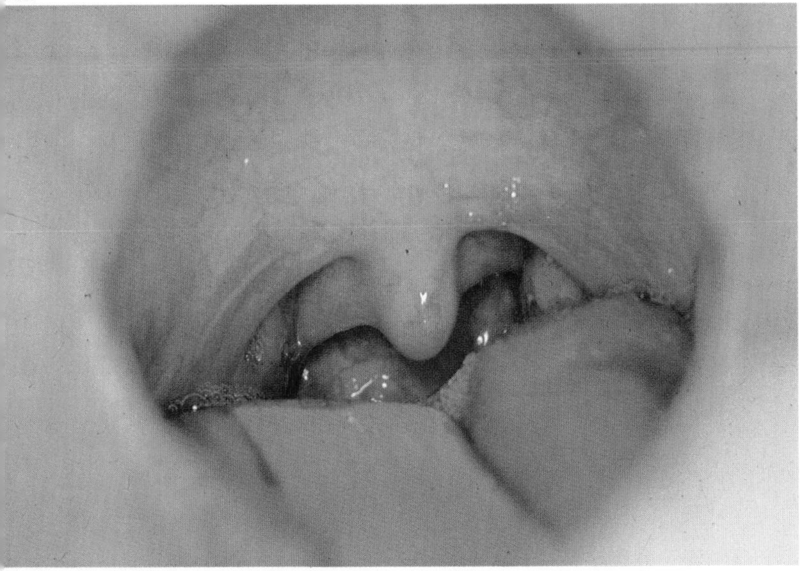

363

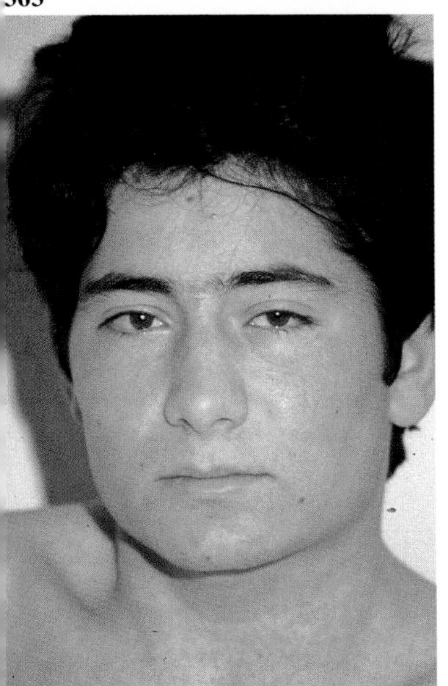

364

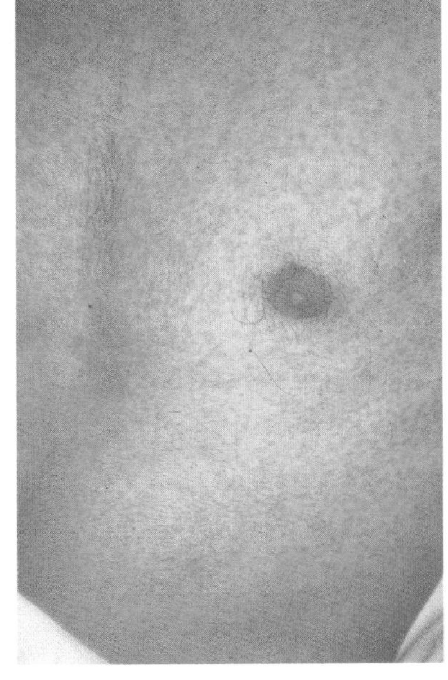

365 Rubella versus measles. Although the typical rash of rubella with its fine pink macules can easily be distinguished from the blotchy, dusky-red, maculopapular rash of measles, the difference is not always so clear-cut. Confusion may arise when the rubella rash has a coarse maculopapular element, but the short duration of the prodromal period and the absence of respiratory catarrh point to the correct diagnosis. When there is doubt, the matter may be settled by demonstrating a four-fold rise in antibody titre between acute and convalescent samples of serum, or by demonstrating rubella-specific antibody in IgM.

366 Rubella rash on second day. The evolution of the rash may be arrested at the macular stage, but more often the individual lesions on the trunk coalesce to produce a pinkish flush, closely resembling the rash of scarlet fever but lacking its punctation.

365

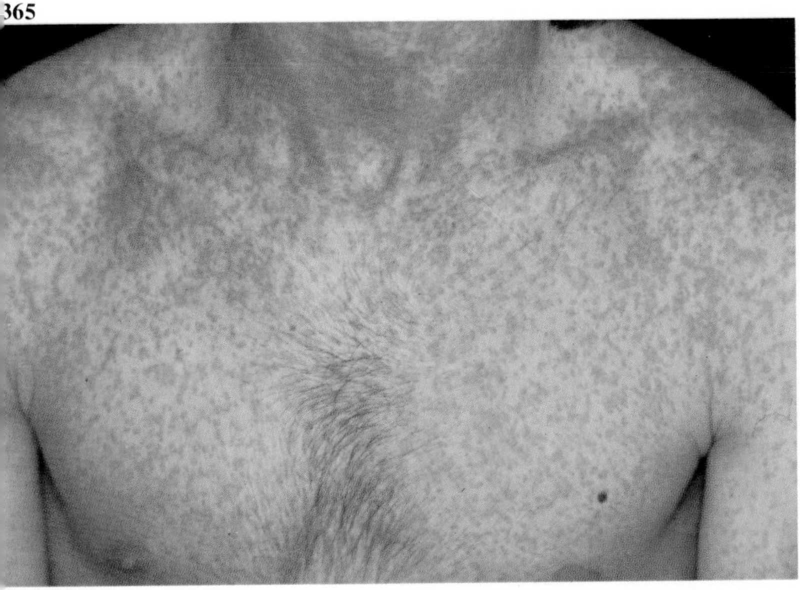

366

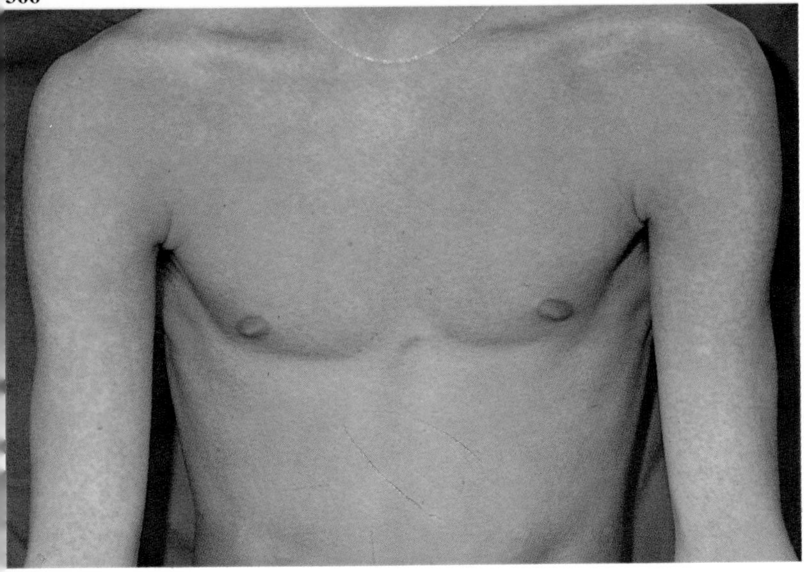

367 Rash on thighs — second day. Although the rash on the trunk may become confluent, the macules on the limbs remain discrete, and fresh lesions may appear on the feet. The rash usually fades on the third day and is not followed by staining or desquamation.

368 Purpura in rubella. A purpuric rash, consisting of petechiae and occasional ecchymoses, may occur during the acute state of rubella or in late convalescence after the exanthem has faded. The condition usually resolves spontaneously.

Congenital rubella

369 Congenital rubella — purpuric rash. A purpuric rash is much commoner in congenital than postnatal rubella. The skin haemorrhages may be present at birth or develop within 48 hours. The rash varies greatly in severity and may be accompanied by bleeding from mucosal surfaces. The initial platelet count is usually low, but in surviving infants it returns to normal within one to four months.

The highest incidence of purpura occurs in infants infected during the fourth to eighth week of pregnancy. Mortality is about 30%.

370 Purpura and hepatomegaly. Purpura is commonly associated with other serious defects. Some infants develop pronounced anaemia with erythroid hyperplasia, which may persist for several months. A high proportion have hepatomegaly, splenomegaly, congenital heart disease, and eye defects. Infection is widely disseminated, and virus has been detected in most organs.

367

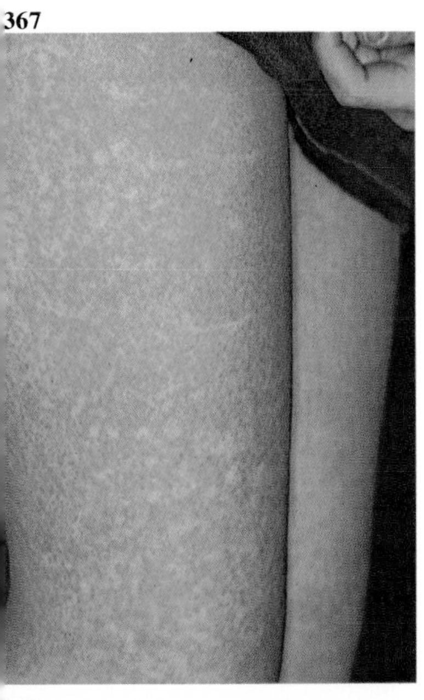

368

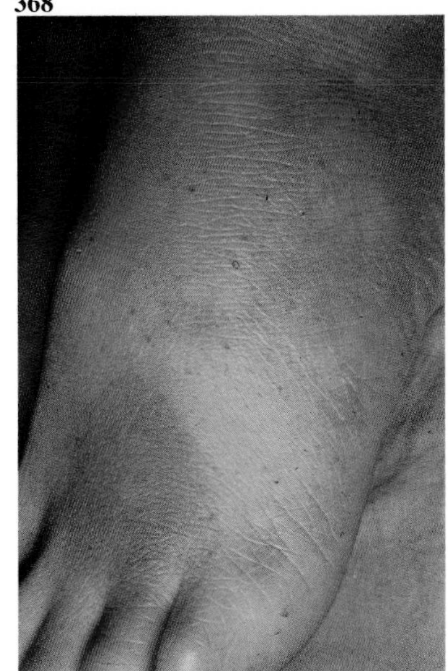

369

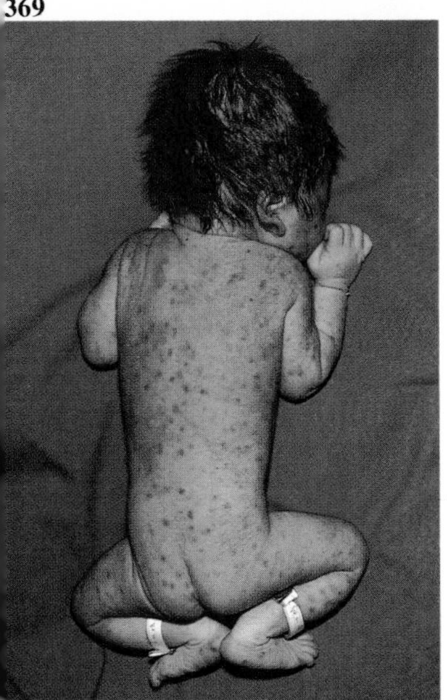

370

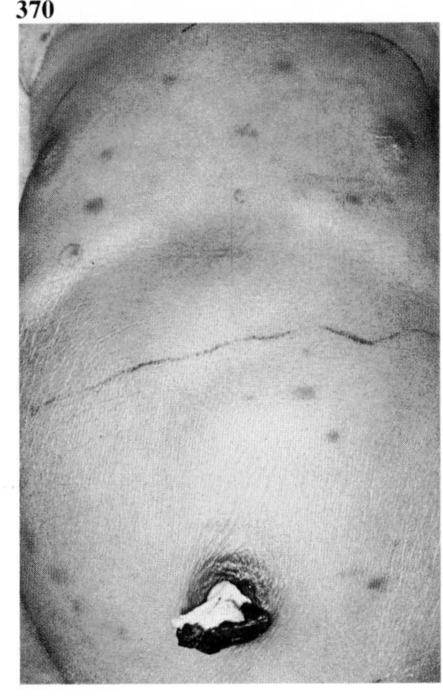

371 Histology of liver in congenital rubella (H and E). Enlargement of the liver is often present in congenital rubella, but may not be detected until the second or third month of life. The spleen may also be enlarged. Jaundice may appear within a few hours of birth and the serum bilirubin reaches high levels of concentration. Anicteric hepatitis may also occur and serum transaminase concentrations may be raised for several months.

Rubella virus has a cytolytic action, and the local inflammatory reaction is minimal. The liver changes may be diffuse or focal. In the section shown here many liver cells have been destroyed, and the surviving parenchymal cells are swollen and have vacuoles in the cytoplasm. The damaged area has been infiltrated by mononuclear cells.

372 Radiograph of chest — congenital heart disease. Several disabling defects may follow an attack of rubella during the second month of pregnancy when the fetal heart is developing. Patent ductus arteriosus, with or without stenosis of the pulmonary valve or artery, is by far the commonest lesion. Cyanotic heart disease is rare and probably a fortuitous association.

The original 'rubella syndrome' of congenital heart disease, cataracts and deafness has been extended to include defects of many other organs, as well as general impairment of growth and development.

373 Histology of heart in congenital rubella (H and E). Electrocardiographic evidence of myocardial damage may be found during life. In fatal cases histological examination of the heart shows extensive myocardial necrosis with no inflammatory response. The muscle fibres become swollen and fragmented. In severely affected areas they may be unrecognisable. The nuclei are pleomorphic and pyknotic.

374 Cloudy cornea in congenital cataract. Corneal haze of varying degree may be present at birth, possibly because of oedema in the stromal layers. It can be distinguished from glaucoma because the diameter of the cornea, the depth of the anterior chamber, and the ocular tension are all normal. The cloudiness usually clears progressively during the first few weeks of life.

371

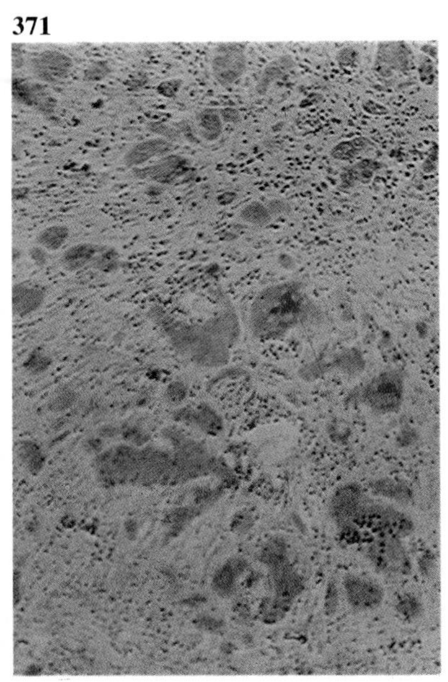

372

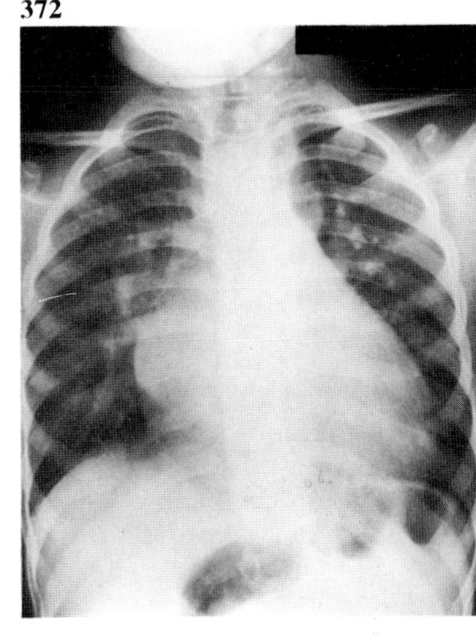

373

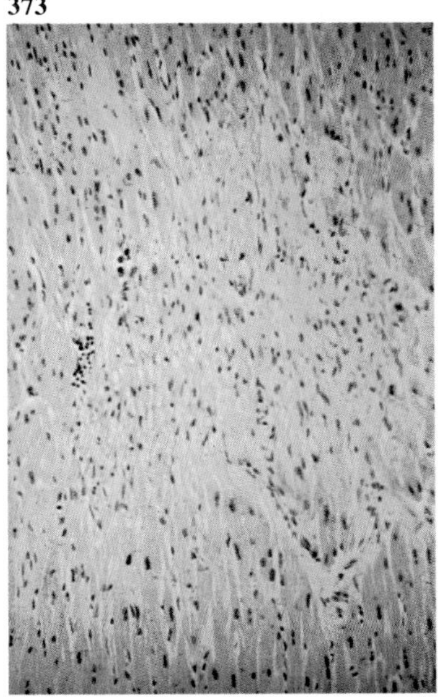

374

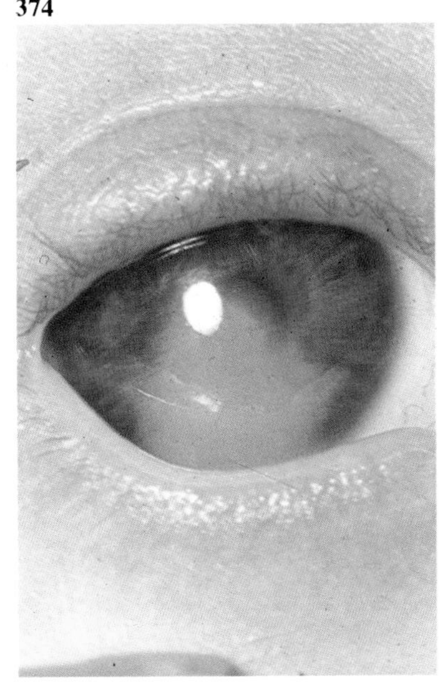

375 Congenital glaucoma caused by rubella. Glaucoma is present in 4% of patients with congenital rubella. The cornea is extremely hazy, and its diameter increased. The anterior chamber is deep, and ocular tension is appreciably increased. Following early operation the tension may be restored to normal and the corneal haze clear. Rubella virus has been isolated from aqueous fluid.

376 Cataract in congenital rubella. Spread of virus into the lens during development gives rise to a cataract. When this occurs between the third and fourth week of pregnancy a dense white opacity results, but when infection takes place later, during the sixth or seventh week, the cataract is small and amorphous and may be difficult to detect without ophthalmoscopic examination. Cataracts may be unilateral or bilateral and are often associated with microphthalmos.

Cataract and pigmentary retinopathy, the eye defects most commonly found in congenital rubella, are often associated with deafness and congenital heart disease — 'rubella triad'. Blindness is a serious handicap to a child with bilateral cataracts, especially when combined with deafness, so surgical treatment should not be delayed unduly after the age of six months.

377 Radiograph of long bone in congenital rubella. On x-ray examination changes are found in the long bones of a high proportion of infants with congenital rubella. Irregular areas of radiotranslucency are present in the metaphyses of long bones, but there is no evidence of periosteal reaction. These changes begin in early intrauterine life and clear completely within six to eight weeks from birth. Rubella virus has been isolated from bone.

The abnormal appearance of the metaphysis is caused by defective deposition and calcification of osteoid, probably secondary to a metabolic or nutritional disturbance. The diaphysis is not affected.

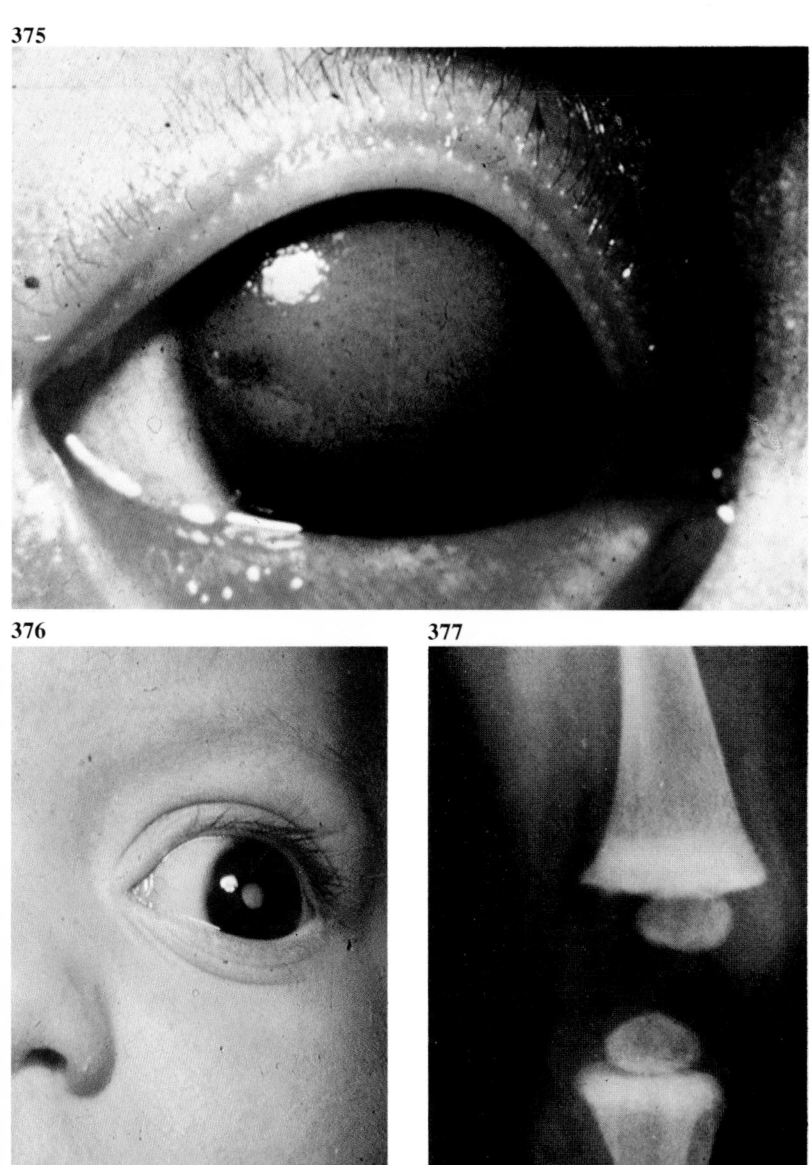
375

376

377

Enterovirus infection

The group name picornaviruses has been given to large numbers of viruses that are small (about 25 nm in diameter), resistant to ether, and composed of a core of ribonucleic acid. The group includes enteroviruses, rhinoviruses and similar viruses of non-human origin.

Enteroviruses include the polioviruses, Coxsackieviruses and ECHOviruses. Members of this family do not fall readily into definable categories but grade into each other. Nevertheless, it is convenient to group together those with close affinities.

Enteroviruses inhabit the intestinal tract, particularly of young children. Infection is transient and usually asymptomatic, but there may be a mild febrile illness. Systemic invasion may cause more serious illness with infection of the nervous system and other organs. These viruses are responsible for a large variety of clinical syndromes and the same symptom complex can result from infection by a number of them.

Enteroviruses are shed in faeces and are also found in secretions from the upper respiratory passages; infection, therefore, may be spread by the faecal–oral route or by inhalation of infected droplets.

Virology

378 Electron micrograph of enterovirus. The enteroviruses are small spheres with a protein shell and an inner core of RNA. They measure 15 to 30 nm in diameter. They are very resistant to ether, chloroform, and bile salts. Enteroviruses differ from rhinoviruses by their ability to withstand a pH as low as 3 and heating to 50°C for one hour in the presence of molar $MgCl_2$. They have been classified into three serotypes of poliovirus, 23 serotypes of Coxsackievirus type A, six serotypes of Coxsackievirus type B, and 30 serotypes of ECHOvirus, but it should be stressed that the division is arbitrary, and the separate categories merge into one another.

378

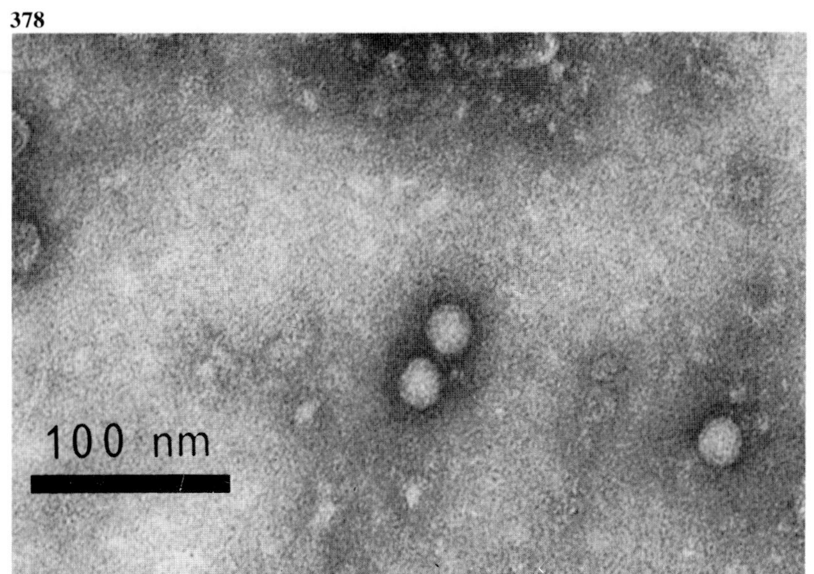

379 Normal monkey kidney cells.

380 Poliovirus in monkey kidney cells. All enteroviruses, with the notable exception of some type A Coxsackieviruses, grow on monkey kidney cells, producing cytopathic effects. These viruses will also grow on other continuous lines of cells derived from normal and malignant tissues. Some type A Coxsackieviruses fail to grow on tissue culture unless specially adapted after primary isolation in suckling mice.

The characteristic cytopathic effect is clearly evident when this illustration is compared with **379**. The uniform cell sheet has been disrupted. The cells are rounded with pyknotic nuclei. At a later stage they separate from the wall of the culture tube.

Exanthematous disease

ECHOvirus infection

381 Petechial rash in ECHOvirus type 9 infection. In ECHOvirus type 9 infections the rash appears shortly after the onset of the illness and consists of pinkish macules, which fade quickly on the trunk but may persist on the face, where they are more blotchy and have a purplish hue. Sometimes the rash has a petechial character as in this illustration.

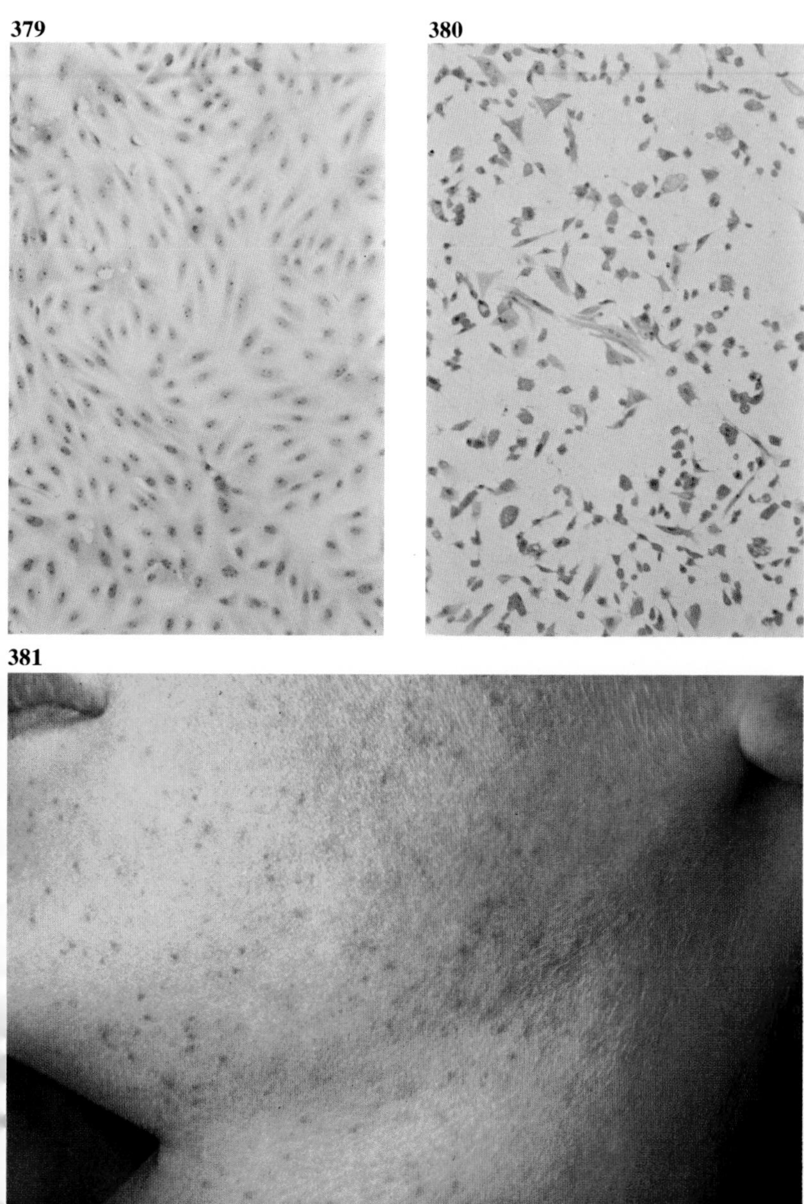
379
380
381

382 Rash on trunk — ECHOvirus type 19. The rash on the trunk of the child has a similar appearance, but is less profuse.

As a general rule, it is not possible to determine the type of ECHO-virus from the nature of the rash. Maculopapular, vesicular, petechial and pleomorphic rashes have been described, but it is seldom feasible to recognise a clinical pattern in the absence of an outbreak. Infections with ECHOvirus 16 are characterised by pinkish maculopapular eruptions, which tend to emerge as other symptoms subside.

383 Maculopapular rash on face in ECHOvirus type 19 infection. Aseptic meningitis is the syndrome most commonly associated with ECHOviruses. Febrile illness with a rash, occurring alone or in conjunction with meningitis, is the next most common manifestation. Paralysis, encephalitis, minor respiratory illness, and diarrhoea have each been linked with ECHOvirus infection.

Maculopapular rashes have been found in infections with ECHO-virus 4, 11, 16, and 19. Such exanthemata may simulate rubella and it may not be possible to arrive at an accurate diagnosis without laboratory tests. A blotchy maculopapular rash is present on the face of this child from whom ECHOvirus type 19 was isolated.

Coxsackievirus infection

384 Maculopapular rash on face in Coxsackievirus infection. Maculopapular, petechial, and vesicular eruptions have been described in infections with Coxsackieviruses, notably A9, A16, A10, A5, B3, and B5. Other types have been implicated in sporadic cases.

A maculopapular rash is seen on the face of a young girl with a febrile illness caused by a Coxsackievirus infection.

382

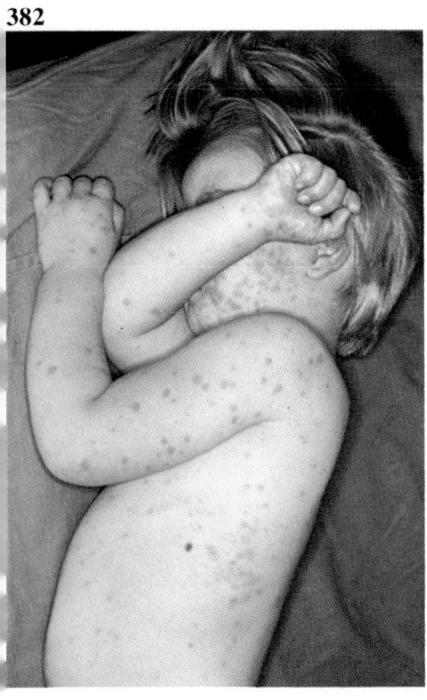

383

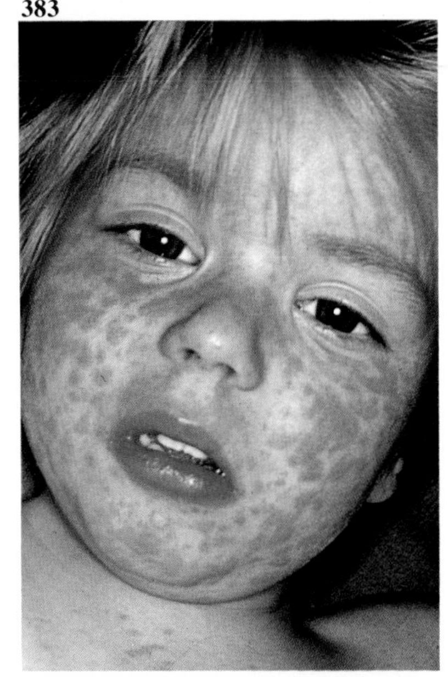

384

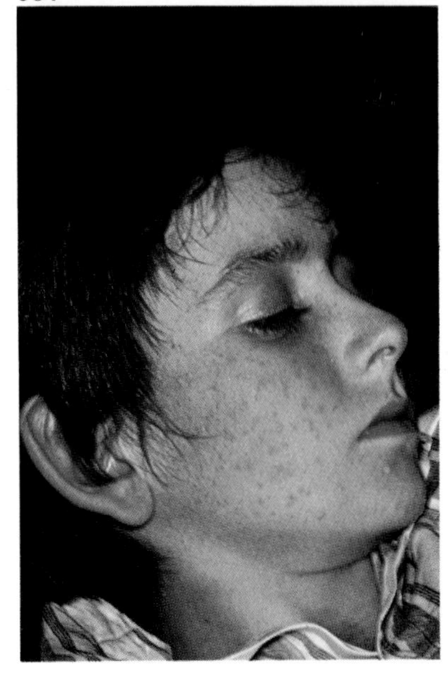

Herpangina

385 Herpangina. Herpangina is predominantly a disease of children and is caused by type A Coxsackieviruses. It is characterised by an acute onset, with fever, sore throat and dysphagia. Headache and myalgia are common symptoms, and abdominal pain may add to the distress.

The throat is inflamed, and small discrete vesicles, each surrounded by a band of erythema, may be seen scattered over the palate, fauces and pharynx. The vesicles rupture and leave shallow ulcers which heal within a week. The original vesicles are small, measuring 1 to 2 mm in diameter, and are replaced by much larger ulcers, measuring up to 5 mm across.

386 Herpes simplex versus herpangina. Herpes simplex may produce similar lesions, but they tend to affect the anterior half of the buccal cavity, whereas herpangina is confined to the posterior.

385

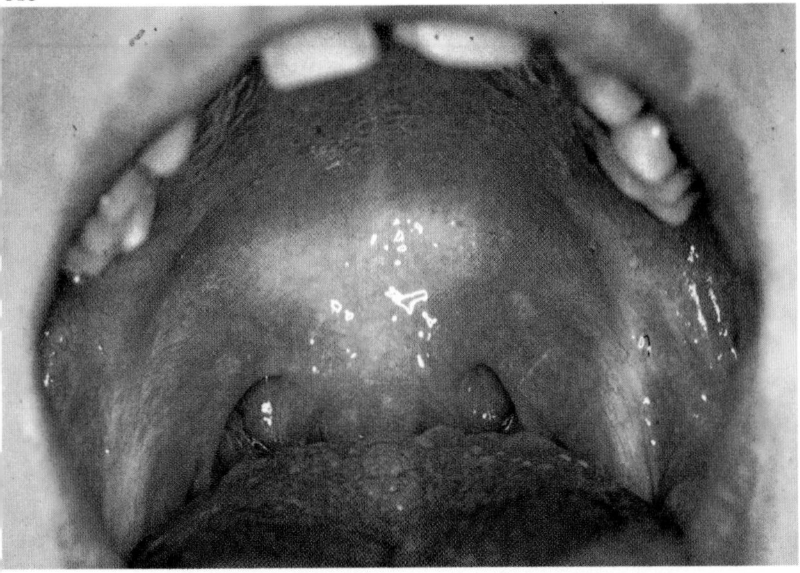

386

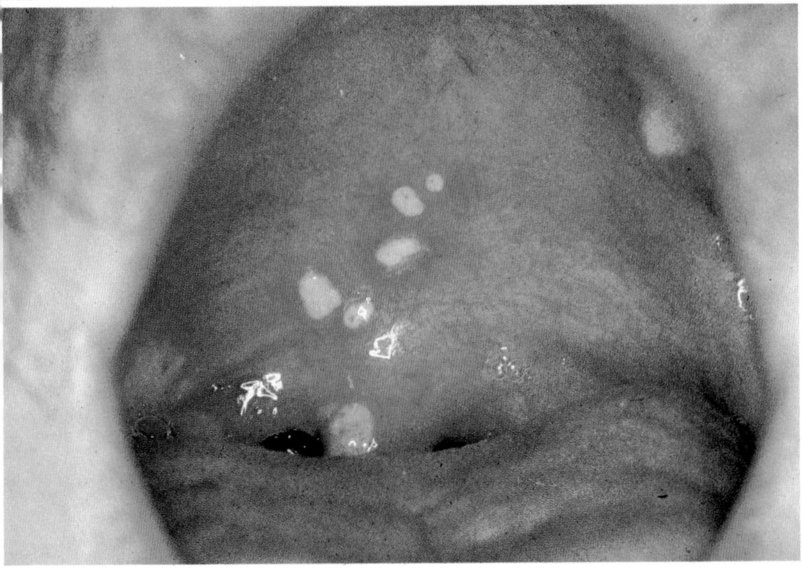

Hand, foot and mouth disease

387 Hand, foot and mouth disease — vesicles on hand. Hand, foot and mouth disease is a mild illness caused by Coxsackieviruses types A16, A10 and A5. Infection occurs in small outbreaks and spreads readily within schools or family groups. After a short incubation period of three to seven days the illness begins with fever, slight malaise and a sore mouth. Characteristic lesions appear in the mouth and on the hands and feet. The syndrome occurs more commonly and with more severity in children than adults.

The lesions on the hands are distributed mainly on the lateral aspects of the fingers but may be found on the palm. The rash is not profuse.

388 Hand, foot and mouth disease — vesicles on finger. The lesions on the skin may consist of bright red macules, small vesicles, thin bullae, or grey ulcers inside a red base.

389 Hand, foot and mouth disease — vesicles on heel. Similar lesions may be found on the feet, particularly on the toes and along the lateral border. Lesions on the feet are seldom seen in children under three years of age.

390 Hand, foot and mouth disease — vesicles on toe. The vesicles are superficial and generally heal within a week. There is very little discomfort.

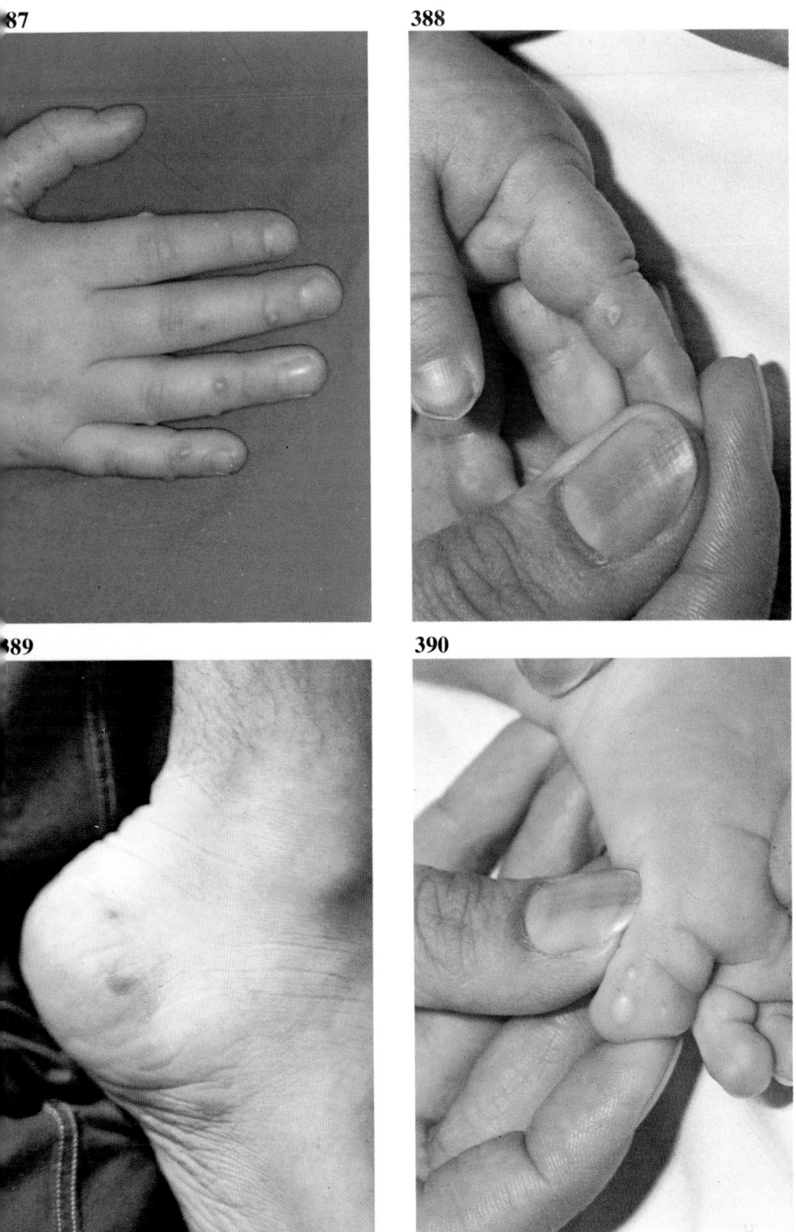

87 388

89 390

391 Hand, foot and mouth disease — lesions in mouth. The mouth lesions are bright red macules, small vesicles on an erythematous base, or painful, shallow ulcers. They may be found on all parts of the mouth but are seldom seen on the tonsils, and only a few lesions are usually present. The pharynx and the skin round the lips are not affected.

392 Hand, foot and mouth disease — rash on buttocks. A maculo-papular rash on the buttocks appears to be part of the syndrome in young children.

91

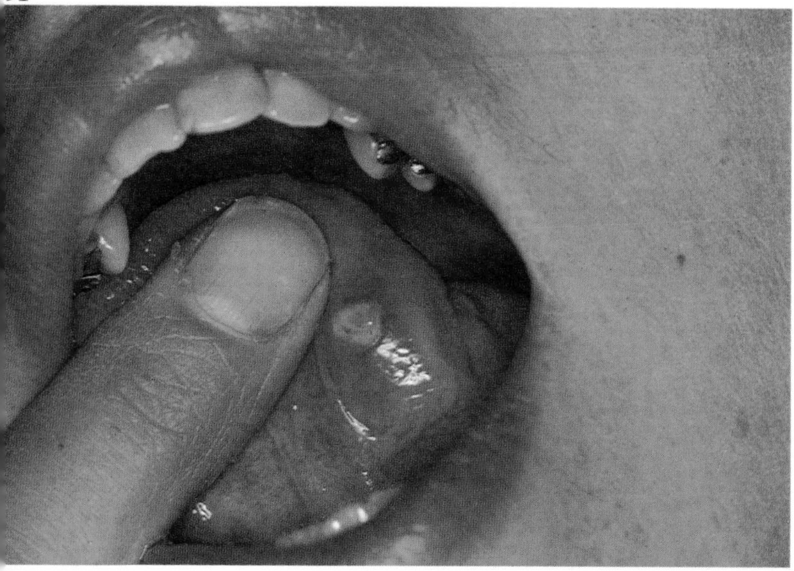

92

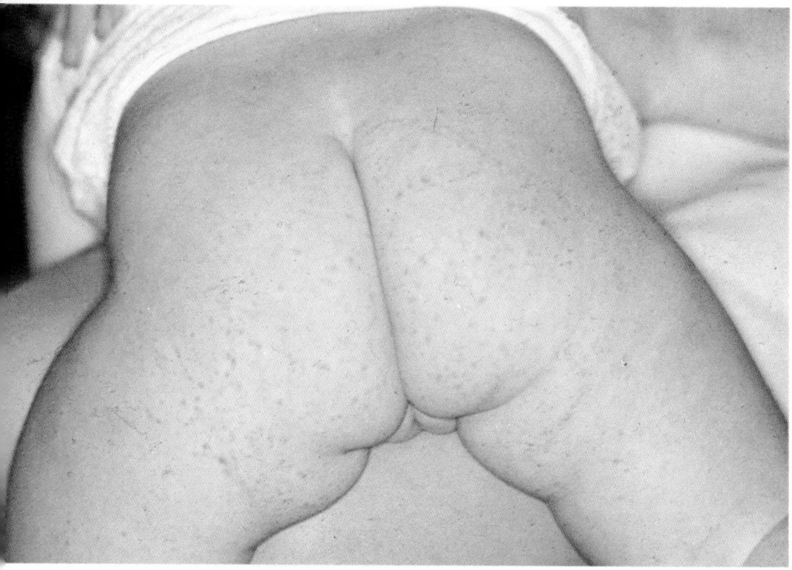

393 Hand, foot and mouth disease versus gonococcal rash. In adults gonococcaemia may be accompanied by a vesicular or pustular eruption on the hands that could be mistaken for hand, foot and mouth disease. Mouth lesions are absent and there is usually a history of urethritis or vaginal discharge. Blood cultures and swabs from the skin lesions may grow gonococci (see **178–180**).

394 Hand, foot and mouth disease versus herpes simplex. Herpetic lesions are usually confined to one finger, whereas the rash of hand, foot and mouth disease is more widespread (see **287**).

Roseola infantum

395 Rash on trunk. Roseola infantum, exanthem subitum, or sixth disease, is believed to be caused by a virus infection with an incubation period of 10 to 15 days. At onset of illness the young child becomes feverish and may have a convulsion. On examination, the throat is inflamed but there is no exudate. After three to four days the fever settles and an erythematous macular rash appears. This persists for 36 hours, then fades. If the child has been given treatment with an antibiotic the rash may be mistaken for drug hypersensitivity. Convulsions are common at onset of illness but other complications are rare.

393

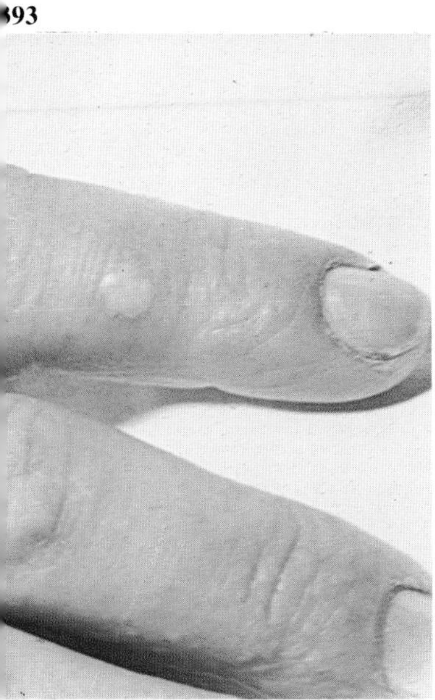

394

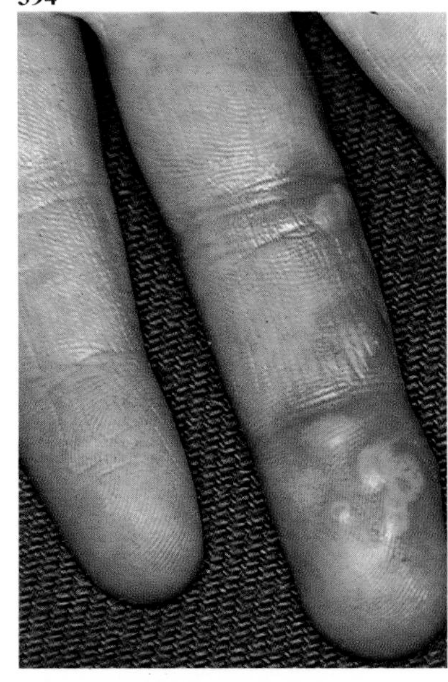

395

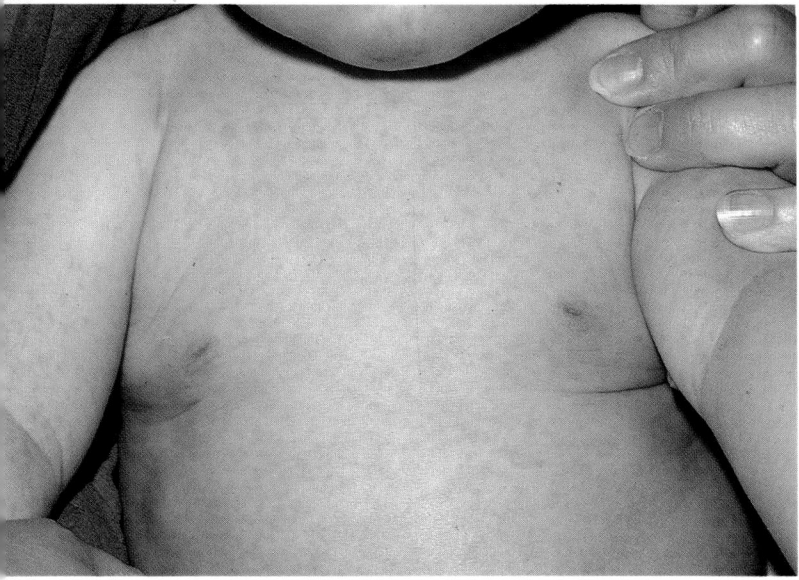

Erythema infectiosum (slapped-cheek syndrome)

Erythema infectiosum, also called fifth disease, is a mild infection caused by a parvovirus. In young children the disease follows a benign course; in adults it is less common, though tends to be more severe with a high incidence of arthritis and post-viral debility.

396 Rash on face. There may be a short prodromal period of mild fever with headache, sore throat, and slight gastrointestinal disturbance, before a rash emerges on the face. In many cases the prodrome is absent. The erythema on the face has a blotchy appearance, suggesting the marks of slapped cheeks, and may be associated with circum-oral pallor.

397 Rash on limb. Either concurrently or within a few days an erythematous rash emerges on the limbs and trunk. It varies considerably in appearance and may be morbilliform, annular, or confluent. The illustration shows discrete macules on the upper limb.

398 Rash on trunk. The rash often takes on a lacy appearance owing to patches of pallor, and has a notable tendency to come and go over a period of a week or more. Recurrence of the rash may be precipitated by hot baths, exercise or emotional upset. As a rule there are no other findings in children, but adults may have lymphadenopathy and may develop arthritis, especially of the wrists and knees.

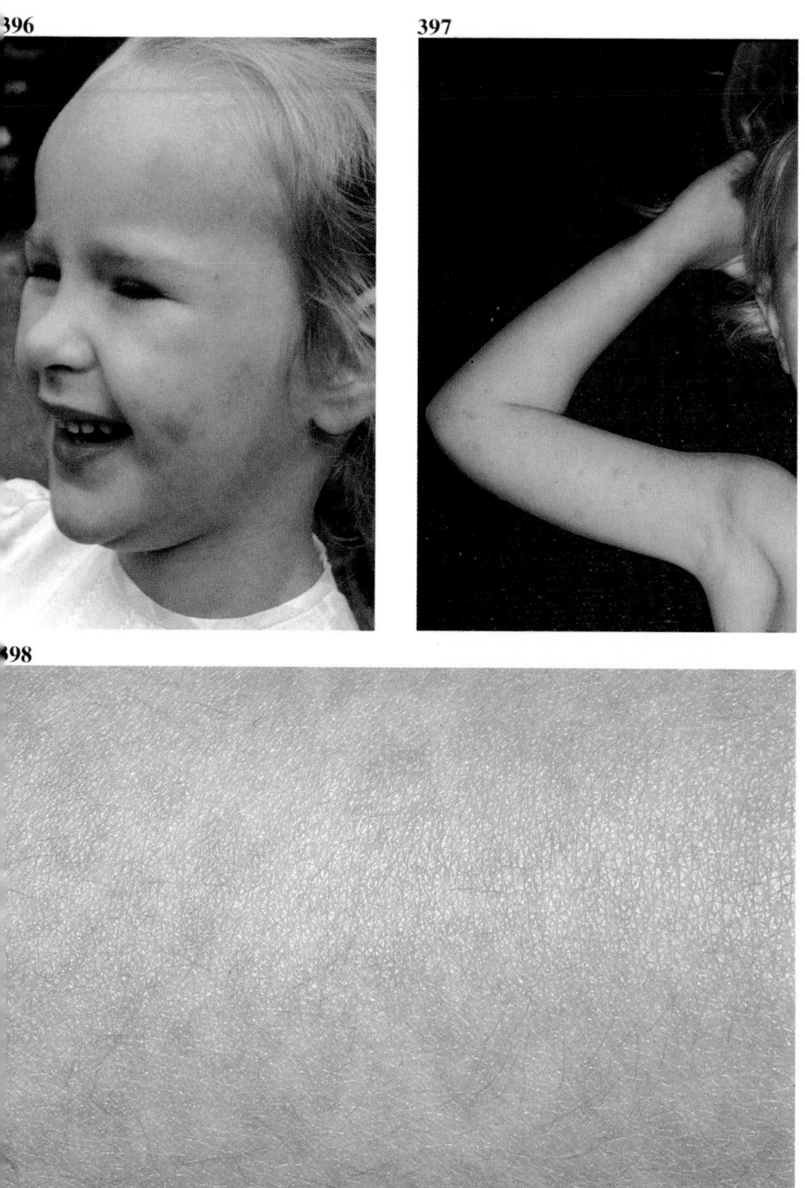
396
397
398

Rabies

Rabies is a viral disease transmitted to man almost without exception by the bite or saliva of an infected dog. Many other animals may be infected, however, and wildlife populations form the chief reservoir of the disease. Rabies is worldwide in its distribution, with the exception of Australasia and Antarctica. Strict control is possible only on islands, such as Great Britain, where control has been effective for many years.

399 Electron micrograph of virus. Rabies virus belongs to a family of single-stranded RNA viruses called rhabdoviruses. The virion measures 75 by 180 nm and is bullet-shaped, being flat at one end and conical at the other. The surface, except at the flat end, is covered with spikes composed of glycoprotein, which protrude through the surface membrane from the nucleocapsid. This glycoprotein is strongly antigenic and generates neutralising antibody. Virulence of rabies virus appears to be associated with the structure of its glycoprotein.

400 Infected dog bite. The virus usually gains access through a bite from an infected animal and may multiply locally before being transported passively within the axoplasm of nerves to the spinal cord and brain. After further proliferation in the central nervous system the virus spreads peripherally along the same nerve pathways to the tissues of the body. Immunisation with vaccine, after exposure, together with immune serum, has been most successful in preventing rabies. The introduction of vaccines prepared on human diploid cells has virtually eliminated the neurological complications associated with the earlier vaccines.

401 Negri bodies. The early clinical picture may not immediately suggest a diagnosis of rabies, although later the illness is usually characteristic. In the past, the only means of confirming the diagnosis was by the demonstration of Negri bodies in nerve tissue, especially the hippocampus and cerebellum. Negri bodies are sharply defined eosinophilic cytoplasmic inclusions, measuring 2 to 10 μm and consisting of viral nucleoprotein. They may not always be detected by routine histological staining, and specific staining with fluorescein-labelled rabies antibody may be required. During life the diagnosis can be made by using this type of antibody to stain infected cells from impression smears of the cornea or from skin biopsies.

399

400

401

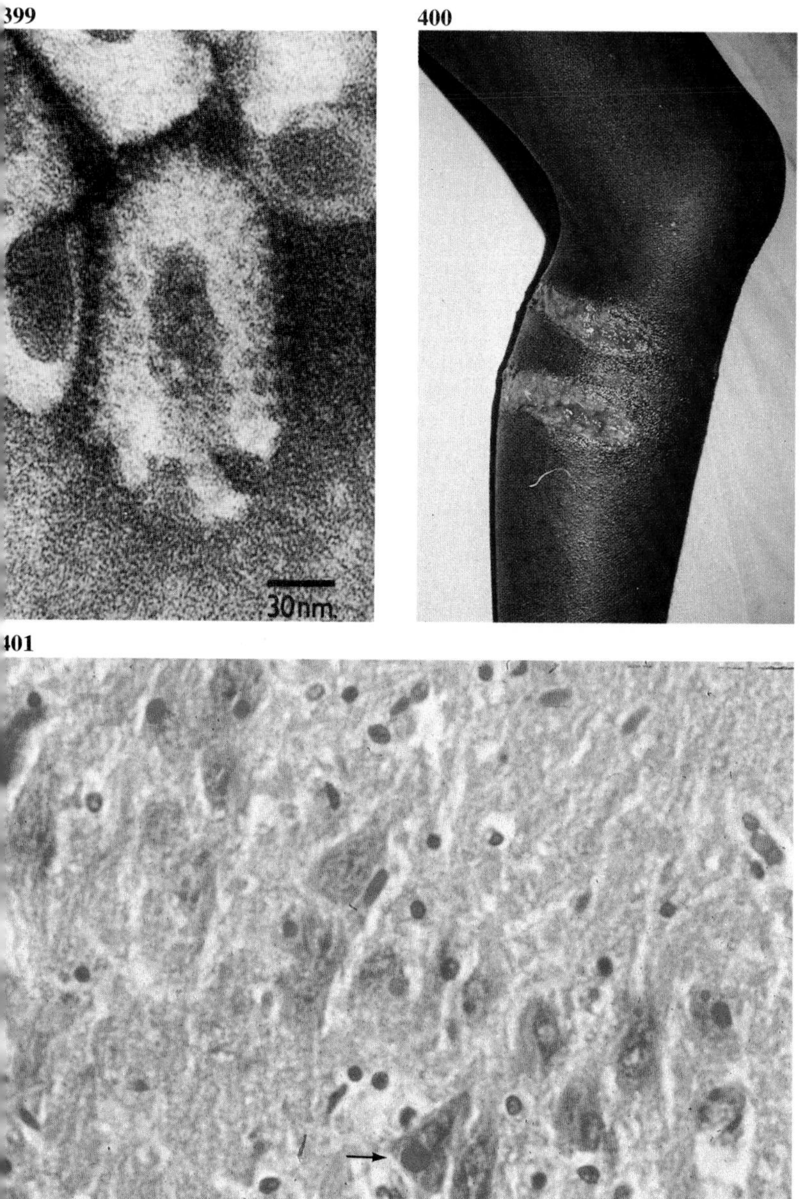

402 Hydrophobia. The initial symptoms are headache, loss of appetite, nausea and vomiting, generally accompanied by mild fever. Some abnormal sensation, such as numbness or tenderness, is a helpful early diagnostic sign. Symptoms of acute anxiety may be present. After three to four days the symptoms become progressively worse; the patient is restless and excited and probably hypersensitive to stimuli. Nevertheless, his mind remains quite clear and he is able to answer questions in an intelligent manner. He may then develop the characteristic feature of hydrophobia. On attempting to drink or even considering it the muscles of swallowing and respiration go into sudden spasm so that any fluid is violently ejected and the head thrown back. Spasms, however, may be induced by a variety of stimuli and may also occur spontaneously as part of a generalised hyperactive state interspersed by periods of calm. Life may be terminated abruptly by respiratory obstruction or cardiac arrest, or gradually by progressive paralysis.

403 'Dumb' rabies. In perhaps 20% of patients hyperactivity is absent and paralysis is predominant, as seen in this child with the expressionless face of 'dumb' rabies.

402

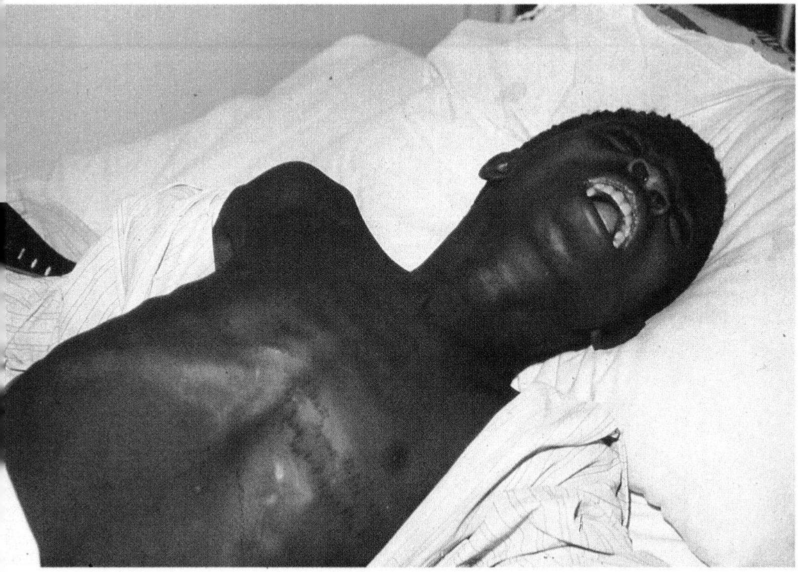

403

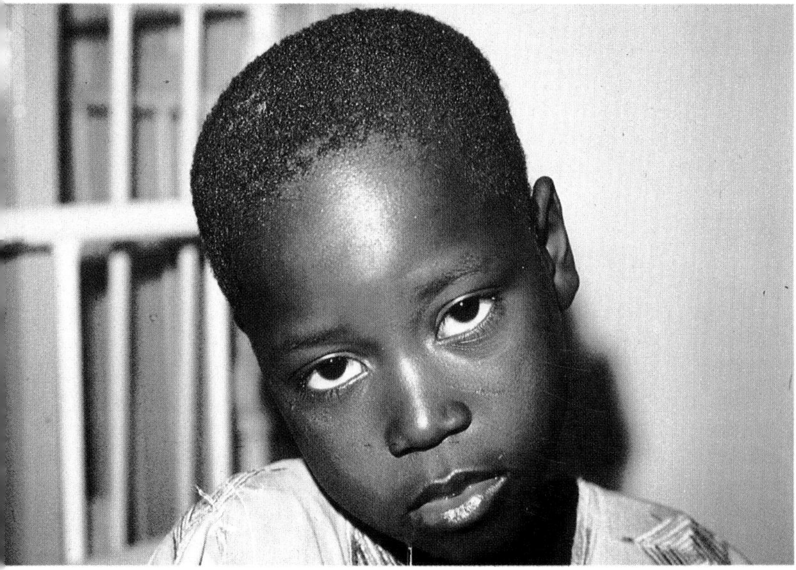

Poxvirus infections

The poxviruses are the largest and most complex of true viruses, causin pox infections in many mammals and birds, myxomatosis in rabbits, an molluscum contagiosum in man. The viruses are oval when hydrated and brick-shaped when dried for electron microscopy. They contai DNA and most have an uneven, mulberry-like surface because of th presence of threads in the surface structure. Sensitivity to ether varie within the group. Multiplication appears to take place entirely withi the cytoplasm of the host cell. Viral particles may be liberated when th host cell disintegrates or may spread directly to contiguous cells.

Orthopoxviruses of man are no longer important since the eradicatio of smallpox in October 1979. A few cases of clinical smallpox have bee recognised in people living on the edges of the tropical rain forests i Africa, but there is little evidence of case-to-case transmission. Th disease has been designated monkeypox, and the virus is closely relate to, but distinct from, smallpox virus. Parapoxviruses are responsible fo such human diseases as orf and paravaccinia (milkers' nodes).

Orf (contagious pustular dermatitis)

404 Orf — electron micrograph of virus. The viruses of orf an paravaccinia have a similar morphology to the poxviruses of the variol group. Orf virus on electron microscopy measures 252 nm × 158 nm an has a coiled or woven appearance. It does not produce lesions on chic embryo but can be grown in a variety of tissue cultures, including huma amnion cells.

405 Orf (contagious pustular dermatitis). Contagious pustular derma titis is a disease of sheep and goats that occasionally spreads to man. It i particularly prevalent in lambs and kids. In animals the infectio manifests with a papulovesicular eruption on the lips and surroundin skin, but may affect non-wool-bearing areas of skin elsewhere. The viru persists in the soil of an affected pasture for some months, and animal probably become infected while grazing. Infection may spread by direc contact to shepherds or butchers handling infected lambs.

404

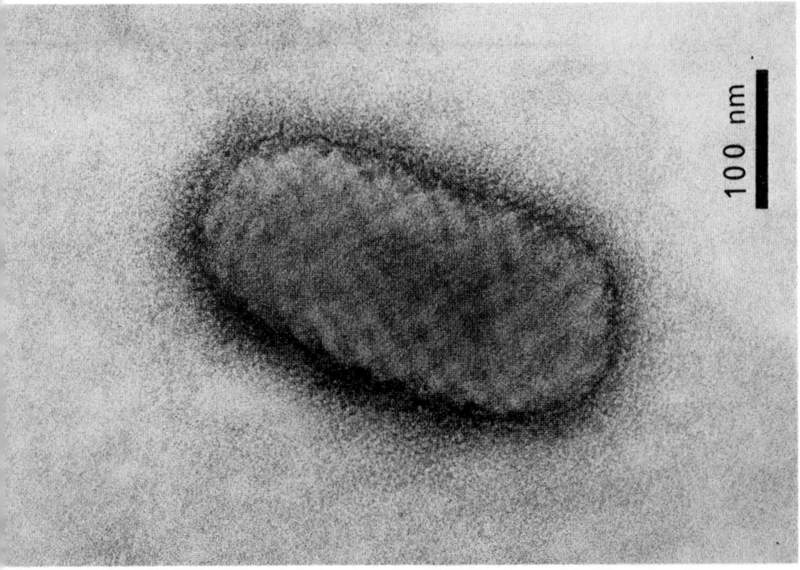

405

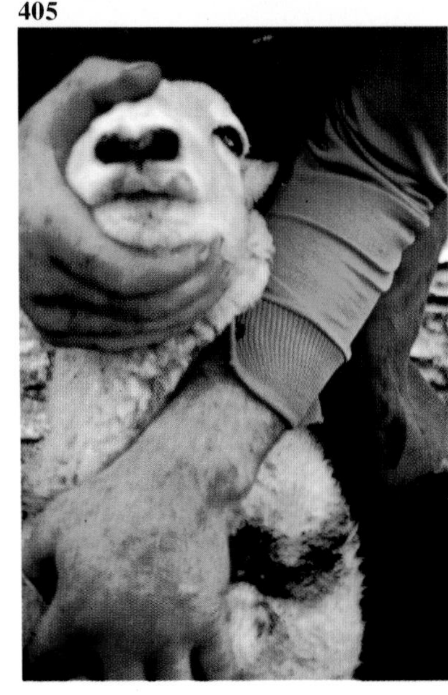

406 Contagious pustular dermatitis — human infection. A lesion may occasionally develop on the face. Although unsightly and slow to heal, it does not usually leave a scar. Virus may be recovered from the lesion by inoculating fluid into tissue culture, or into the scarified skin of a sheep.

407 and **408 Contagious pustular dermatitis — lesions on forearm and hands.** In most patients a single papule appears on the skin of the hand, wrist, or forearm and slowly develops into a large, flat vesicle or bulla, which may be haemorrhagic. The surrounding tissues are indurated and inflamed, but the lesion is remarkably free from pain. There is no constitutional disturbance.

406

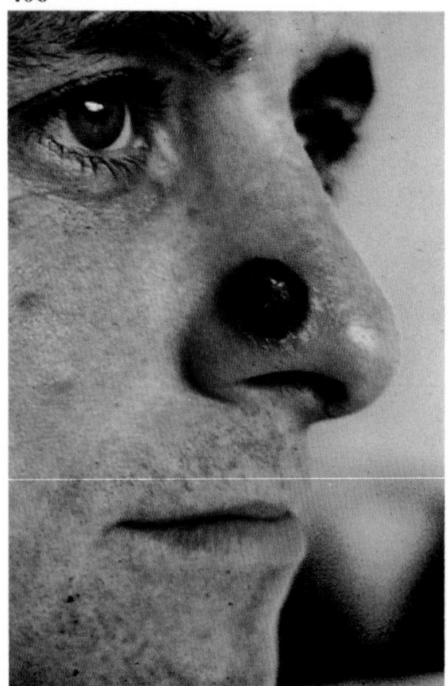

407

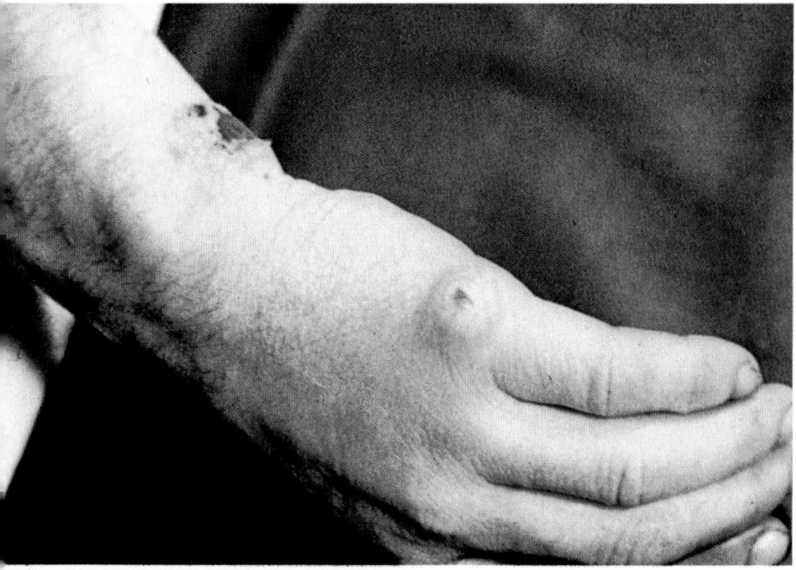

408

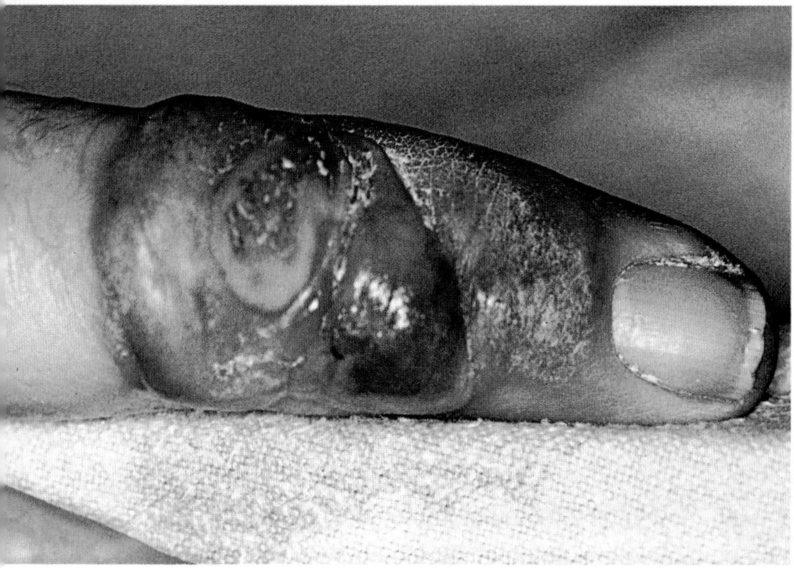

Milkers' nodes (paravaccinia)

409 Milkers' nodes — rash on hands. This condition is distinct from cowpox and orf. The virus responsible is closely related to that of orf. It cannot be propagated on chick embryo but can be cultured serially in bovine cells. Human infection is acquired from milking infected cows.

In man, papular lesions appear on the fingers or hands and increase slowly in size over a period of one to two weeks. The nodules are bluish-red in colour and painless. Vesiculation does not occur. The lesions heal without forming a scar. Fever is usually absent, but there may be severe allergic rashes.

410 Milkers' nodes — allergic rash. Nodular lesions are present on the swollen hands, and there is an allergic rash on the face and neck. Note the absence of toxaemia. The regional lymph nodes are seldom enlarged.

409

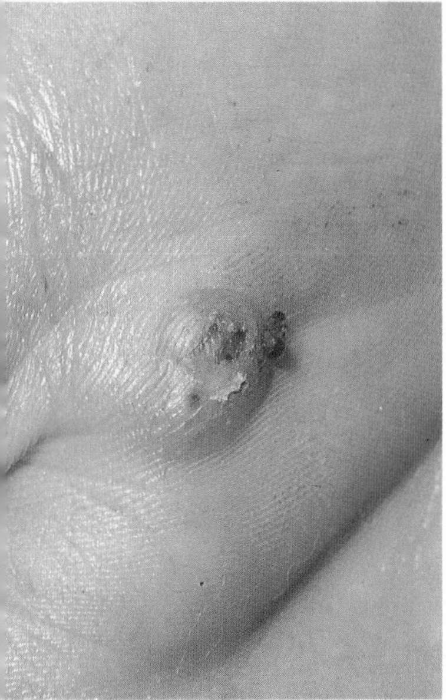

410

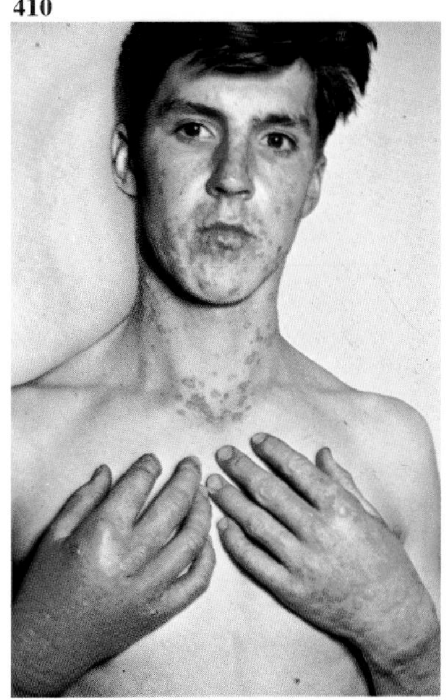

Molluscum contagiosum

Molluscum contagiosum is a worldwide human infection caused by an unclassified poxvirus. Infection is transmitted by direct contact or by fomites. Any age group may be affected.

411 Electron micrograph of virus. The virus contains DNA and measures roughly 300 × 220 nm. It causes a benign infection of the epidermis of man and may be found in high concentration in the superficial epithelial cells, where it causes ballooning degeneration and the formation of large hyaline, acidophilic, granular, intracytoplasmic inclusions (molluscum bodies). These contain virus particles similar in appearance to those of orf. With negative staining, the particles resemble balls of yarn on electron microscopy. The virus has not been propagated serially in tissue culture, and no serological tests are available.

412 Skin lesions. The number of lesions varies from one patient to another; any part of the body may be affected except the palms and soles. The lesion begins as a small, firm, shiny, pearly nodule measuring 1 to 5 mm in diameter.

413 Skin lesions. These slowly enlarge and become umbilicated. Caseous material may be discharged or expressed from the lesions. After a few months the lesions spontaneously regress and heal without scarring.

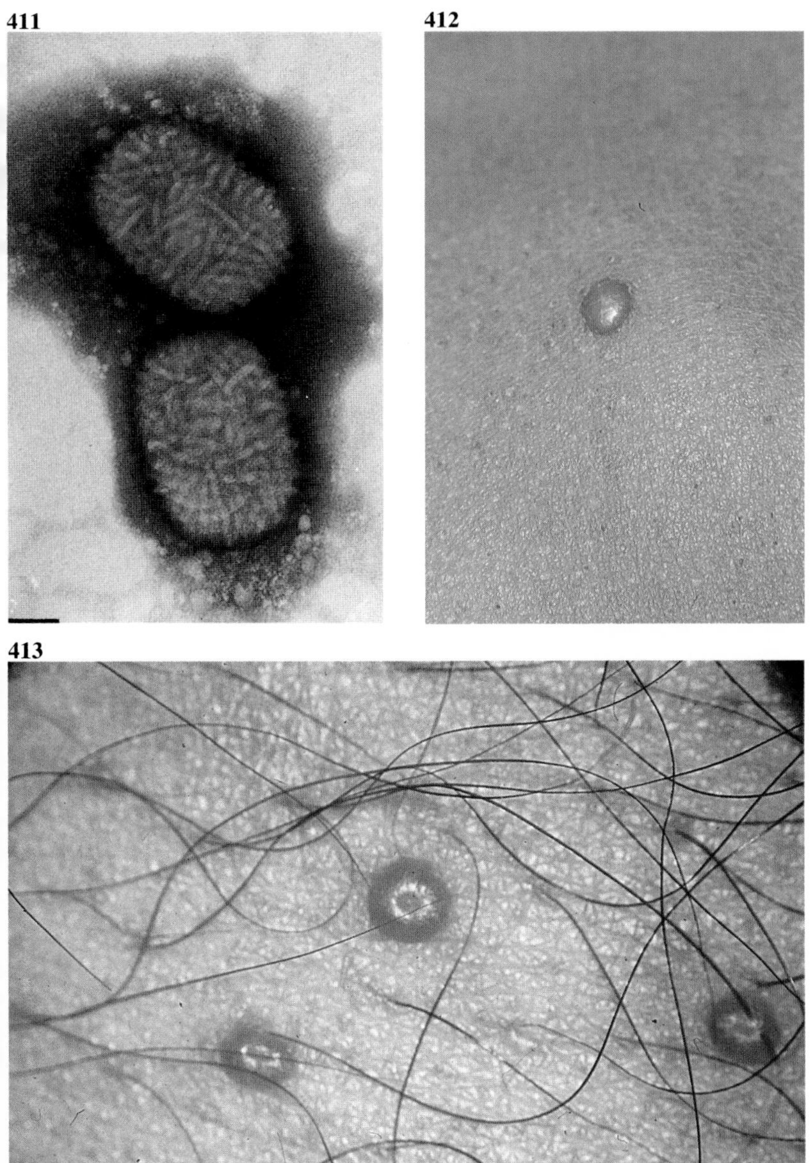
411
412
413

414

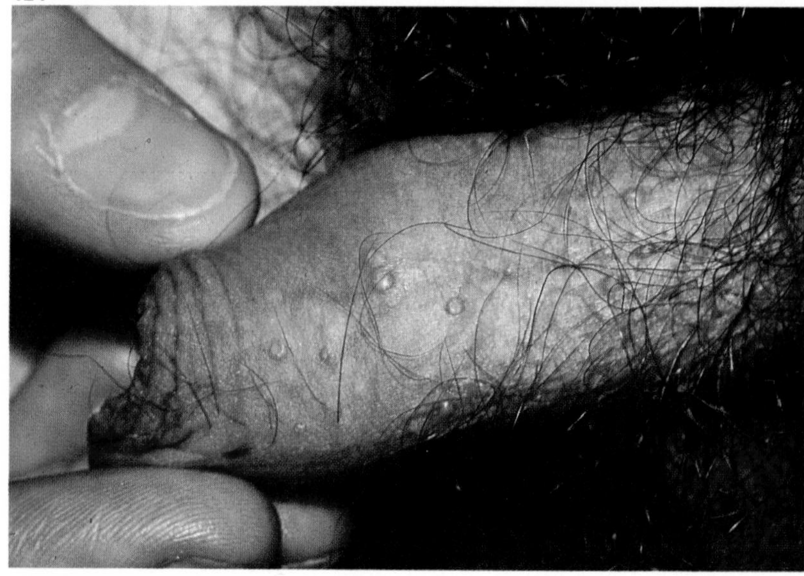

414 Penile lesions. There is increasing evidence that molluscum contagiosum may be transmitted sexually.

Probable virus infections

Cat-scratch disease

Cat-scratch disease is generally acquired as a result of a scratch, lick or bite from an apparently healthy cat. Within a few days a primary lesion develops at the site of injury and usually takes the form of a reddened papule, but may be vesicular or crusted. Occasionally there is no local reaction. After an interval of 10 to 30 days the regional lymph nodes become enlarged and there may be slight constitutional disturbance. The subsequent course of the illness is variable and may be prolonged, but ultimate recovery is the rule and death unknown.

The nature of the infective agent has not been determined. Elementary bodies resembling those of psittacosis have been found in stained preparations of pus, but the Frei test is negative and complement-fixation tests for psittacosis and ornithosis negative or only weakly positive. The diagnosis may be suspected clinically, but final proof rests with the specific skin test. The antigen consists of sterilised dilute pus from a bubo.

415 Histology of lymph node (H and E). Initially there is hypoplasia of the reticulum, but necrotic foci soon appear in the germinal follicles and break down to form micro-abscesses, which coalesce and may discharge on the surface of the skin. The foci of necrotic material are surrounded by a layer of epithelioid cells interspersed by giant cells of Langhans type. The necrotic areas in the lymph node section shown here have stained a bright pink.

416 Enlarged supraclavicular and infraclavicular lymph nodes. During the early stage of lymphadenitis constitutional disturbance is common but seldom severe. When suppuration is absent the swelling may subside in two or three weeks, but in patients with gross suppuration the illness is prolonged, and regression may take two or three months. The nature of the infection may be overlooked when the primary component is missing, but the possibility of cat-scratch disease should always be considered when there is a history of exposure to cats in a patient with unexplained lymphadenitis.

417 Enlarged epitrochlear and infraclavicular lymph nodes. The epitrochlear, axillary, and cervical groups are most commonly affected. The swollen nodes are mobile and vary in consistency with the degree of suppuration; some are tender. The overlying skin is usually normal but may be inflamed and sometimes breaks down to form a discharging sinus. Lymphangitis is not a feature.

415

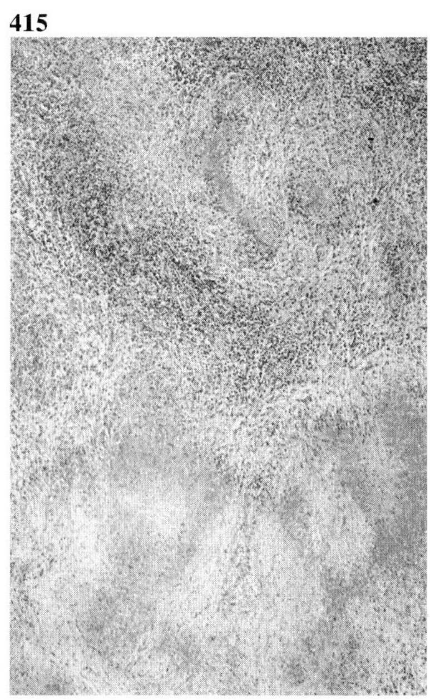

416

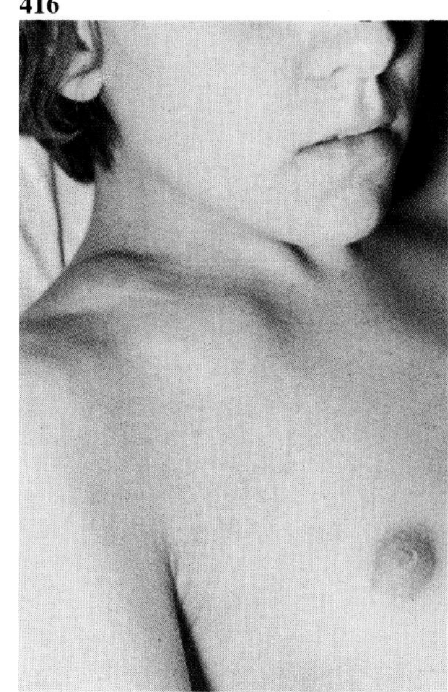

417

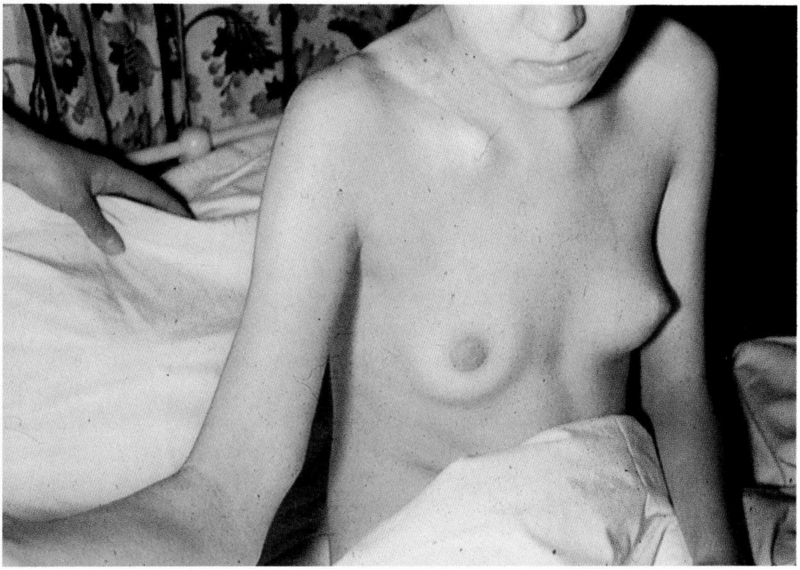

Pityriasis rosea

Pityriasis rosea is thought to be caused by a viral infection, but the agent has not yet been identified. The main eruption is often preceded by a 'herald' patch that may appear a week or 10 days before the rash occurs elsewhere. In the early stages of the illness there may be slight redness of the throat and minimal enlargement of the cervical lymph nodes, but general distrubance is trivial. The rash disappears within four to eight weeks from onset.

418 Pityriasis rosea — 'herald' patch and general rash. A typical 'herald' patch is present on the skin over the buttock. The rash elsewhere consists of scaly oval macules and rounded follicular papules. The roseolar rash of secondary syphilis may simulate pityriasis rosea, but the presence of a 'herald' patch, and the absence of mucosal lesions indicate the correct diagnosis.

419 and **420 Pityriasis rosea — generalised rash.** Older children and young adults are predominantly affected. The illness is usually heralded by a solitary scaly red macule with little or no constitutional disturbance. About a week later a general rash appears on the trunk and proximal parts of the limbs. Over the thorax the long axes of the oval macules tend to follow the lines of the ribs. Lesions are scanty on the periphery of the limbs.

418

419

420

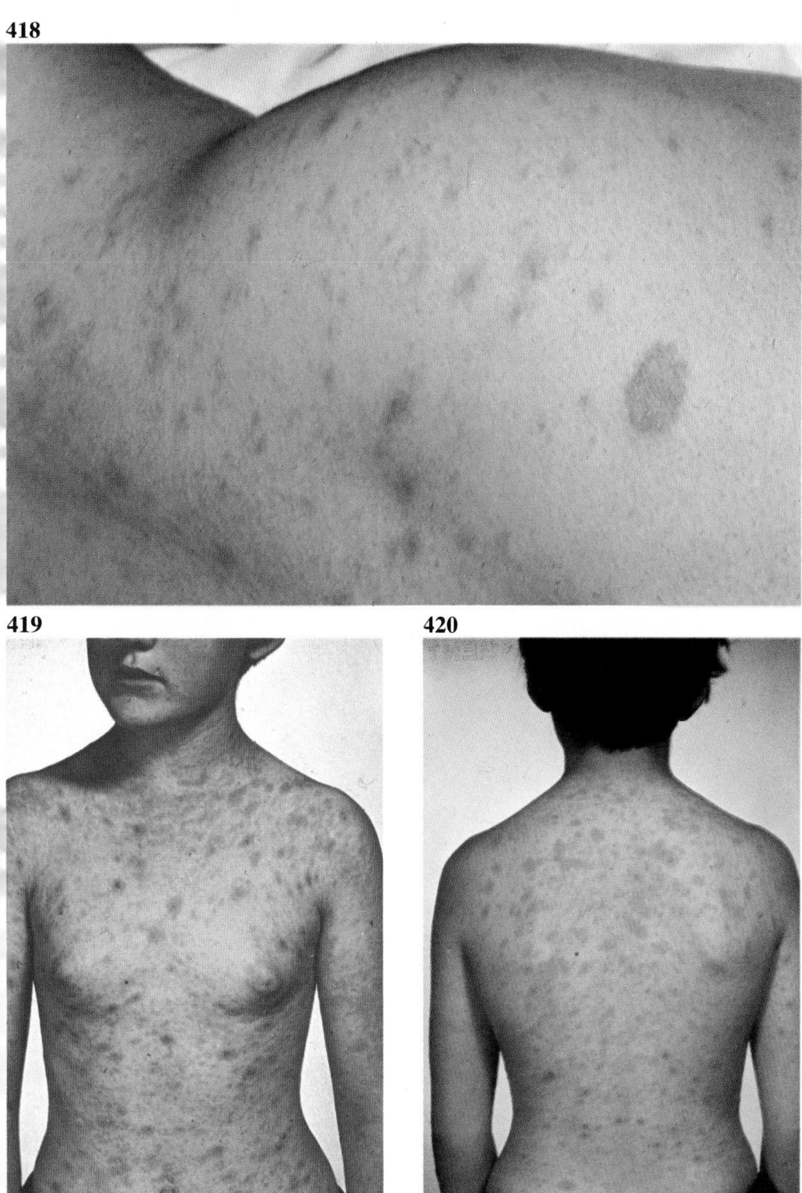

421 Pityriasis rosea — 'herald' patch. The 'herald' patch usually appears on the trunk but is sometimes found on the upper parts of the limbs or on the neck. It begins as a red scaly macule that enlarges rapidly and may eventually measure 3 to 4cm in length. There may be temporary loss of pigment in dark skins.

422 Pityriasis rosea — components of rash. The rash is composed of two types of lesion: small red papules and characteristic pink oval macules, measuring 1 to 2cm in length. After a few days the macules begin to desquamate from the centre outwards and form a collarette of scales with the free edges towards the centre. The rash is variable and the papular elements sometimes dominate; there may be slight itching.

421

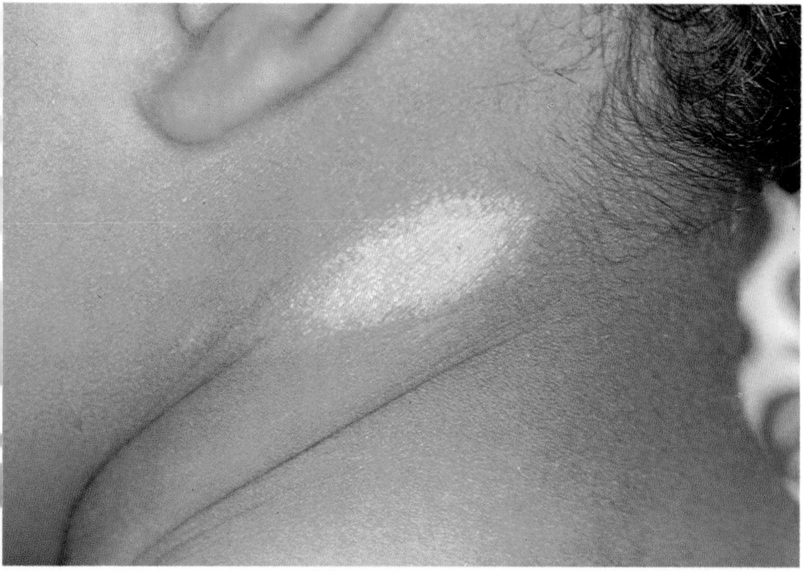

422

PROTOZOAL INFECTIONS

Amoebiasis

Amoebiasis is infection with the protozoan parasite *Entamoeba histolytica.* Man is the only host, and infection is usually transmitted by water. The parasite exists in two forms: the vegetative form, capable of division but sensitive to the outside environment; and the cyst, which is incapable of division but is resistant to the environment. Under certain circumstances, not properly understood, the vegetative form may become invasive, penetrating the mucosa of the large bowel and replicating in the submucosa to produce symptoms. In a small proportion of infected individuals amoebae may reach the liver or other organs, replicate, and produce localising symptoms.

423 *E. histolytica* cyst. Diagnosis of amoebiasis is most often made by finding cysts in the stool, usually in an asymptomatic person. The amoebic cyst measures more than 10 μm in diameter, and four nuclei can usually be identified, distinguishing it from the cyst of the non-pathogenic *E. coli* with eight nuclei.

424 *E. histolytica* trophozoite. The trophozoite is not found in the stool unless the patient is symptomatic; diarrhoea with or without blood, absence of abdominal pain, and lack of constitutional upset are characteristic features. On microscopy the trophozoite, measuring 20 to 30 μm, is motile and contains ingested erythrocytes. It moves in a characteristic manner with protrusion of a pseudopod, into which the cytoplasm and any ingested red blood cells flow, like a 'bag of marbles' rolling along. The stool is remarkably lacking in inflammatory cells, thereby distinguishing amoebic from bacillary dysentery.

425 Appearance of large bowel. In the submucosa of the large bowel amoebic trophozoites multiply and cause tissue necrosis. This produces the undermined ulcer seen on sigmoidoscopy. Only occasionally do the amoebae penetrate more deeply into the bowel wall and cause perforation. (A = amoeba.)

At necropsy the bowel may be ulcerated from end to end with multiple perforations. The wall may be extremely friable, with the consistency of wet blotting paper. Such extensive ulceration causes death, especially in the elderly, debilitated and malnourished.

423

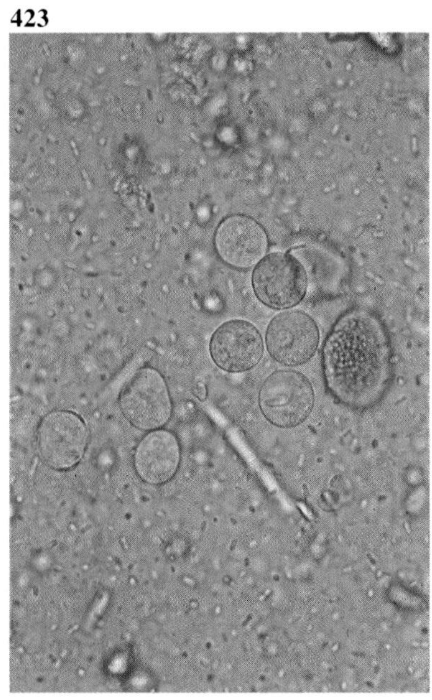

424

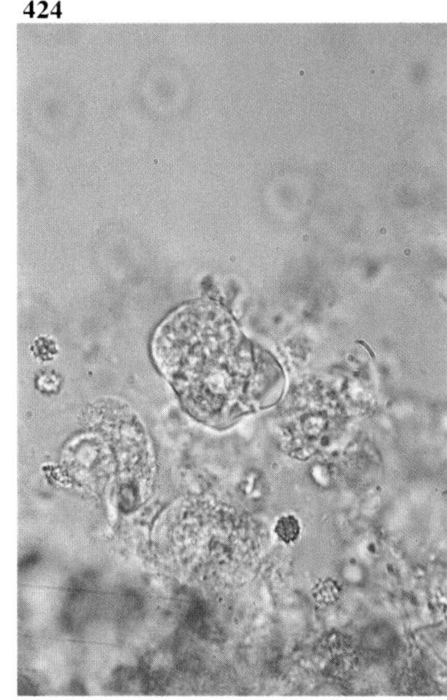

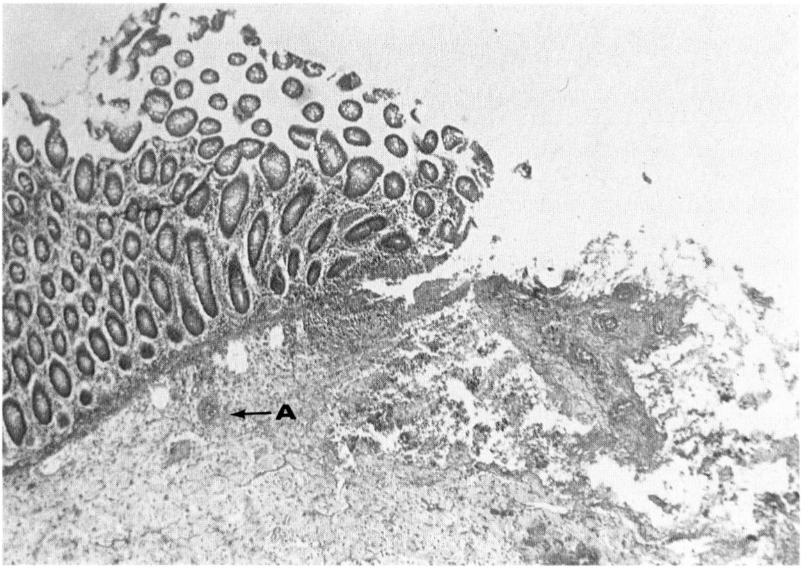

426 Liver abscess — ultrasonography. Ultrasonography of the liver confirms the presence of a cavity and distinguishes between an abscess and a cyst. Amoebic abscesses are most commonly found in the right lobe of the liver and may appear multiple on examination. The size and exact location of the abscess may be determined from the scan. (A = abscess.)

427 Liver aspiration. Aspiration was the only method of diagnosis before the invention of scanning. If amoebic material was encountered then aspiration continued as part of treatment; this has now been replaced by chemotherapy. When rupture of an abscess seems imminent or when the response to chemotherapy is slow, aspiration may, however, be beneficial. In parts of the world where scanning and serological tests are not available aspiration is still important for diagnosis and treatment.

426

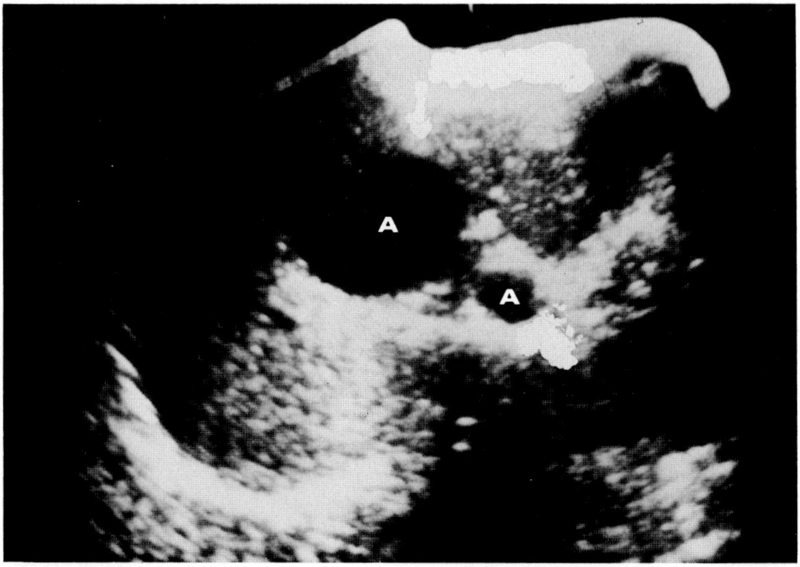

427

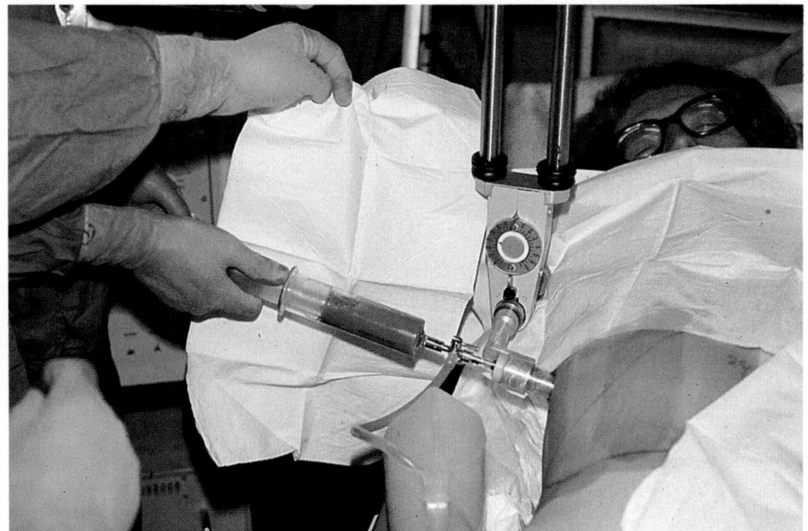

428 Liver aspirate. The material aspirated from an amoebic liver abscess has a characteristic appearance and smell. Although described as 'anchovy sauce', the material often has a more reddish tinge. It is not pus in the strict sense of the term, as neutrophils are not present; it consists of necrotic liver tissue, the result of proteolytic enzymes of the trophozoite. The smell of the aspirate is not unpleasant, and culture yields no bacterial growth. Secondary bacterial infection in an amoebic abscess is rare.

429 Amoebiasis of the skin. This was a serious complication in the days before effective treatment. It occurred at the site of rupture of an amoebic abscess or in the perineum of debilitated patients with amoebic colitis. Here a misdiagnosed empyema has been drained surgically; the correct diagnosis was liver abscess, which had ruptured through the diaphragm into the pleural cavity.

430 Radiograph of chest. X-ray examination of the chest may suggest amoebic liver abscess. The radiological features are elevation of the diaphragm, a small pleural effusion, and some linear collapse at the right base. On screening there is reduced or paradoxical movement of the right hemidiaphragm.

428

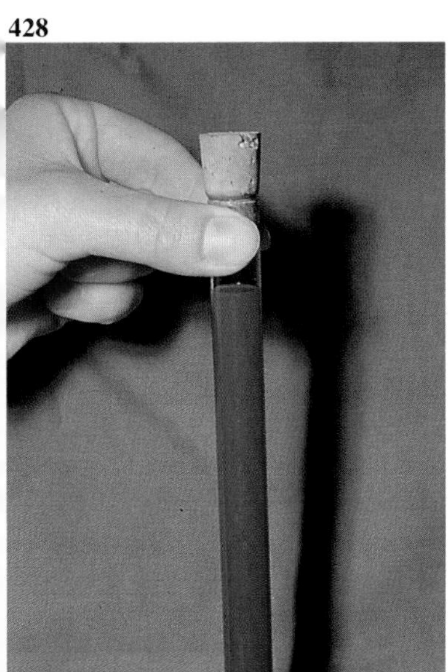

429

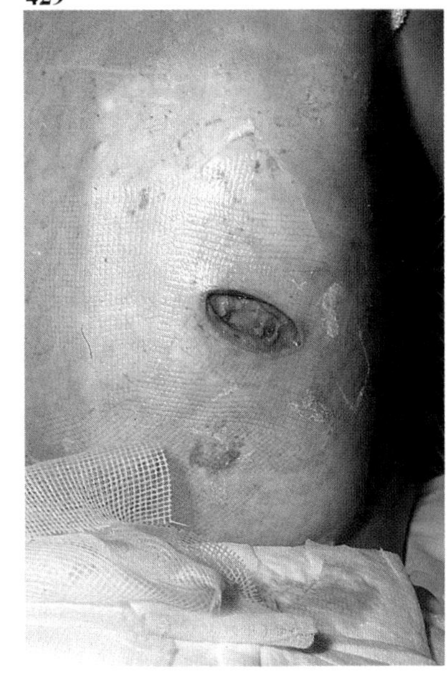

430

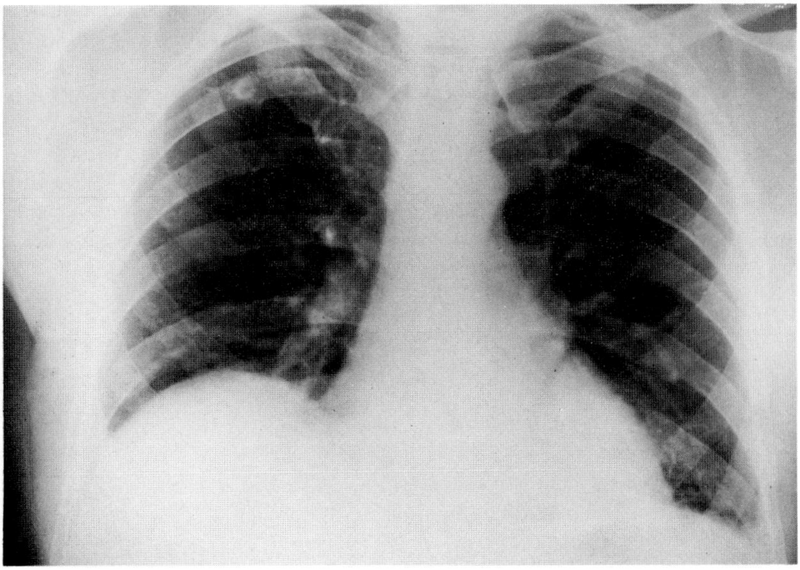

Malaria

Malaria is caused by protozoan parasites of the genus *Plasmodium* transmitted to man by the bite of female anopheline mosquitoes. Malarial infections are confined to man, who is the intermediate host. The definitive host is the mosquito, in which the sexual forms of the parasite are found. Malaria is almost entirely restricted to the tropics and subtropics; occasionally, however, an infected mosquito may be transported to a non-endemic area and infect man, or an infected person from an endemic area may be the source of infection for a mosquito in a temperate part of the world.

431 Liver schizont. Sporozoites inoculated by the biting mosquito spend a short time in the peripheral blood before localising in the liver. Depending on the species of parasite, the products of the liver schizont are released early or late into the peripheral blood, where they parasitise erythrocytes. The parasites of malignant tertian or falciparum malaria and those of quartan malaria are released early, whereas those of vivax and ovale may be released weeks, months, or even years later.

432 *Plasmodium falciparum* — small rings. The parasite of malignant tertian malaria appears within peripheral erythrocytes as small rings or merozoites. More than one parasite may be seen within a single red blood cell, and the parasitaemia (proportion of red blood cells parasitised) may even be as high as 20%. Further development of the parasite takes place in deep visceral rather than surface vessels.

433 *Plasmodium falciparum* — gametocytes. These sexual forms of the parasite appear in the peripheral blood days or weeks after the asexual forms are first seen and are infectious for mosquitoes. Those of *P. falciparum* are characteristically crescent-shaped.

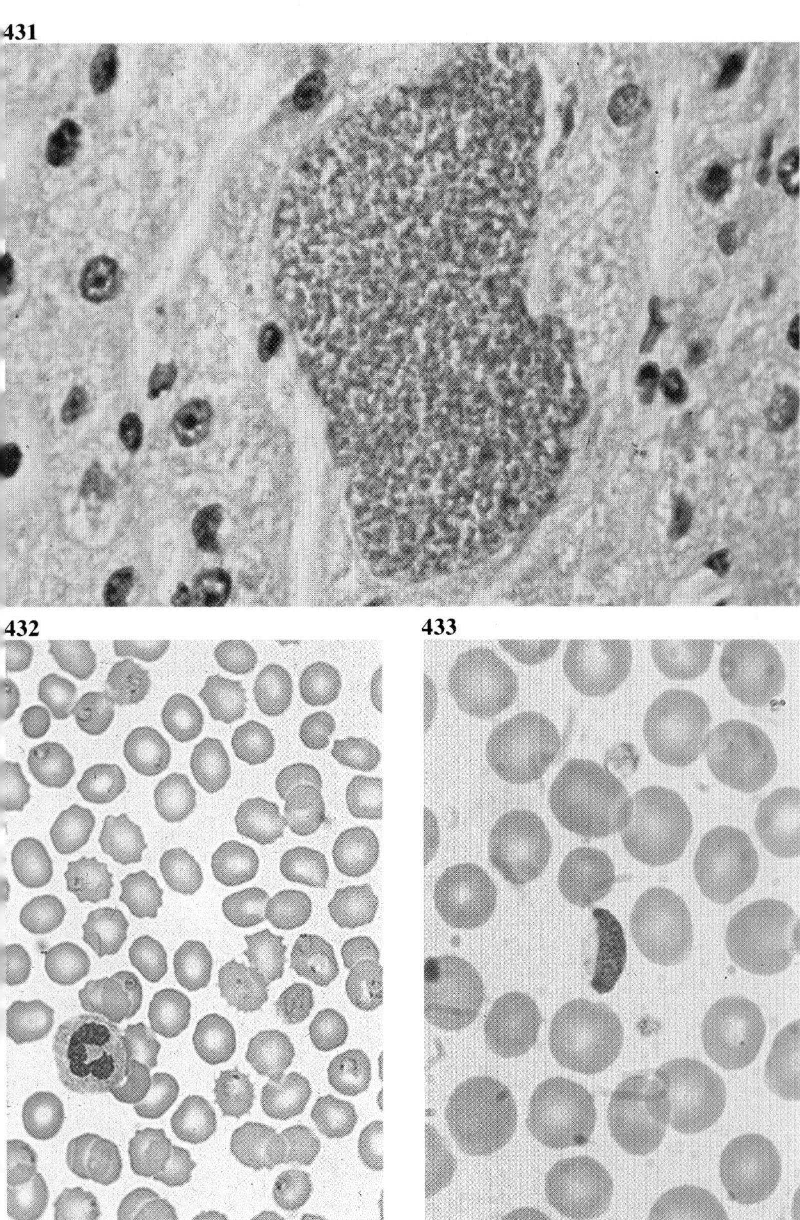
431
432
433

434 ***Plasmodium vivax.*** This species is readily recognised in peripheral blood films, as it fills and enlarges the invaded erythrocyte. Note the characteristic Schüffner's dots. Parasitaemia is seldom greater than 1%, and gametocytes are rarely seen.

435 ***Plasmodium ovale.*** *P. ovale*, seen in peripheral blood films, is similar to *P. vivax*, but the filled red blood cells tend to be oval and have a somewhat crenated surface. Gametocytes are rarely seen.

436 ***Plasmodium malariae.*** The parasite of quartan malaria produces febrile paroxysms with a 72-hour periodicity and generally gives a low parasitaemia. Recrudescences resulting from the persistence of blood forms, rather than liver forms, may occur years after the initial infection. The 'band' form seen here is characteristic of *P. malariae*.

437 **Nephrotic syndrome.** The nephrotic syndrome is a complication of malaria, especially in children infected with *P. malariae*. It differs from the nephrotic syndrome of children in temperate climates in that it occurs at a later age (three to five years), responds less well to corticosteroids, and has a worse prognosis. Furthermore, it does not respond to antimalarial treatment.

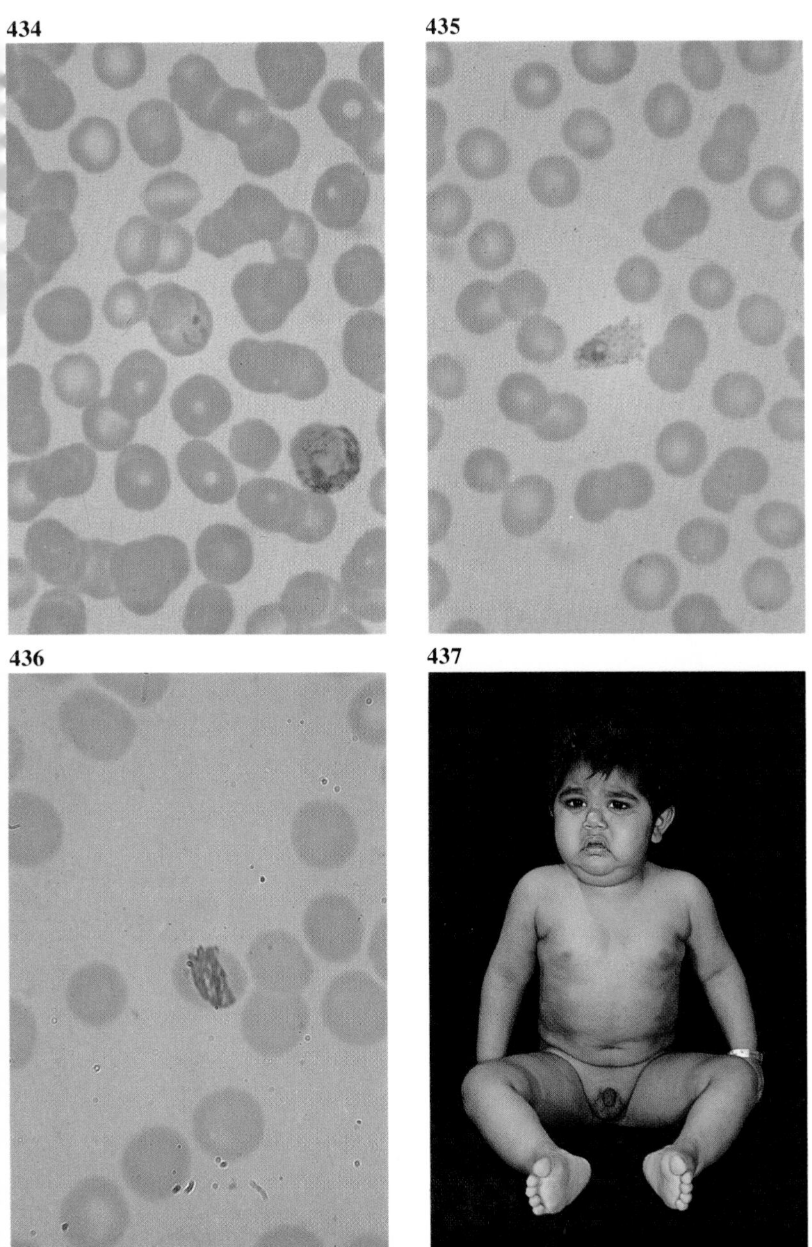
434
435
436
437

438 Jaundice. Fever, rigors and sweating are usually the sole abnormal physical findings in an attack of malaria. In falciparum infections, which are responsible for complicated malaria, there may be other signs, including jaundice. This is caused partly by haemolysis and partly by liver damage. When jaundice is pronounced it is often associated with other features of complicated malaria, including cerebral symptoms, renal failure and haemorrhage.

439 Haemorrhage. Thrombocytopenia is common in falciparum malaria but is usually not severe enough to produce bleeding. Occasionally, however, subconjunctival haemorrhage may occur.

438

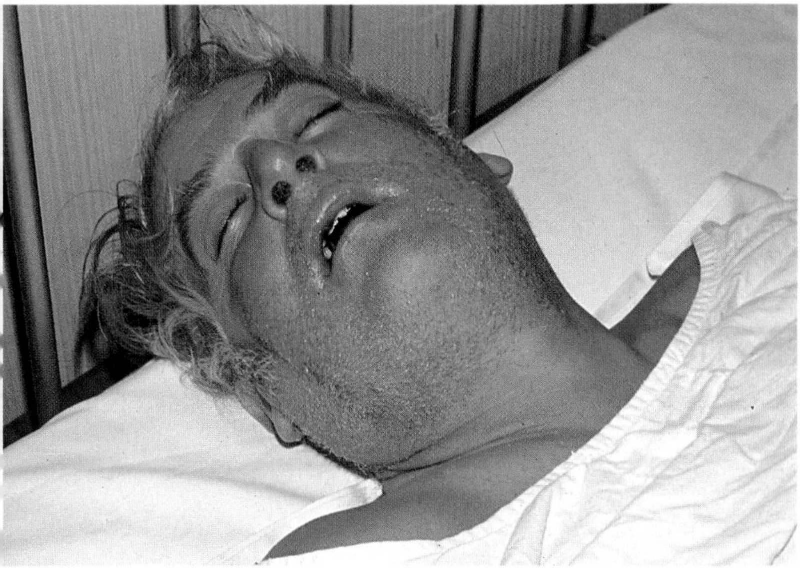

439

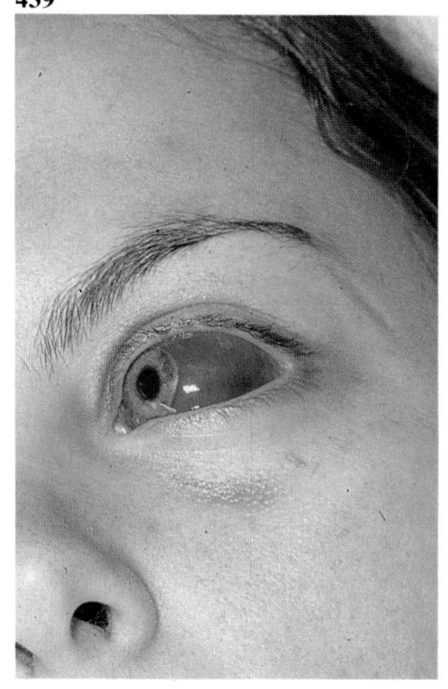

440 Histology — cerebral malaria. Only falciparum malaria is fatal. Deterioration may be sudden and can occur even when the patient is taking antimalarial drugs by mouth. Death is due to the effects of occlusion of visceral vessels packed with parasitised erythrocytes. Cerebral malaria is a manifestation of such occlusion. In the section of brain shown here there is pigment, and the erythrocytes contain dividing parasites (schizonts).

441 Histology – liver. Malarial pigment is prominent in liver sections from fatal cases and in liver biopsy samples from patients living in endemic areas. (A = pigment.)

440

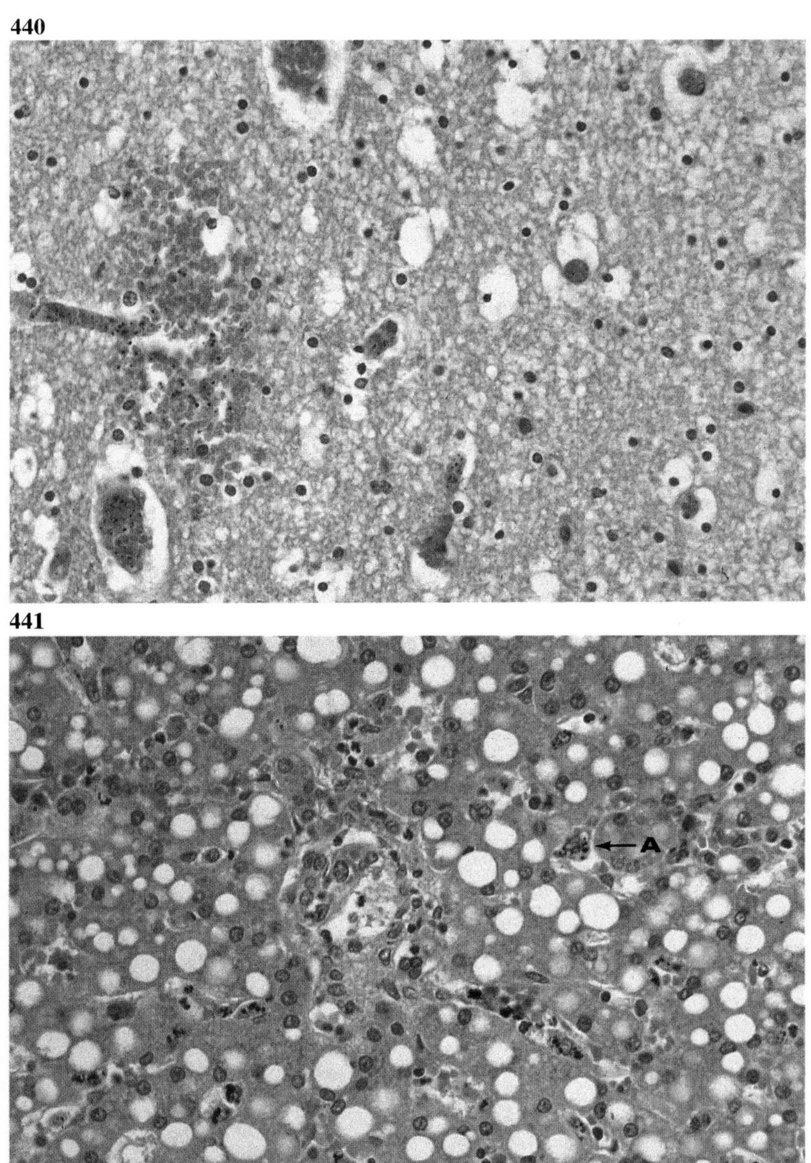

Toxoplasmosis

Infection with the protozoon *Toxoplasma gondii* is widespread in birds and many mammals, including man. The incidence in human populations varies considerably throughout the world and is highest in the tropics. Human toxoplasmosis acquired after birth generally results in subclinical infection or a benign lymphadenitis, but may occasionally cause encephalitis or a highly fatal generalised disease. During pregnancy maternal toxoplasmosis readily spreads to the fetus causing death, or serious damage to the eyes or brain.

In acquired toxoplasmosis the common pattern of disease is benign lymphadenitis closely resembling the glandular variety of acute infectious mononucleosis. Examination of the blood may show a lymphocytosis with atypical cells, but results from Paul–Bunnell testing are invariably negative. The main features of the illness are fatigue and slight lymphatic enlargement, which may be generalised or confined to one region. Convalescence is protracted, but complete recovery is the rule. The diagnosis is established by the Sabin–Feldman dye test.

The toxoplasma exists in three main forms: trophozoite, tissue cyst, and faecal cyst. The trophozoite, or free form, spreads within the host causing disease. It is a nucleated cell with a crescent or pear shape and is approximately 5 μm in length. It multiplies within the cytoplasm of a host cell by a process of internal budding called endodyogeny. Eventually the host cell becomes distended with trophozoites and ruptures, releasing the active parasites to infect other cells.

As immunity develops the free forms are destroyed, and the parasite enters a cystic phase in the tissues of the eye, central nervous system, and skeletal muscle. These cysts contain zoites and may persist for many years without provoking a host reaction. It is likely that infection is transmitted by eating uncooked meat containing cysts.

A sexual cycle of reproduction has been discovered in the intestines of infected cats. Gametes form within the mucosal cells, and a fertilised macrogamete is shed as an oocyst. This undergoes further maturation in the soil to form a mature faecal cyst containing four sporozoites. After ingestion by any warm-blooded animal the cyst wall is digested, and the sporozoites penetrate the mucosal cells where they change to trophozoites and invade the host.

Organism

442 Trophozoites within cytoplasm of host cell (Leishman's stain). Trophozoites may be found within the cytoplasm of any nucleated cell but are particularly common in cells of the reticuloendothelial system. They are crescent- or pear-shaped with rounded or pointed ends. With Leishman's stain the cytoplasm of the trophozoite is blue and contains a rounded red-stained mass of chromatin, the nucleus. The sizes can be gauged relative to the faintly outlined red blood cells. Reproduction is asexual by longitudinal binary division. Eventually an intracellular colony (pseudocyst) of 16 to 32 trophozoites is formed.

443 Trophozoites released from cell (Leishman's stain). The host cell ruptures, releasing the trophozoites, which spread throughout the body, invading and multiplying within cells of the reticuloendothelial system until immunity develops, and the free forms are destroyed.

444 Tissue cyst in cerebellum (H and E). As immunity rises cysts form, and the parasite enters another phase of its cycle. These cysts are separated from the host tissues by a tough elastic membrane and do not provoke an inflammatory reaction unless they leak. The young cyst is small and contains only two zoites, which resemble small trophozoites, but the cyst gradually grows as the zoites multiply until it may eventually reach 100 μm in diameter and contain many thousands of zoites.

Tissue cysts are scanty, and many tissue sections may be examined before one is found. Shrinkage during fixation has caused the unstained halo round this cyst in the cerebellum. (Arrow = cyst.)

Pathology

445 Section of infected lymph node showing active germinal centres (H and E). The histological appearance of an infected lymph node is not pathognomonic, and parasitic cysts are seldom found. The lesion is a non-necrotising granuloma with numerous small clusters of large epithelioid macrophages scattered amongst lymphoid tissue. There are no giant cells. A similar appearance is found in early tuberculosis and in sarcoidosis. (Arrow = large epithelioid macrophages.)

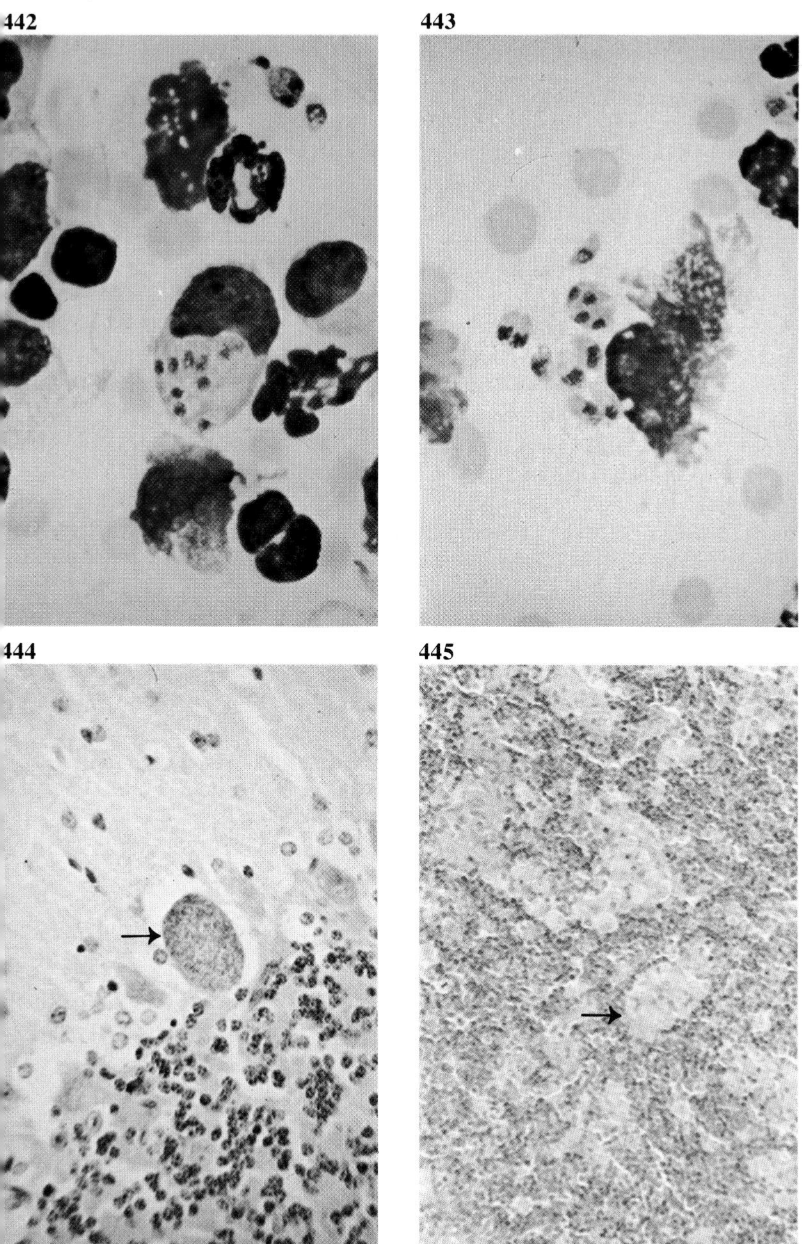
442
443
444
445

Clinical features

446 Acute choroidoretinitis.

447 Chronic choroidoretinitis. Clinical or subclinical infection during pregnancy may result in invasion of the fetus by trophozoites. The extent of the damage depends on the age of the fetus and the virulence of the strain of toxoplasma. In early pregnancy infection may cause abortion, but in the later stages evidence of damage may not appear for several weeks after birth. The reticuloendothelial system and muscles are heavily infected initially, but ultimately the parasite tends to localise in the central nervous system, where it may cause severe and lasting damage. The classical triad of hydrocephalus, cerebral calcification, and choroidoretinitis is found in 60% of cases.

Choroidoretinitis is a common manifestation of congenital toxoplasmosis and may be present at birth or develop a few weeks later. In most patients both eyes are affected. Although the eye changes are usually confined to the choroid and retina, adjacent structures may be affected, and the eye grossly damaged. When severe, the defect will be obvious shortly after birth. In such cases a white 'reflex' is present, and it may not be possible to inspect the fundus. When infection is less severe it may be overlooked until attention is drawn to the eye by the presence of squinting and nystagmus. Changes in the fundi may be discovered on routine examination of school children with defective vision. Occasionally older children and adults have acute exacerbations accompanied by haziness of the vitreous and diminished visual acuity.

Once the acute stage has subsided the necrotic tissue is absorbed, leaving an avascular scar through which the sclera often shows. These scars vary in size and may be multiple. They are surrounded by black choroidal pigment.

446

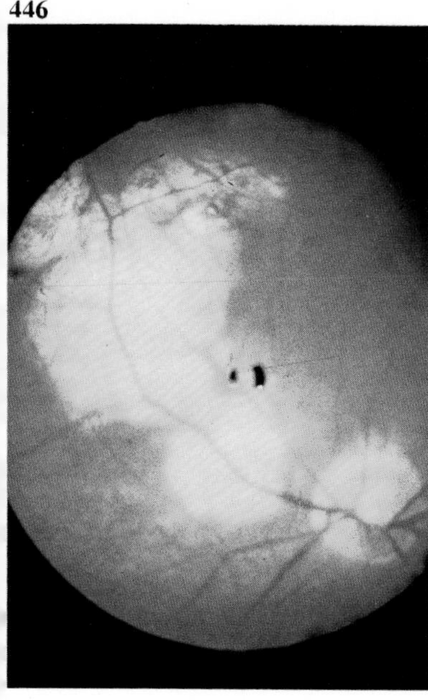

447

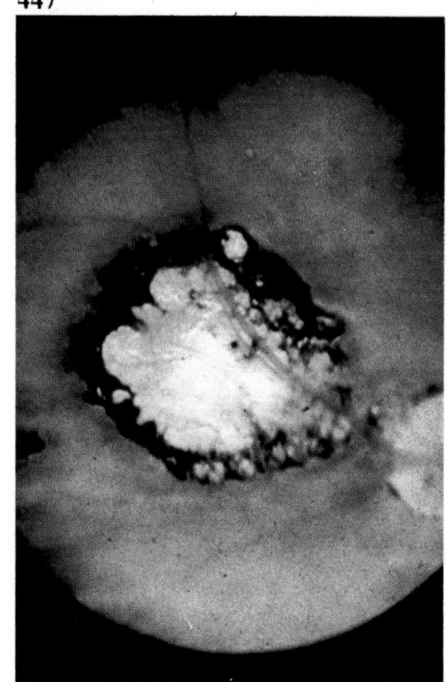

448 Hydrocephalus. Cerebral damage is common but may be difficult to recognise during the first few months of life. In the average attack mental retardation is usually present, often accompanied by epilepsy. The cerebrospinal fluid is xanthochromic with increased protein and cells, predominantly mononuclear.

Inflammatory foci with areas of necrosis are scattered throughout the brain and spinal cord but are particularly numerous in the subependymal layer of tissue in the walls of the lateral ventricles. Necrotic fragments may be shed into the ventricles and block the aqueduct, or acute inflammatory oedema may compress the walls of the aqueduct, leading in both cases to obstructive hydrocephalus.

Destruction of brain tissue in the fetus may be so extensive that the brain is shrivelled, and the greater part of the cranial cavity filled with yellow cerebrospinal fluid. 'Pseudocysts' may be present within the areas of necrosis and are a diagnostic feature. Painstaking search may occasionally reveal trophozoites lying free in the brain, but they can be detected more readily by inoculating cerebrospinal fluid into young mice.

449 Radiograph of skull showing intracranial calcification. During healing, calcium salts are deposited in the necrotic tissue and may be detected by x-ray examination. Calcification is sometimes present at birth but may be delayed for several months.

On x-ray examination linear streaks may be found parallel to the walls of the lateral ventricles and irregular opacities detected in the subcortex and basal ganglia. It should be appreciated, however, that only 50% of children aged under one year with cerebral calcification or choroido-retinitis have toxoplasmosis.

448

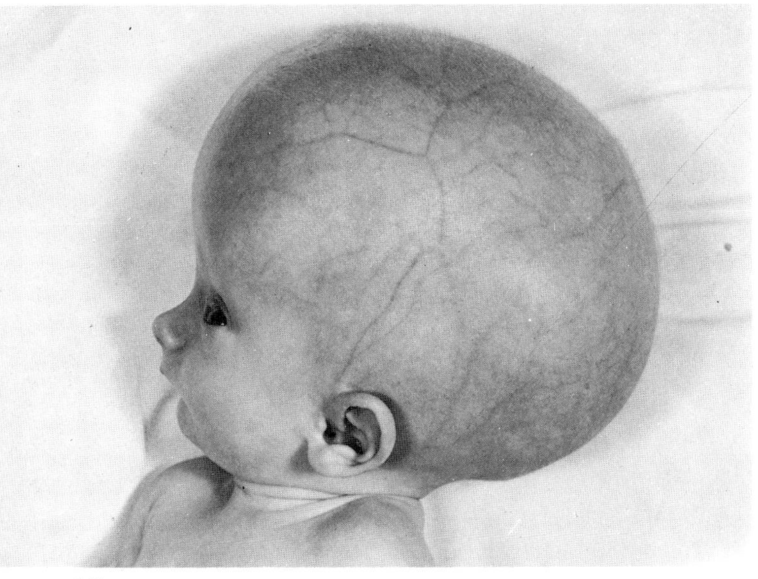

449

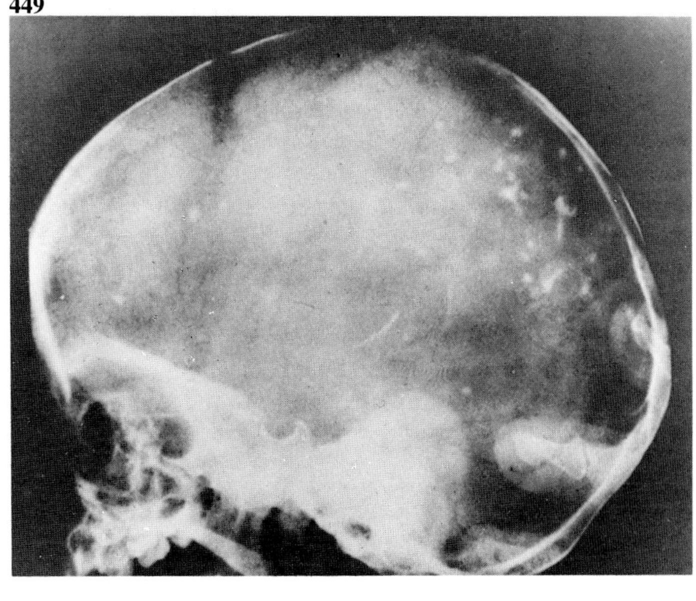

MISCELLANEOUS CONDITIONS

Mycoplasma infection

Mycoplasmas, formerly known as pleuropneumonia-like organisms (PPLO), are very small parasitic or saprophytic micro-organisms that are widely distributed in nature. They are responsible for respiratory disease in man and many animals. *Mycoplasma pneumoniae* (Eaton's agent) has been incriminated as a cause of respiratory illness in man, while *Mycoplasma hominis* type 1 has come under suspicion as a possible cause of non-specific urethritis and other genital tract infections. Many species are found as commensals in the mouth and genital tract of man and animals.

Organism

450 Mycoplasma colonies on agar medium. Mycoplasmas are very small pleomorphic organisms, varying in diameter from 0·125 to 0·3 μm. They contain both DNA and RNA but lack a rigid cell wall. Most species will grow aerobically on a cell-free serum-enriched medium but some require additional carbon dioxide. Growth begins with a granule (elementary corpuscle) that enlarges and then divides by multiple fission into fresh granules or filaments. Granules may remain attached to the parent cell, so many different shapes may arise. On solid agar medium the granules are drawn by capillary action into the interstices of the gel and then grow upwards to the surface where a thin layer spreads outwards from the centre of the colony in the film of water on the surface of the agar. The heaped-up, granular centre surrounded by the thin transparent border produces the typical 'fried egg' appearance. The colonies grow slowly but are visible to the naked eye after seven to 12 days. The morphology of the colony varies with the species. Specific antisera labelled with fluorescein can be used to stain the colonies for identification.

451 Beta-haemolysis caused by *M. pneumoniae*. Some species of mycoplasma produce lysis of sheep or guineapig red blood cells. The haemolysis may be of α or β type and extends for 2 to 5 mm around the colonies. Fermentation of sugars can be used to distinguish *M. pneumoniae* from commensal strains found in man. Each species of mycoplasma appears to be antigenically distinct.

450

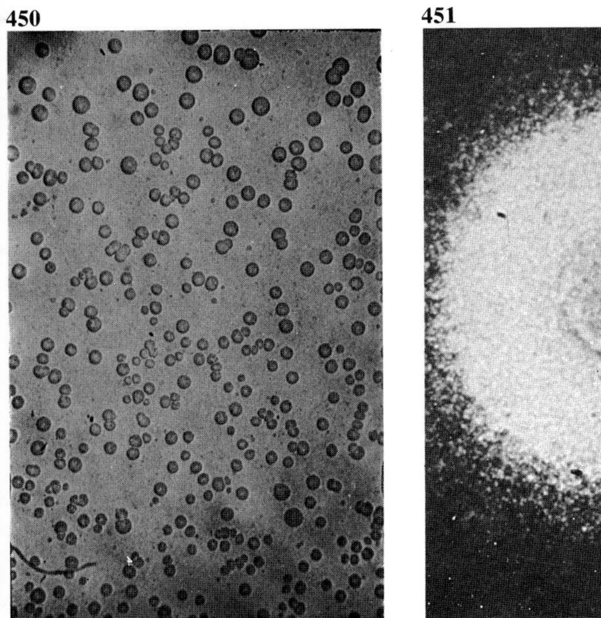

451

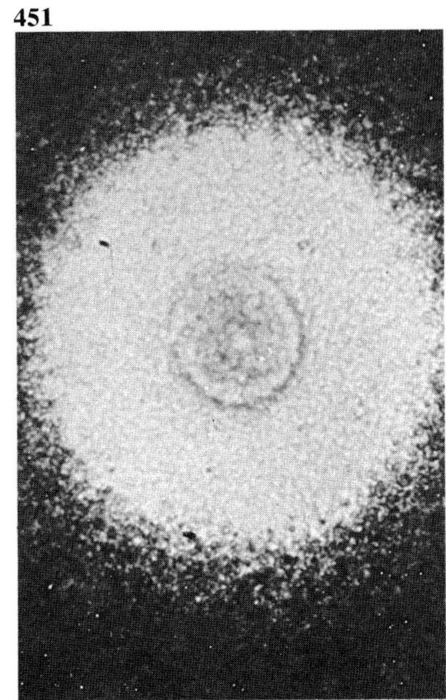

452 Mycoplasma colony. The colonial morphology is distinctive and may be used for preliminary identification. On cross-section the colony has the outline of a drawing pin. The central portion is dense, partly because of the growth of organisms in the interstices of the agar gel and partly because of heaping of organisms on the surface. The peripheral zone is thin and confined to the surface of the agar.

Diseases associated with *Mycoplasma pneumoniae*

Acute respiratory disease

Mycoplasma pneumoniae may cause outbreaks of acute respiratory disease, particularly in enclosed communities. Epidemics may occur at irregular intervals among the general population. Stevens–Johnson syndrome may be associated with mycoplasmal infection. Myringitis bullosa is a rare manifestation in which haemorrhagic bullae are found on the ear drum.

During the course of the illness antibodies against the mycoplasma develop and can be demonstrated by complement fixation, neutralisation, or immune fluorescence. In addition, many patients produce agglutinins that react with *Streptococcus MG* and with human group O erythrocytes at low temperatures.

453 Histology of lung in mycoplasmal pneumonia (H and E). During the acute stage there is widespread inflammation of the lung parenchyma, and the alveolar walls are thickened with infiltrate. Bronchitis and bronchiolitis are prominent features, and there may be ulceration of the mucosa. Plugs of mucopus and debris may block the lumina of bronchioles, causing collapse of some alveoli and compensatory distension of others. The inflammatory exudate consists mainly of mononuclear and red blood cells. The section opposite shows a characteristic appearance in the late stage of the disease, with numerous lymphoid follicles adjacent to a bronchiole. (A = bronchus, B = lymphoid follicle, C = alveolus.)

452

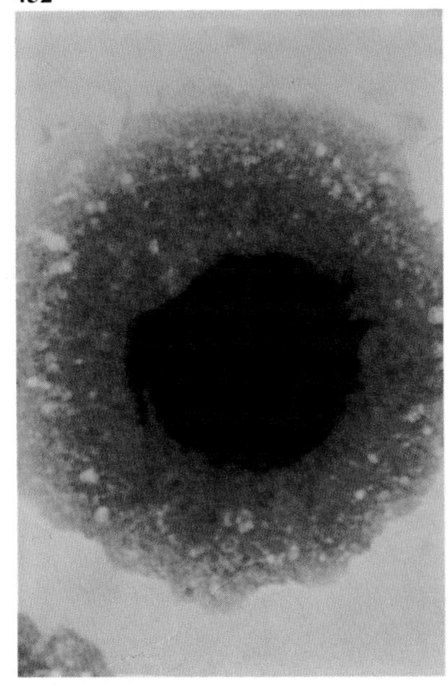

453

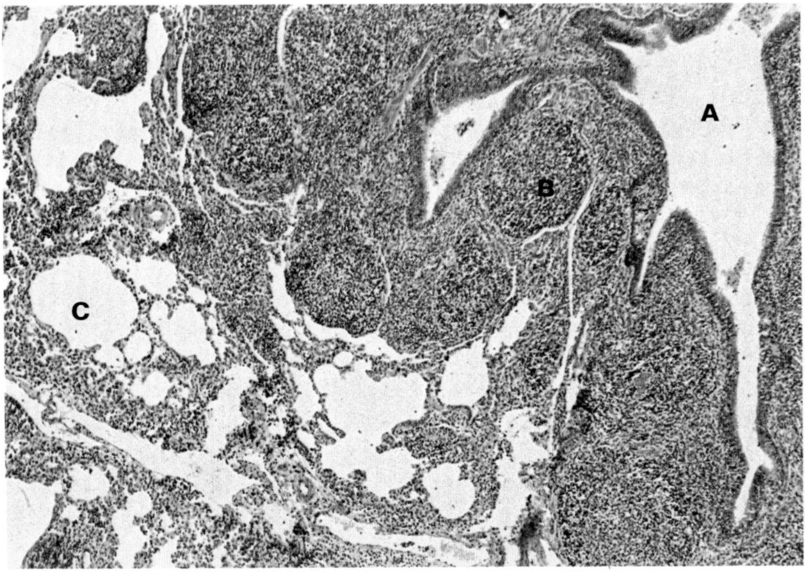

454

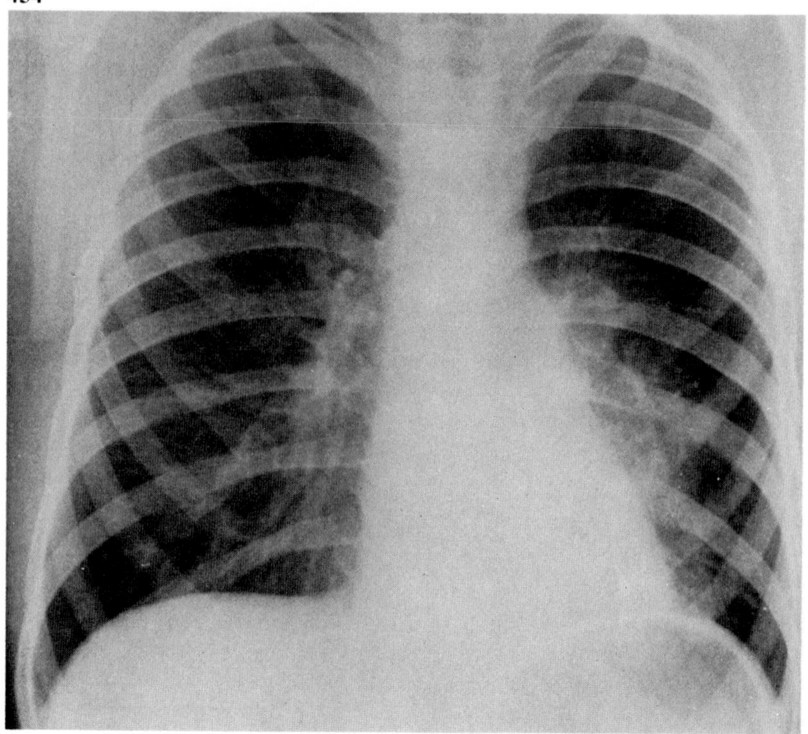

454 Radiograph of chest — peribronchial congestion. Onset of illness is gradual with general symptoms of headache, shivering, myalgia, and notable lassitude. Within a day or two the patient develops signs of an upper respiratory infection with an inflamed throat, followed by a distressing cough and retrosternal discomfort from tracheobronchitis. The sputum is scanty and may be mucoid or mucopurulent. Occasionally there may be streaks of blood. Radiography of the chest in such patients may show streaky shadowing from peribronchial congestion.

455

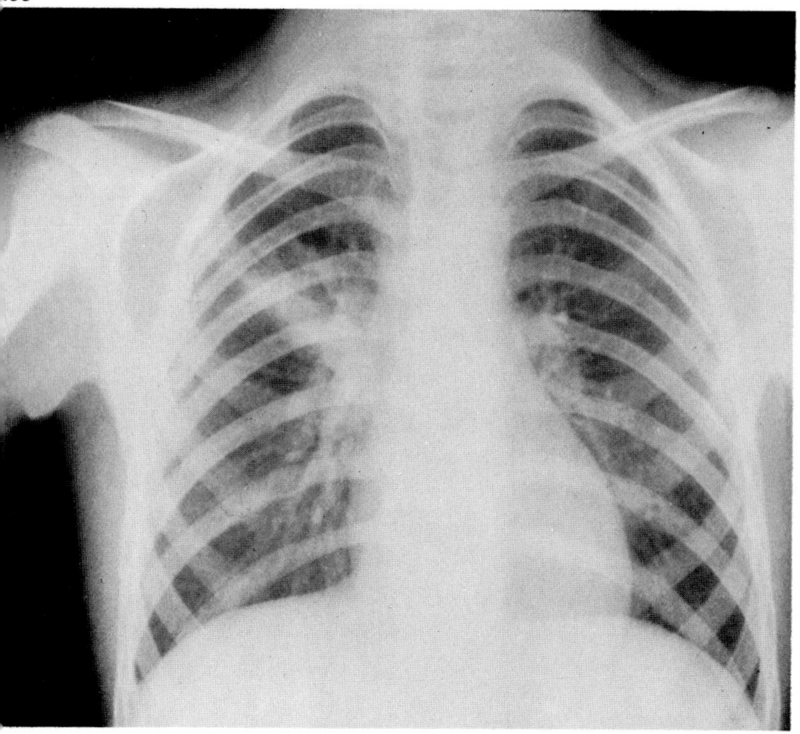

455 Radiograph of chest — lobular infection. The severity of the illness and the extent of pulmonary infection vary greatly. The main features are fever, malaise and undue tiredness. Respiratory distress is unusual and little can be found on clinical examination of the chest, apart from a few crepitations. Blockage of bronchioles, resulting in small areas of atelectasis, and spread of inflammation into the lung tissue around the bronchioles, are manifest as soft miliary shadowing or fine nodular mottling on chest radiographs.

456 Radiograph of chest — hilar flare. In some cases radiography will show opacities with a ground-glass appearance fanning out from the hilum. This finding is not confined to mycoplasmal infection but can be caused by the psittacosis/ornithosis agent, *Coxiella burnetii*, and a number of viruses, including respiratory syncytial virus, adenovirus, para-influenza virus, and influenza virus. For a definitive diagnosis it is necessary to demonstrate a four-fold rise in antibody against the suspected agent. Complement-fixation tests are commonly used; although not as sensitive as other antibody tests in mycoplasmal infections, they have the advantage of simplicity. Up to 50% of patients with mycoplasma pneumonia develop cold agglutinins against human type O red blood cells and over 60% may also possess agglutinating antibody against *Streptococcus MG*.

456

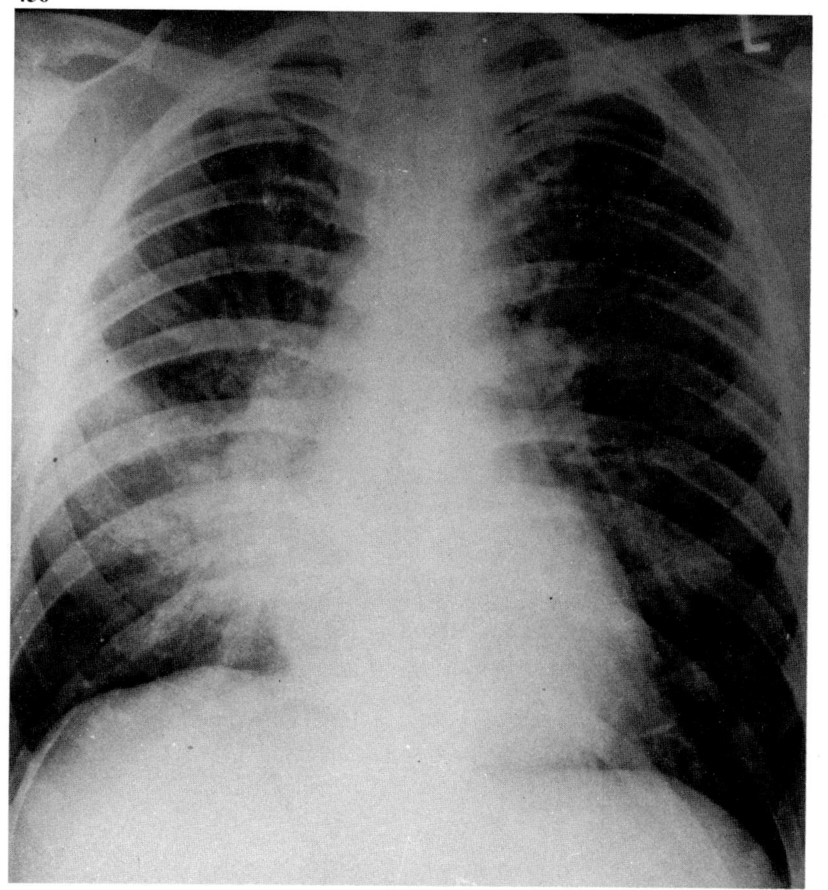

457 Radiograph of chest — lobar infection. The appearance of the lungs on x-ray examination varies considerably and does not match the clinical state. The shadows may be discrete and scattered throughout both lungs or may be confluent and confined to one lobe, especially the lower. Occasionally, the shadows migrate from one area to another.

The white blood cell count is usually normal but may be increased to 15×10^9/l. In at least 40% of cases the erythrocyte sedimentation rate exceeds 80mm/h. Although the illness usually follows a benign course, recovery is slow and radiological changes may persist for weeks. Death is rare and complications uncommon.

457

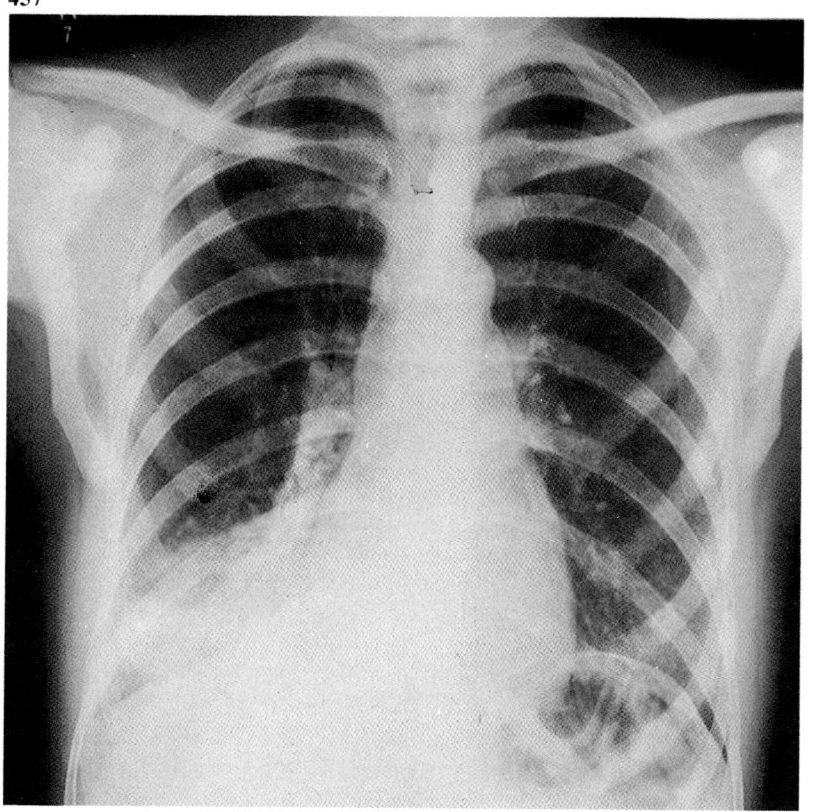

Stevens–Johnson syndrome

458 Mycoplasma and Stevens–Johnson syndrome. *Mycoplasma pneumoniae* may give rise to Stevens–Johnson syndrome with or without evidence of pulmonary infection. The fully developed syndrome consists of conjunctivitis, stomatitis, vulvitis or urethritis, and a pleomorphic rash (see **460** to **463**).

The conjunctivae are acutely inflamed, and the eyelids may be stuck together with congealed pus. When the mouth is severely affected there may be extensive ulceration and swallowing is painful. Towards the end of the second week the mucocutaneous lesions begin to heal, and the patient's general condition improves rapidly.

459 Mycoplasma and Stevens–Johnson syndrome. *Mycoplasma pneumoniae* has been recovered from patients with Stevens–Johnson syndrome. Because the dermis and epidermis are both affected there is considerable variation in the clinical appearance of the lesions. There is notable oedema of the dermis and heavy infiltration with neutrophil and eosinophil leucocytes. The small blood vessels are dilated and surrounded by lymphocytes. Vesicles may form both in the epidermis and in the dermis. Subepidermal vesicles may coalesce to form large bullae. The centre of the lesions may be discoloured by haemorrhage.

The typical target appearance is seen in the two skin lesions in this illustration. A large bulla rests on an erythematous base, and a dark area of haemorrhage is present in the centre.

458

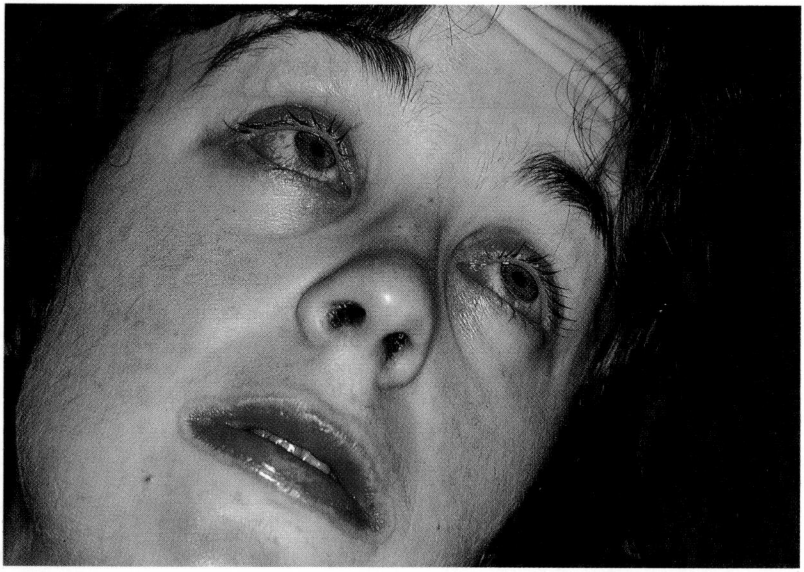

459

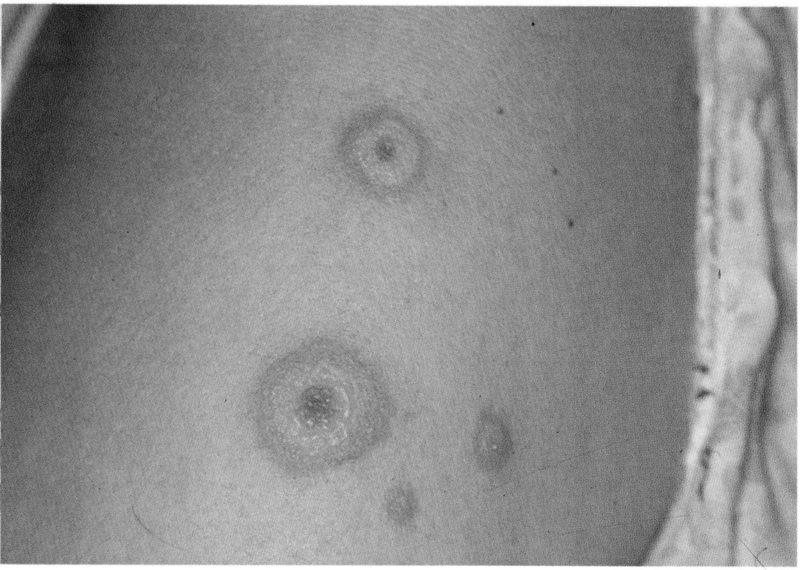

Stevens–Johnson syndrome

The Stevens–Johnson syndrome consists of a combination of a pleomorphic rash with severe ulceration of the mouth and inflammatory lesions of the eye and urethra. It is a condition of acute hypersensitivity and probably a severe variant of erythema multiforme. The precipitating factor may be an infection, particularly of the throat, or the syndrome may follow the use of drugs, such as sulphonamides or antibiotics (see also page 374).

460 Stevens–Johnson syndrome — mouth and buccal cavity. The illness usually begins with fever and some general malaise, followed by lesions on mucous membranes and skin. The stomatitis is particularly distressing since the mouth ulcers are painful and tend to bleed. The lips are often black with congealed blood and there may be difficulty in opening the mouth. When the buccal cavity and pharynx are severely ulcerated swallowing becomes an ordeal. Ulceration may extend into the trachea and bronchi and may be accompanied by pneumonia.

461 Stevens–Johnson syndrome — eyes. There is intense inflammation of the conjunctiva and the eyelids are often stuck together with pus.

Urethritis causes pain on micturition and lesions are usually present on the external genitalia. The patient remains acutely ill for a week or ten days before the disease gradually resolves.

460

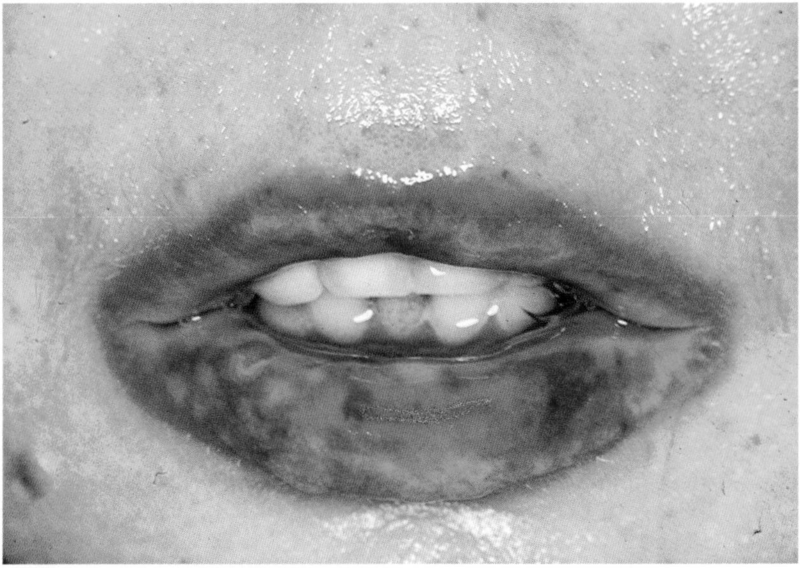

461

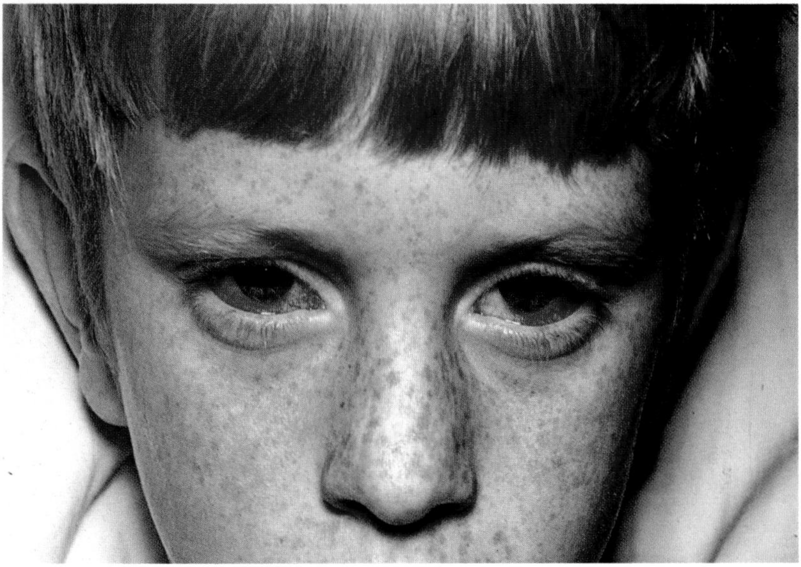

462 Stevens–Johnson syndrome — rash on trunk. The rash may precede or follow the other features. In mild cases the eruption appears on the extensor surfaces of the limbs and on the dorsum of the hands and feet; in more severe cases it involves the trunk, neck and head and even the palms and soles. The scalp is rarely affected. Centrifugal distribution of the rash may closely resemble that of smallpox and used to cause difficulty in differential diagnosis. Some rashes are morbilliform but they do not evolve from above downwards; extensor surfaces are much more heavily affected than in measles (see **348** and **355**).

463 Stevens–Johnson syndrome — close-up of rash. The typical eruption consists of circular erythematous lesions with concentric rings of different colours. These target or iris lesions measure about 1 cm in diameter and appear chiefly on the extremities. The rash is very variable and may consist of erythematous patches, vesicles, pustules and bullae in different combinations. Blood may escape into some of the lesions, altering the colour.

On histological examination of the skin the small blood vessels are congested and surrounded by mononuclear cells. Fluid exudate disrupts the cell layers, producing papules, vesicles and bullae.

464 Stevens–Johnson syndrome — arthritis. Many other structures may be affected in addition to the skin and mucous membranes. Pneumonia is a common complication, and myocarditis, pericarditis, encephalitis, and enteritis occur occasionally. This patient with Stevens–Johnson syndrome had painful swelling of the small joints of her hands during the acute stage of the rash. The arthritis persisted for a few weeks and then subsided, leaving no residual disability.

462

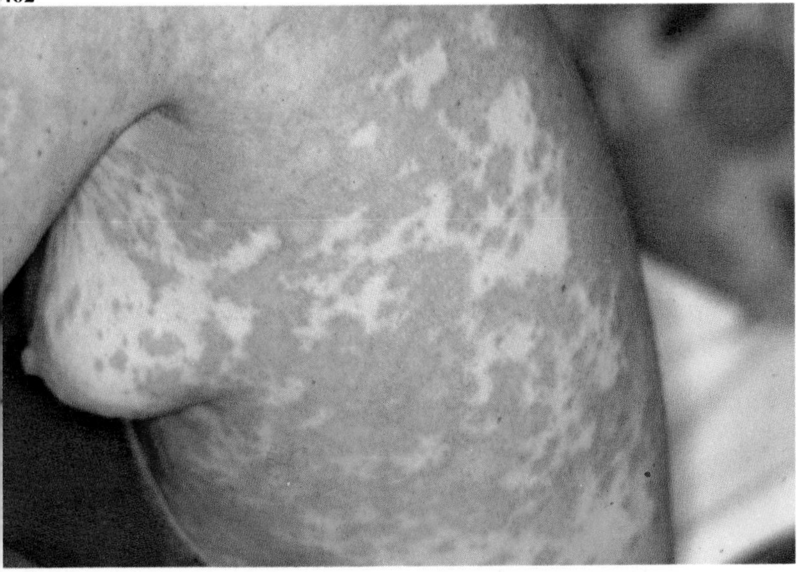

463

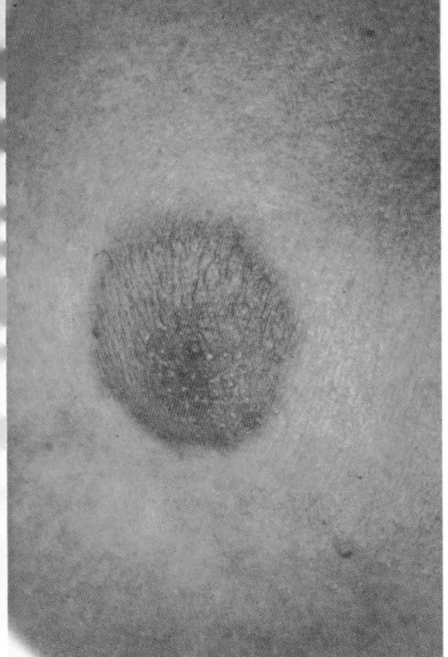

464

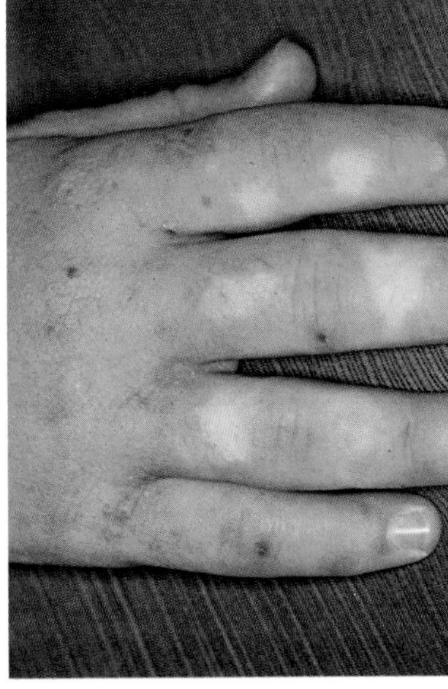

Scalded-skin syndrome (toxic epidermal necrolysis)

Scalded-skin syndrome (toxic epidermal necrolysis), resembles Stevens–Johnson syndrome but differs in respect of skin lesions. These are extremely painful and consist of large patches of necrotic epidermis, which slide off the underlying skin at the slightest pressure, leaving extensive raw areas. The overall picture is that of scalding.

There appear to be two types of scalded-skin syndrome: one induced by drugs and the other by infection with *Staphylococcus aureus*, usually of phage group II. The cleavage in necrolysis induced by drugs takes place in the subepidermal layers, whereas in staphylococcal infection it occurs within the epidermis. The staphylococcal form affects younger age groups and has a lower mortality. The strains of staphylococci associated with scalded-skin syndrome are those causing impetigo, pemphigus neonatorum, and Ritter's disease (see **55** and **56**). The staphylococcus may be present on the skin or other sites and produces an exotoxin (exfoliatin), which is responsible for the necrolysis.

465 Scalded-skin syndrome — lesions on face. The skin has a scalded appearance. The surface layer of the epidermis has separated and slid over the deeper layer, producing a wrinkled effect. The lips are acutely inflamed and crusted.

466 Scalded-skin syndrome — destructive effects. Necrolysis in the subepidermal layers may result in permanent damage to the skin. This child had a severe attack during which her right eyebrow slid on to her forehead before separating with the necrotic skin. The patient survived the acute stage, but the hairs of the eyebrows did not regenerate and keloid scars developed elsewhere.

467 Scalded-skin syndrome — face of Indian woman. The intense conjunctival congestion may be accompanied by keratitis, which may leave scarring and impaired vision. The surface epidermis has sheared off the skin on the eyelids; the lips are ulcerated and covered with dark scabs, where they have bled. The buccal cavity was extensively ulcerated.

465

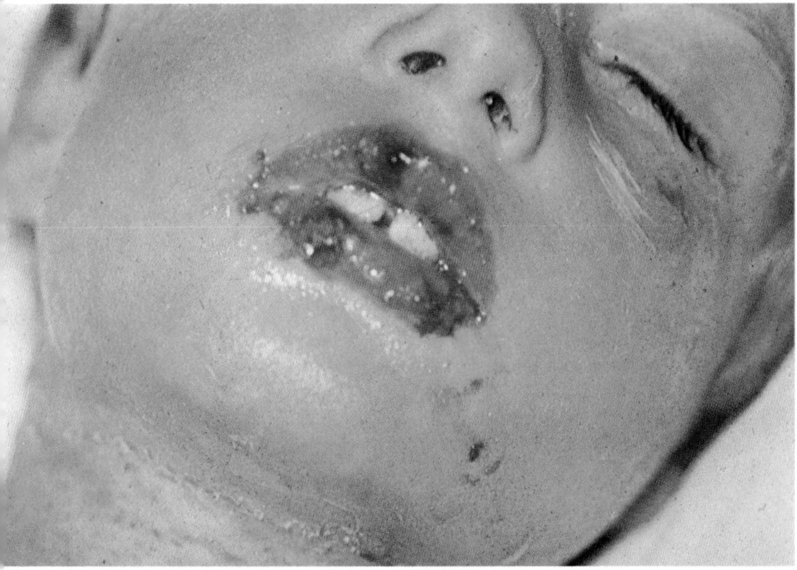

466

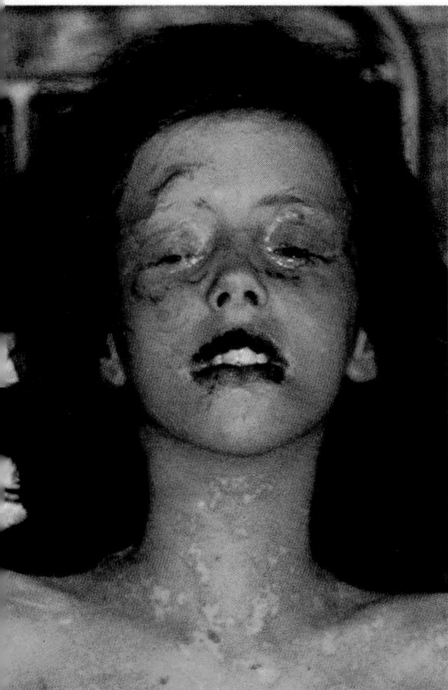

467

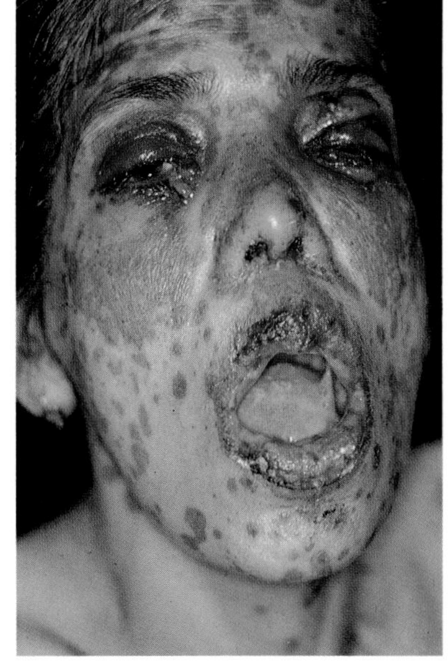

468 Scalded-skin syndrome — lesions on trunk. The surface pigmented layers may be shed during the acute stage in dark-skinned patients, but the colour of the skin is restored to normal during convalescence.

469 Scalded-skin syndrome — close-up of skin. The necrotic epidermis slides off the underlying skin at the slightest pressure. This constitutes Nikolsky's sign, which is not pathognomonic but may be found in other skin diseases, such as pemphigus.

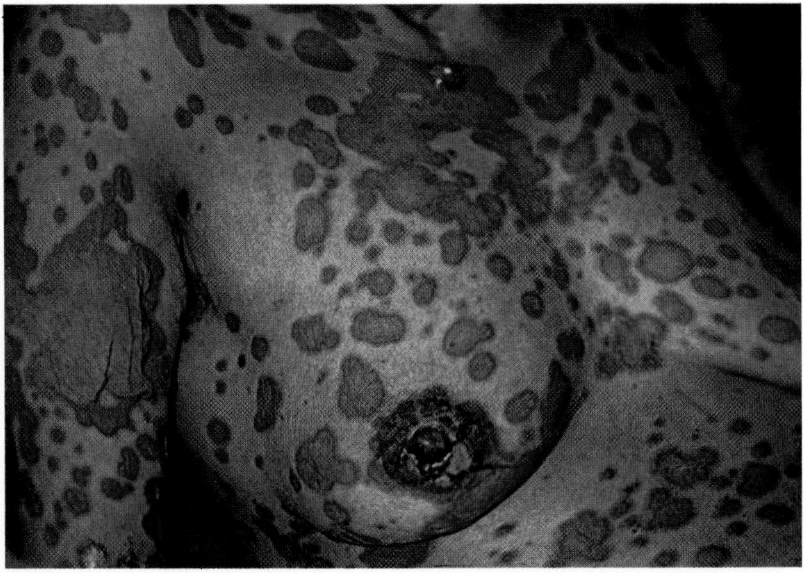

469

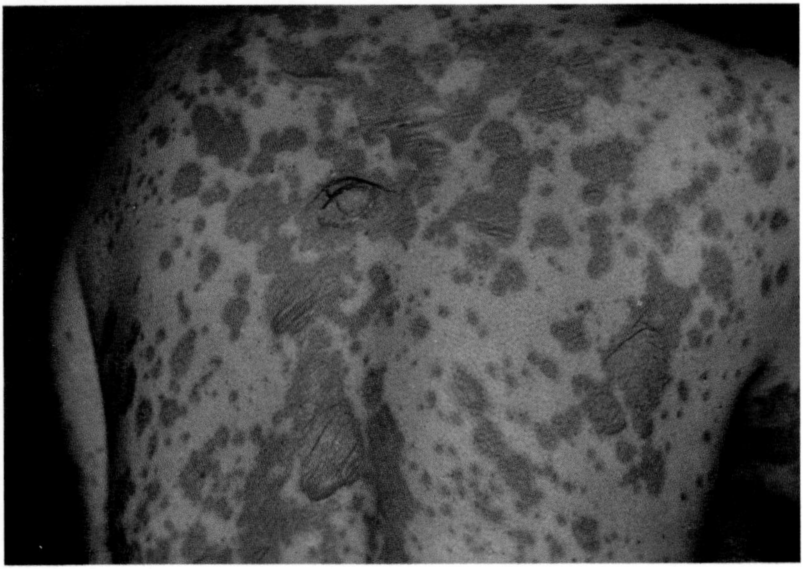

Kawasaki disease

Kawasaki disease, also called mucocutaneous lymph node syndrome, affects children and has been reported from many countries, but particularly Japan, where it was first described. The aetiology is unknown though the disease is believed to be caused by an infectious agent. There are no specific tests and the diagnosis is established clinically when five out of the following six criteria have been met:

1 Fever of unknown aetiology
- Lasting for five days or longer
- Unresponsive to antibiotics

2 Conjunctivae — bilateral congestion

3 Lips and mouth
- Lips dry with redness and fissuring
- Tongue — 'strawberry' appearance
- Oropharynx — diffuse redness of the mucosa

4 Periphery of limbs
- Early stage — redness of palms and soles with accompanying oedema of the dorsum of the hands and feet.
- Late stage — membranous desquamation beginning round finger tips

5 Exanthem — pleomorphic rash most prominent on trunk, absence of vesicles and crusts

6 Lymphadenopathy — acute non-suppurative enlargement of cervical nodes

470 Kawasaki disease — conjunctiva. Bilateral conjunctivitis is present in about 90% of cases. The bulbar conjunctivae are most severely affected but the palpebral conjunctivae may also be slightly congested.

471 Kawasaki disease — lips. The same proportion (90%) of patients have dry, reddened, cracked lips.

470

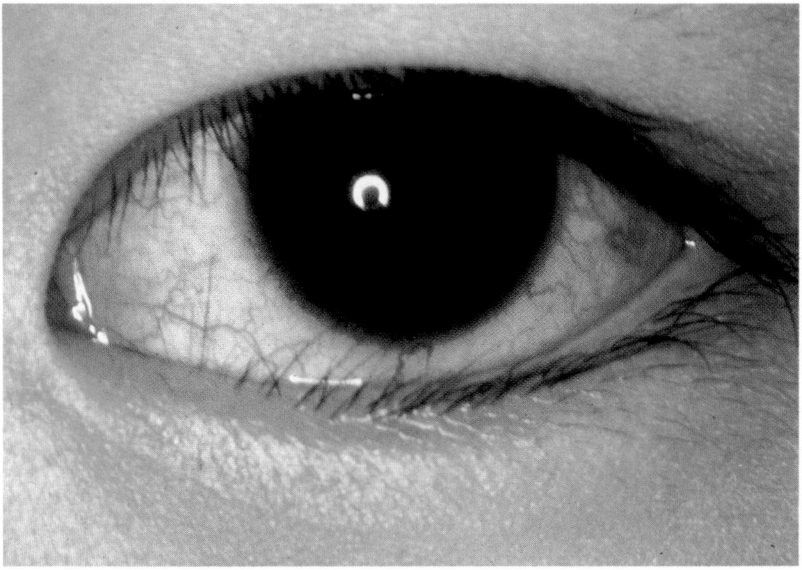

471

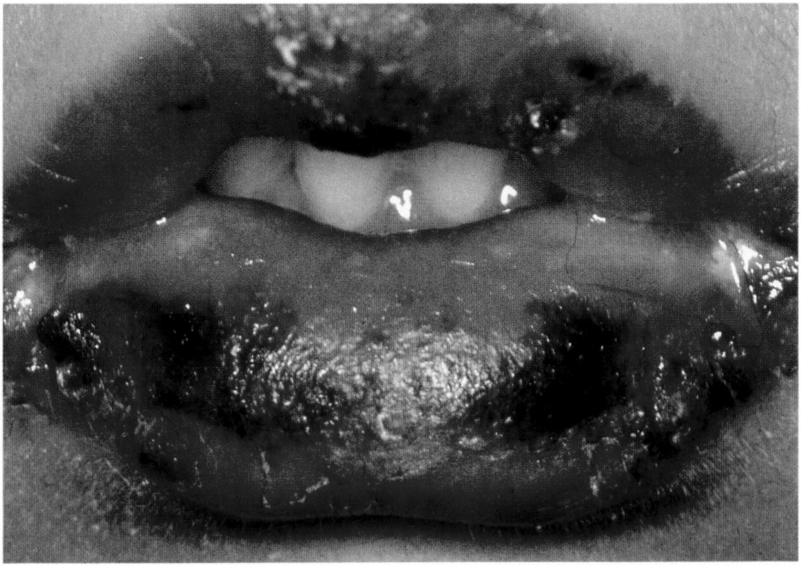

472 Kawasaki disease — tongue. The mucous membrane of the mouth and throat is reddened and dry, and the tongue with prominent red papillae closely resembles the peeled strawberry tongue of scarlet fever.

473 Kawasaki disease — lymph nodes. The cervical lymph nodes are enlarged, firm, and slightly tender. They do not suppurate.

474 Kawasaki disease — exanthem. A rash appears within a few days of onset of fever and usually persists for about a week. It is most prominent over the trunk, but may extend to the face and limbs. It is erythematous and may simulate the exanthem of measles or erythema multiforme.

472

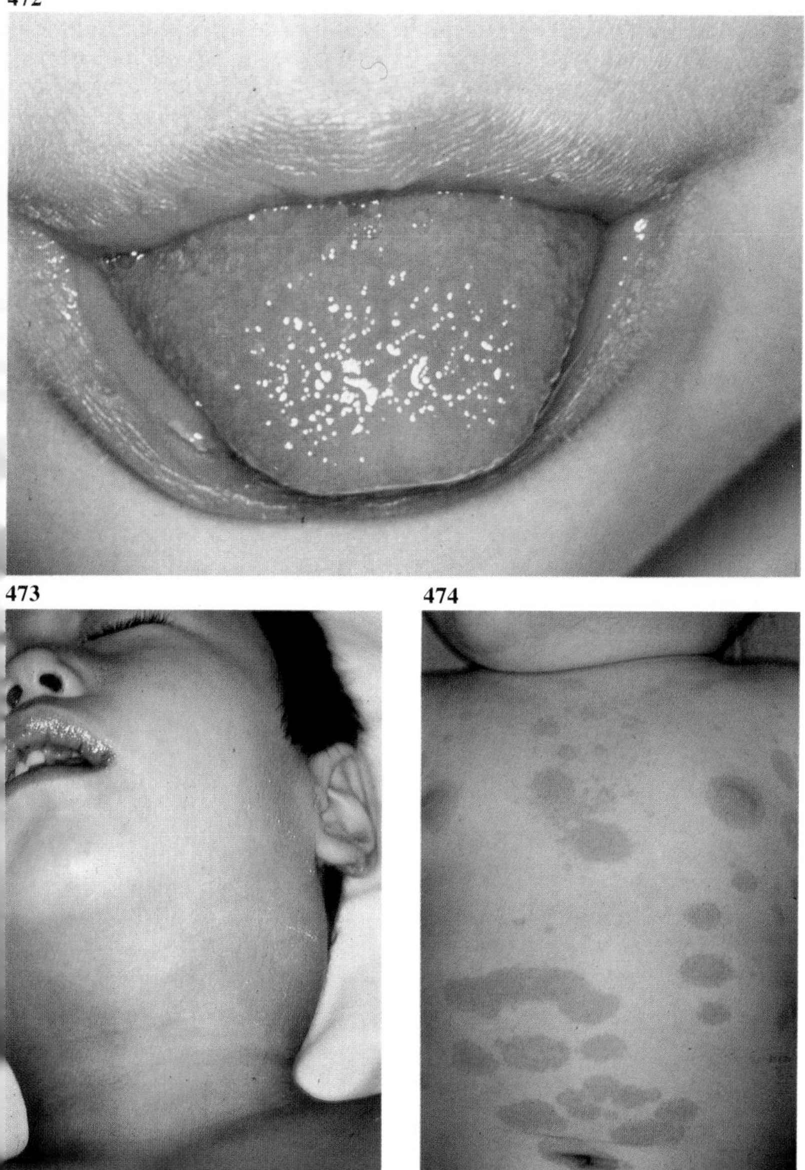

473

474

475 Kawasaki disease — extremities. Indurative oedema of the dorsum of the hands and feet is an early feature and may be accompanied by flushing of the palms and soles.

476 Kawasaki disease — membranous desquamation. During the second or third week of illness the skin begins to peel around the nail folds, and large strips of skin may separate from the fingers.

475

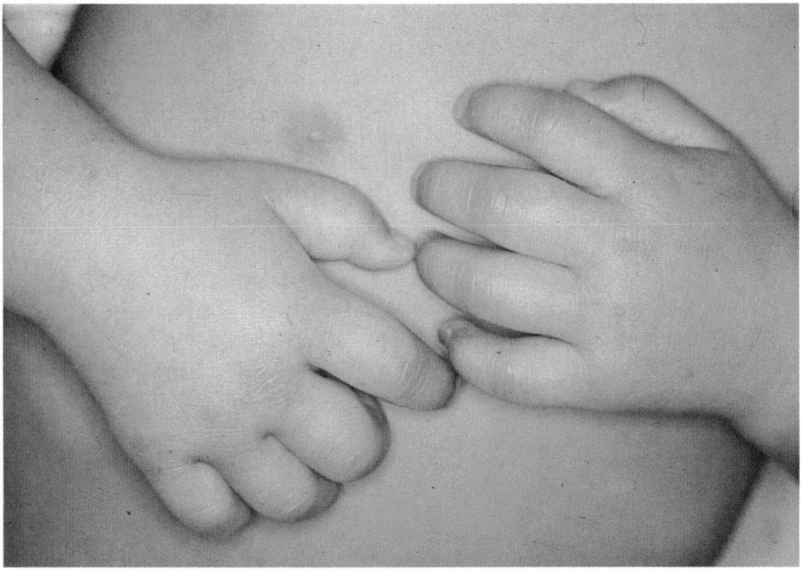

476

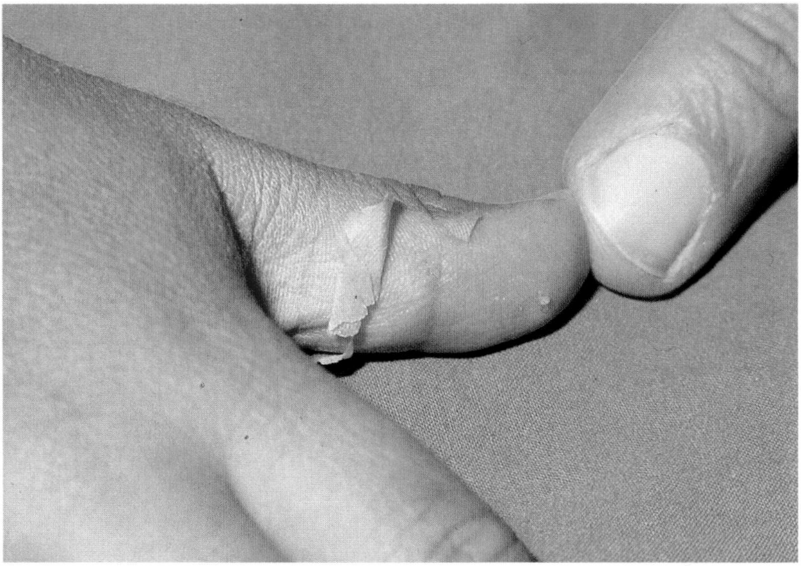

477 Coronary artery thrombosis. Carditis is a common finding and the main cause of death. It may be associated with angiitis of the coronary vessels resulting in aneurysm and thrombosis. The prognosis is worst in boys under one year of age, who have prolonged fever and a rash accompanied by a very high erythrocyte sedimentation rate. Pronounced thrombocytosis is common during the second and third weeks of illness and may predispose the patient to thrombosis. Mortality is between 1 and 2%.

478 Coronary angiography. Abnormal coronary arteries were shown in about 60% of the patients studied in one series. Some patients were found to have aneurysms; others were found to have irregular, tortuous, or stenosed arteries. The angiographic appearances returned to normal in a few patients.

477

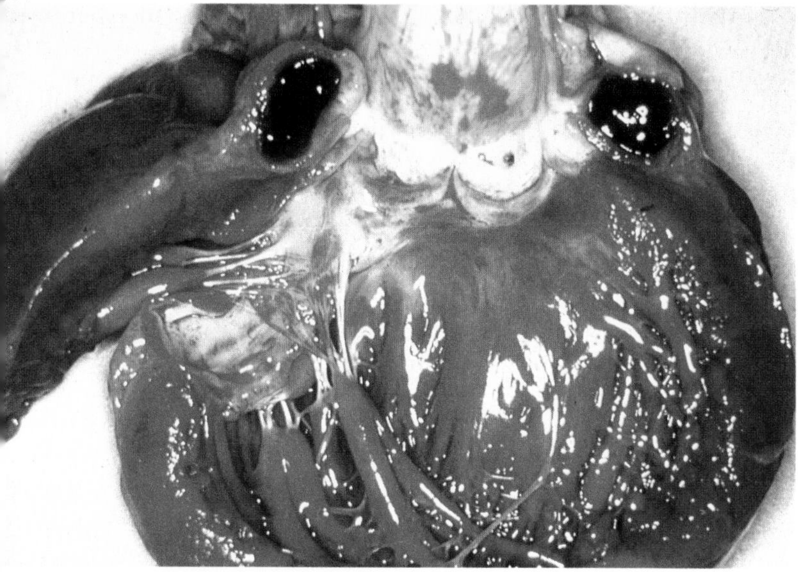

478

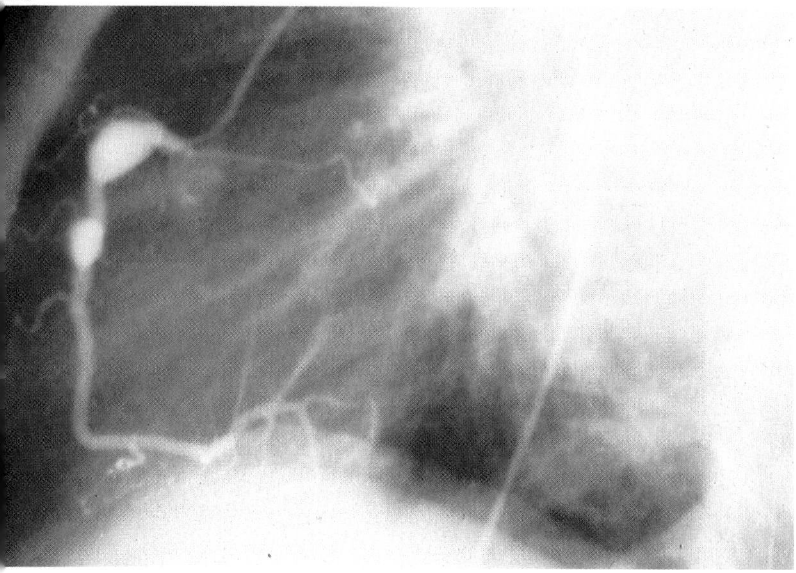

479 Hydrops of the gallbladder. Diarrhoea and abdominal pain may occur at any stage of the illness. In some patients the abdominal discomfort may be associated with hydrops of the gallbladder, which has been demonstrated here by ultrasonography. In this child the hydrops resolved spontaneously. Other features found occasionally include meningitis, arthritis, urethritis, and otitis media. (A = liver, B = gallbladder, C = kidney.)

479

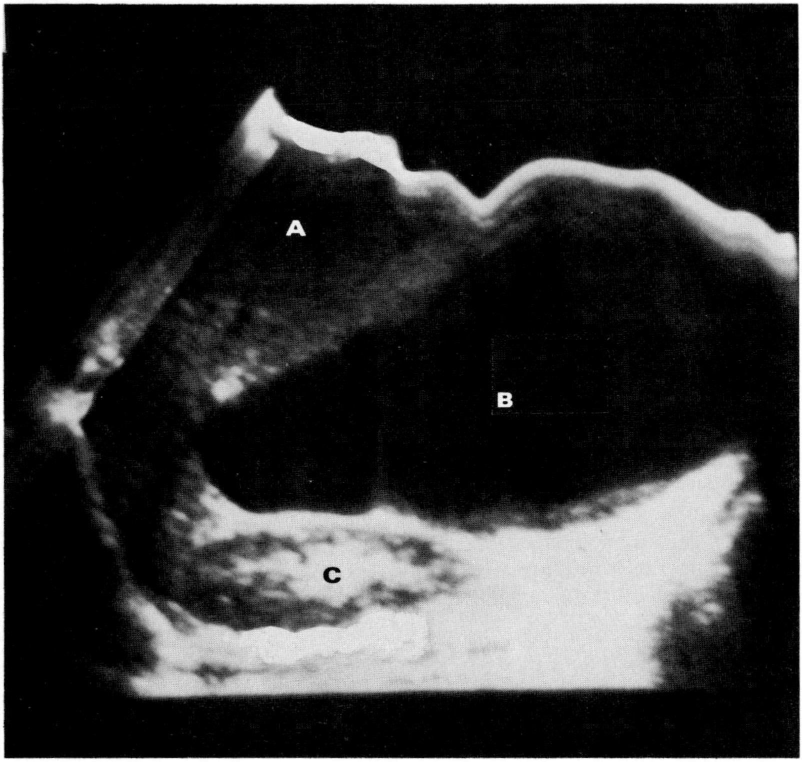

INFECTIONS IN PATIENTS WITH DISTURBED IMMUNITY

There is no sharp distinction between pathogens, commensals, and saprophytes because host immunity plays a decisive part in controlling infection by micro-organisms. When immunity is defective opportunist invasion by commensals and saprophytes may cause serious illness or even death. Increased susceptibility to infection may result from primary disorders of the immune mechanisms, or may be secondary to other disease processes and to immunosuppressive treatment. Opportunist infections have been highlighted by the increasing use of antimicrobial drugs and cytotoxic preparations, and by the emergence of the acquired immune deficiency syndrome (AIDS), caused by HIV (LAV/HTLV III).

480 Hodgkin's disease and varicella. Patients with diseases affecting the reticuloendothelial system are especially vulnerable to infection and may succumb to otherwise trivial conditions. This patient with Hodgkin's disease contracted chickenpox from her children and quickly became very ill. Despite treatment with hyperimmune serum the rash continued to crop, her condition deteriorated, and she died after three to four weeks. Note the large size of the pustules, which proved to be sterile on culture. Blood cultures likewise did not yield bacteria.

Susceptible patients with leukaemia, Hodgkin's disease, and other lymphoproliferative disorders should not be exposed to chickenpox or herpes zoster.

481 Herpes zoster and carcinomatosis. Roughly 8% of patients admitted to hospital with herpes zoster are found to have underlying disease, such as leukaemia, Hodgkin's disease, myelomatosis, or carcinomatosis. Attacks may also be precipitated by radiotherapy or immunosuppressive drugs. Depression of immunity in these circumstances permits latent virus to spread with unpleasant and sometimes disastrous consequences.

The zoster lesions are often haemorrhagic and necrotic, and the generalised rash profuse. Death may follow from uncontrolled growth of the virus and widespread cellular destruction.

480

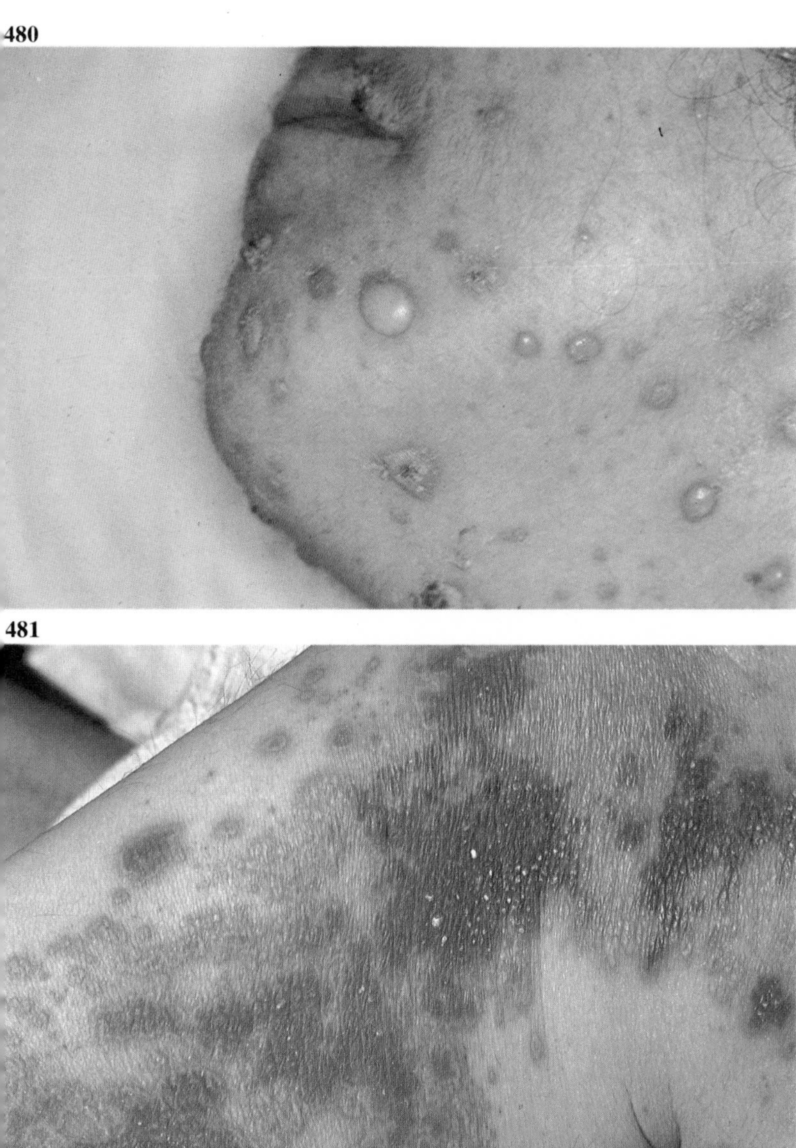

481

482 Cytomegalovirus infection and immunosuppressive treatment. Generalised inclusion disease may occur in patients with reticulosis or those receiving immunosuppressive drugs after transplant surgery. The lungs and kidneys are commonly involved and virus may be recovered from the throat and urine (see **297**). It seems likely that the immunity disturbance permits reactivation of latent virus.

Typical large intranuclear inclusion bodies can be seen in the epithelial cells lining the dilated tubule in the centre of the kidney section opposite. (Arrow = renal tubule lined with large cells containing inclusions.)

483 Infection of pressure sore — carcinomatosis. Immunity drops during the terminal stages of carcinomatosis and Gram-negative organisms from the environment may invade the tissues or bloodstream causing death. Enterobacteria and pseudomonads may colonise pressure ulcers in such debilitated patients. Spread may occur to other patients. In the last hours of life dying patients may shed pathogenic staphylococci.

484 Tuberculosis and corticosteroid treatment. Corticosteroid treatment may cause reactivation of latent tuberculous infection with dissemination. This section of brain shows the typical histological appearances of tuberculous meningitis. There is a granulomatous reaction in the meninges with caseation, round cell infiltration, and giant cell formation. (A = brain tissue, B = tubercle in meninges, C = giant cell.)

482

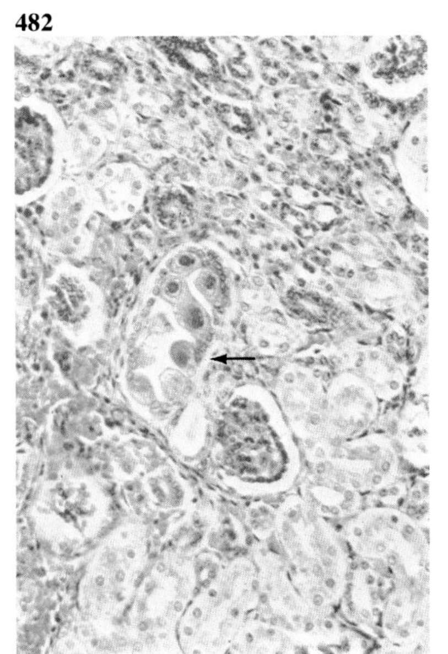

483

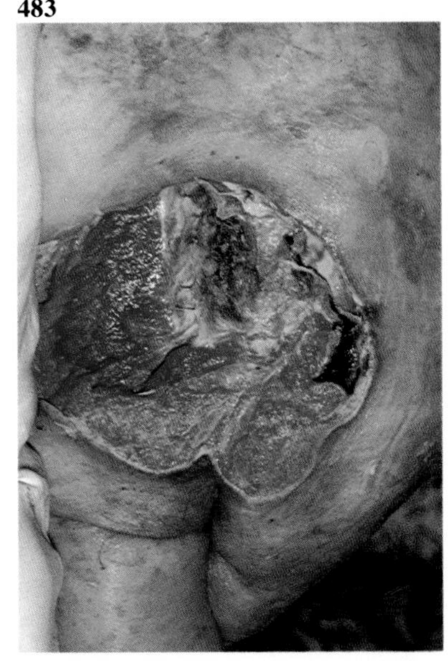

484

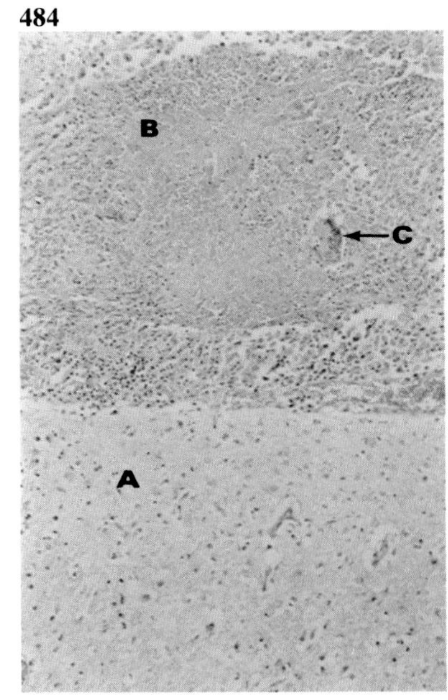

485 ***Cryptococcus neoformans*** **— nigrosin stain.** *Cryptococcus neoformans* is a true yeast that reproduces by budding and does not form mycelia. The cells are spherical in shape and measure 5 to 20 μm in diameter. The organism is Gram-positive and has a thick gelatinous capsule, which is clearly visible in Indian ink or nigrosin preparations. Cryptococci grow slowly on selective media, such as Sabouraud's glucose agar or tellurite malt agar. Pathogenicity can be established by inoculating mice.

486 Cryptocococcal meningitis and reticulosis. *Cryptococcus neoformans* causes sporadic infections in man and animals. The source of infection in man is uncertain, but the yeast is commonly present in mammals and birds and withstands drying in soil and dust. Pigeon droppings are the most abundant known source of virulent strains. The mode of transmission is equally uncertain but it is likely that the organism gains access through the respiratory or alimentary tracts.

The cryptococcus rarely causes trouble in healthy individuals, in whom it may occasionally be found on the skin or in the contents of the bowel. Pulmonary infection is often a benign incidental finding. Cryptococcal disease of the brain and meninges usually runs a subacute or chronic course with a very high mortality.

Patients with reticuloses are especially vulnerable to cryptococcal meningitis. The onset is insidious, and the course of the illness similar to tuberculous meningitis, but the protein, sugar, and chloride concentrations in the cerebrospinal fluid often remain normal until the disease has reached an advanced stage. There is generally an increase in lymphocytes. Many yeast cells are present and may be mistaken for lymphocytes, endothelial cells, or red blood cells, unless a smear is made and suitably stained.

Cryptococci may invade tissues and multiply by budding without initially provoking an inflammatory reaction but eventually their presence in larger numbers leads to infiltration with round cells and macrophages. Granulomatous lesions form and are conspicuous round the base of the brain. In this section of cerebral cortex arrows point to capsulated spheroidal cryptococci.

485

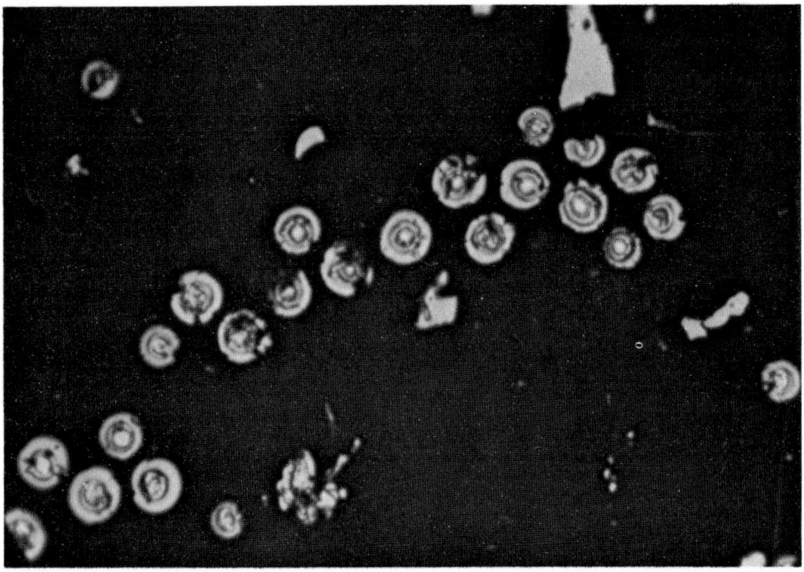

486

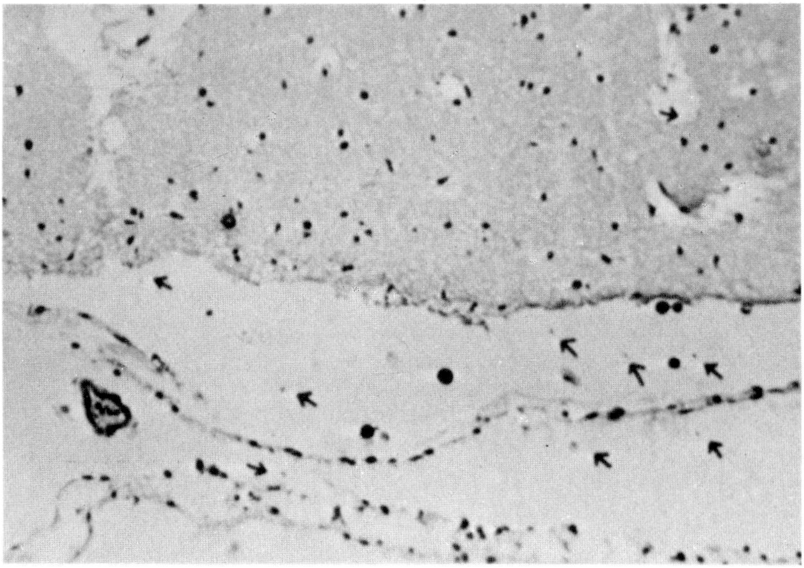

487 Pneumocystis infection — section of lung (H and E). *Pneumocystis carinii* is a protozoon that is often found in animals and not uncommonly in man. Human infection is usually latent but the protozoon may give rise to interstitial plasma cell pneumonia, particularly in premature babies, or in older children and adults with chronic debilitating diseases or disorders of immunity. Fatal pneumonia, however, has occasionally occurred as a primary illness. The mode of transmission is uncertain, but small outbreaks among neonates have suggested that infection may be airborne. Pneumonia caused by *Pneumocystis carinii* is a very common presentation of acquired immune deficiency syndrome (AIDS). In patients with AIDS, infection of the lungs by pneumocystis may occur alone or in conjunction with other opportunistic infections, such as cytomegalovirus, mycobacteria, or cryptococcus.

At necropsy the lungs are distended, and the cut surface grey and airless. The interlobular septa are thickened and infiltrated with histiocytes, lymphocytes and plasma cells. The alveoli are distended with a foamy, semi-liquid substance — when suitably stained this is found to be teeming with organisms. Plasma cells may be diminished in number or absent in patients with agammaglobulinaemia or hypogammaglobulinaemia. Pneumocystis infection is particularly common in children with thymic aplasia. (A = alveolus distended with foamy material, B = histiocyte, C = plasma cell, D = lymphocyte.)

488 *Pneumocystis carinii* pneumonia. Section of lung stained by Grocott's silver-impregnation method. The parasite is found in the lungs as a small cyst, containing two to eight uninucleated bodies. These are very small, measuring 2 to 4 μm in length, are oval or crescent-shaped and divide by binary fission. The protozoon stains with many dyes but not with haematoxylin/eosin. The organism is difficult to detect in secretions from the respiratory passages, but the diagnosis may be confirmed by endobronchial brushing, transtracheal or translaryngeal aspiration, lung biopsy, or by serological tests, if available. (Arrows = protozoa.)

487

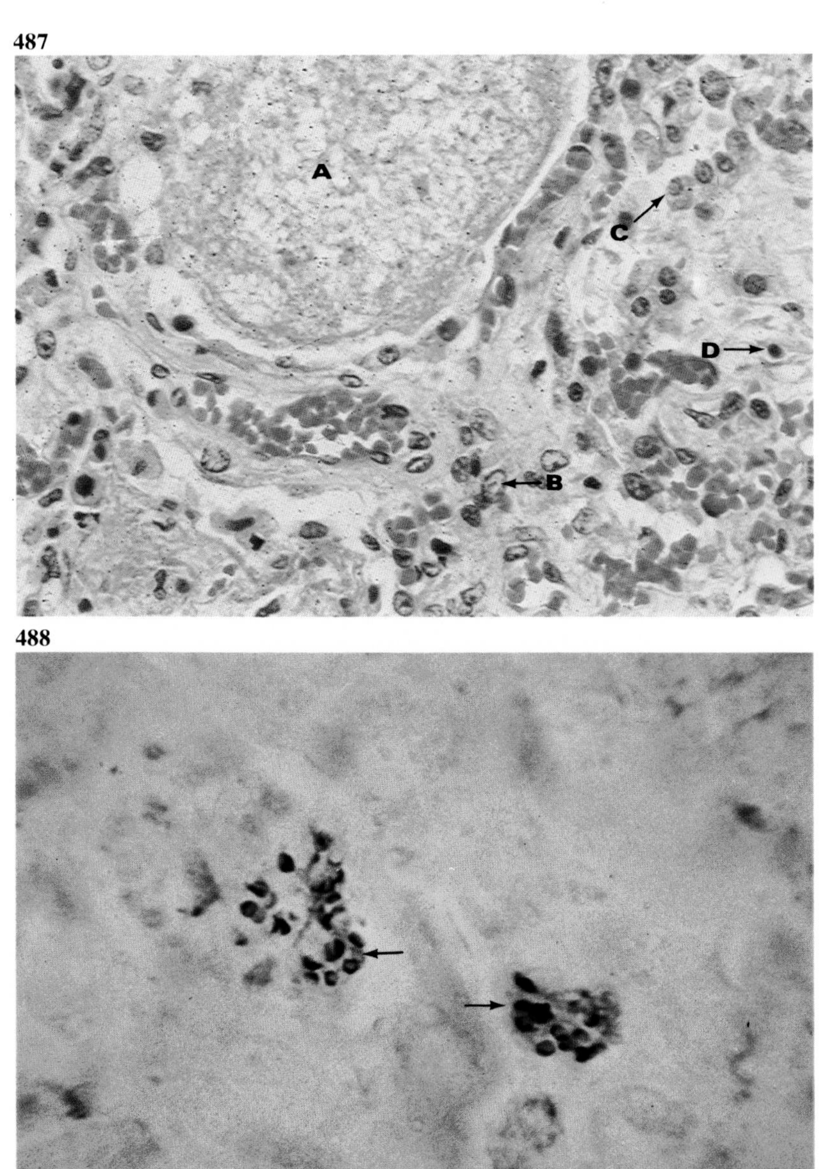

488

489 Radiograph of chest in pneumocystis pneumonia. The possibility of *P. carinii* pneumonia should always be considered in newborn infants or patients with altered immunity who develop respiratory distress out of proportion to the chest signs. The onset of illness may be gradual or abrupt and fever may not be present. The patient becomes progressively more dyspnoeic and may develop a persistent non-productive cough. The initial chest radiograph may be clear, but usually shows interstitial lung shadowing. Blood gas analysis commonly indicates notable hypoxia, even if the appearance of the chest x-ray is normal. It is not possible to make a diagnosis from the radiographic signs and lung biopsy is usually necessary. Serological tests are sometimes helpful.

489

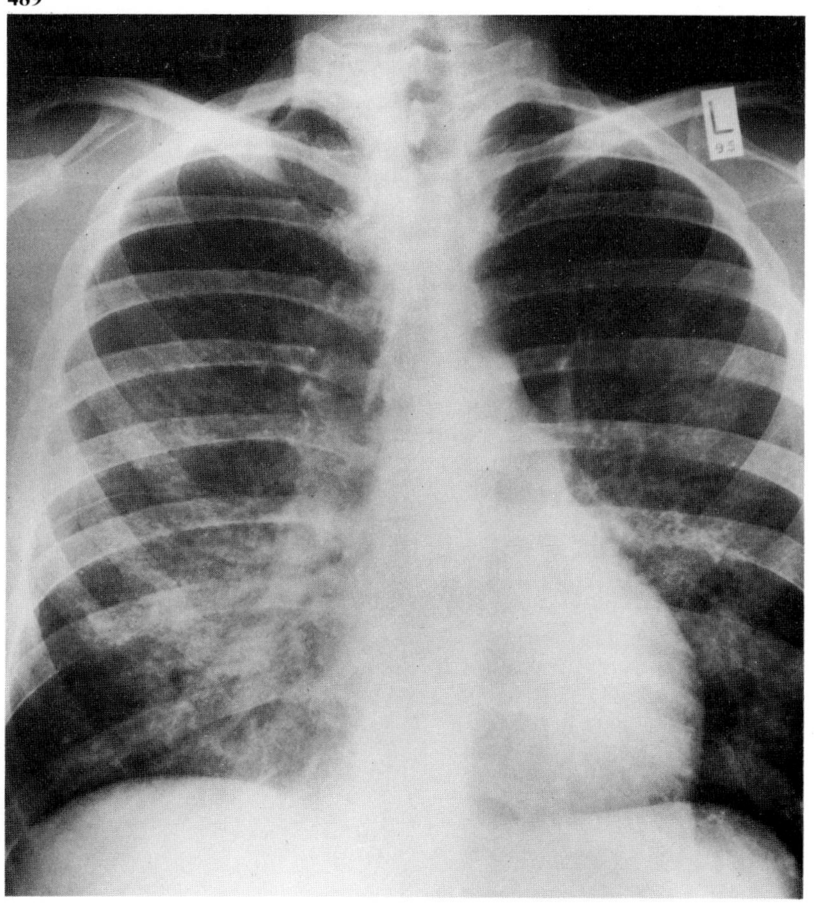

490 Kaposi's sarcoma — skin lesion. Patients with acquired immune deficiency syndrome (AIDS) may present with a wide range of opportunistic infections and a few rare malignancies. Among the commonest presentations are pneumocystis pneumonia in 60% of patients, and Kaposi's sarcoma in 25%. The skin lesions in Kaposi's sarcoma usually appear first on the legs as discrete, bluish-red macules or papules, which later become pigmented.

Histologically, the lesion consists of lobulated masses of highly vascular cellular tissue lying deep within the corium and separated by fibrous trabecula. The tumour is probably an angiosarcoma derived from lymphatic endothelium. At a later stage there is a strong tendency to haemorrhage.

491 Kaposi's sarcoma — skin lesions. The skin lesions have a predilection for the extremities. Individual lesions may coalesce, some may resolve with scarring, others may enlarge slowly and eventually ulcerate. Lymphoedema and purpura may develop in the later stages.

492 Kaposi's sarcoma — mouth. There may be spread to the regional lymph nodes or to almost any organ of the body. The gastrointestinal tract is commonly affected with resultant melaena or frank haemorrhage. Lesions may be found on the hard palate or adjacent gums. The lesions in the buccal cavity of this patient with AIDS were associated with thrush. Some early lesions regressed and healed, and new lesions appeared elsewhere in the mouth. None ulcerated or bled.

490

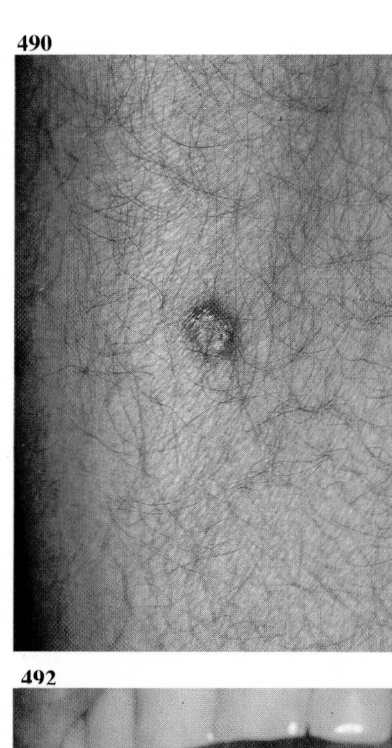

491

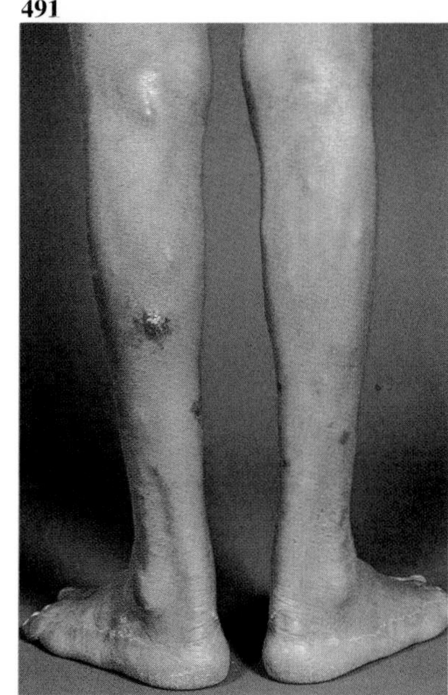

492

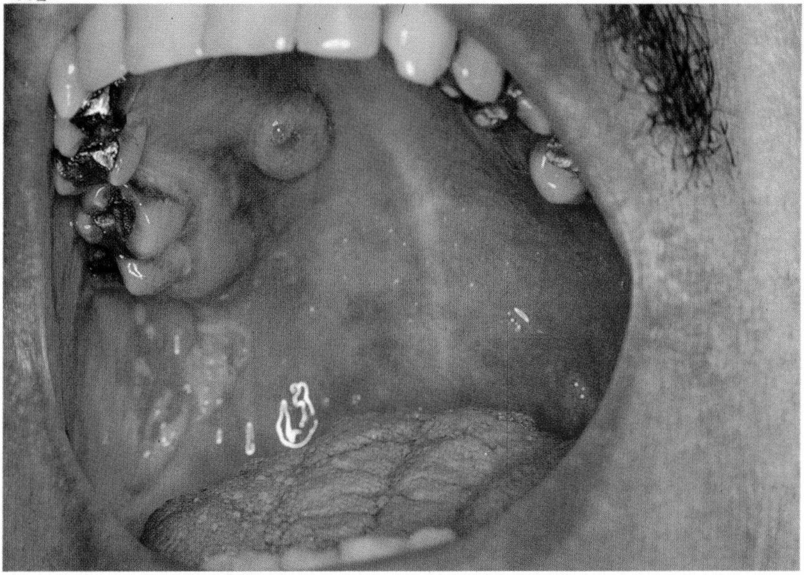

493 Cryptosporidiosis — direct smear of stool stained by Ziehl–Neelsen method. Cryptosporidiosis is a protozoal infection of the bowel derived from domestic animals, including dogs and cats, meat or meat products, and infected individuals, especially children. In healthy people cryptosporidiosis is a benign infection, but in immune-deficient patients, especially those with AIDS, it may cause intractable diarrhoea. The diagnosis is made by detecting the oocysts in a direct smear of stool stained by auramine, Giemsa, or modified Ziehl–Neelsen. Concentration of the stool specimen may be necessary.

493

INDEX

(*The references printed in* **bold** *type are to picture and caption numbers, those in light type are to page numbers.*)